# Free Health Care, Free Medical Information and Free Prescription Drugs

by

**Matthew Lesko**

with

Mary Ann Martello

and

Andrew Naprawa

Research: Caroline Pharmer
Julie Paul

Production: Terry J. Seamens

FREE HEALTH CARE, FREE MEDICAL INFORMATION AND FREE PRESCRIPTION DRUGS,
 Printed in the United States of America. Published by Information USA, Inc., P.O. Box E, Kensington, MD 20895.

FIRST EDITION

Cover Illustration: Mark Dagenais

---

Library of Congress Cataloging-in-Publication Date

Lesko, Matthew

Free Health Care, Free Medical Information and Free Prescription Drugs

ISBN # 1-878346-34-2

---

T O

all the federal and state bureaucrats who

eagerly share information that empowers us

to pursue our goals and dreams

Other books written by Matthew Lesko:

*Getting Yours: The Complete Guide to Government Money*

*How to Get Free Tax Help*

*Information USA*

*The Computer Data and Database Source Book*

*The Maternity Sourcebook*

*Lesko's New Tech Sourcebook*

*The Investor's Information Sourcebook*

*The Federal Data Base Finder*

*The State Database Finder*

*The Great American Gripe Book*

*Lesko's Info-Power II*

*Government Giveaways for Entrepreneurs*

*Free College Money, Termpapers and Sex(ed)*

*1001 Free Goodies and Cheapies*

*Free Stuff for Seniors*

# WARNING TO READERS

If you begged for, borrowed, stole or even purchased this book, I want to thank you. But I must warn you that this book comes with certain limitations.

## 1) THIS BOOK IS OUT OF DATE

Although by publishing my own books, I am able to go from manuscript to printed book in as little as 6 weeks instead of 12 to 18 months it took when I used New York publishers, there is still a problem with timeliness. Life around us changes so quickly that it is almost impossible to have a book 100% perfect by the time the reader uses it. Phone numbers change, organizations move, and publications go out of print. If you telephone a source in this book and instead get some pizza parlor, don't distress. At least you know such an organization exists, somewhere. You can get help in locating the source's new telephone number by calling any or all of the following:

- The Information Operator in the city where the organization is located (dial the area code followed by 555-1212)
- The U.S. Government Federal Information Center (listed in the blue pages of your telephone book under U.S. Government or call your local information operator)
- For state government offices contact the state government operator located in the state capitol.

## 2) YOU HAVE TO BE NICE

This book will not work for you unless you know how to be nice to a bureaucrat. The sources in this book are staffed by public servants whose motives differ from professionals in the private sector. The paycheck of professionals in the private sector is dependent upon how much work they do for you. However, public servants get the same paycheck whether they work for you for two weeks for free or if they hang up on you right after you say hello. So the amount of help and information you derive from a public servant is directly related to how much they WANT to work for you. And this is a function of how well you treat them.

## 3) LIFE AIN'T EASY

We designed this book so that most users can look up their health problem, make a single phone call, and get the information they need to solve their problem. But some problems may take three calls, seven calls, a dozen, or more. Much of our salesmanship culture wants us to believe that our problems can be solved with just one phone call, but deep down we know that most of life doesn't work that way. Finding the help and information you need can take a bit of effort, but the help is very likely to be there, and there's no magic to getting to it. You'll just have to make a few more phone calls.

Matthew Lesko
Information USA, Inc.

# Table of Contents

**C —**

**D —**

**G —**

**T —**

# Introduction

The importance of health care in our society doesn't have to be explained here. Better people than me are doing a very good job of letting the public know how important health care is, how costly it has become, and how much it has to be changed.

What I want to share in this book is how to use the tools of our information society to get:

- the **best treatment** for any health problem whether you're rich or poor,
- the **latest information**, for free, on any health related topic, and
- **free prescription drugs** when you have trouble paying your bills.

## Money Isn't Everything

Money doesn't always buy you the best treatment, the latest information, or even get you justice in our health care system. We live in a large, complex, information-oriented society, where the answers to our questions are changing daily. In this environment, some of the obvious sources of help and information are often the worst.

Health care practitioners who barely have enough to time to care for patients, certainly don't have time to keep up on the mountains of information, data and studies that are generated daily by health care researchers. As a result, they aren't always the ones who can tell you what the latest causes, treatments and cures are to a particular illness. Hospitals that are struggling to survive financially are not likely to advertise the fact that there are federal laws that require most of them to provide a certain amount of their services for free, or that some doctors get government money to perform procedures and operations for free.

## Learn To Use The World's Largest Source Of Free Health Care

The government now represents approximately 37% of everything in our country. More people now work in government in our country than they do in manufacturing. Uncle Sam is a force to be reckoned with, no matter what subject you are talking about. But government has a bigger impact on health care than on any other sector of our society. In 1995, the budget for the U.S. Department of Health and Human Services is more than twice that of the Department of Defense. Even if you take the cost of Social Security out of the U.S. Department of Health and Human Services budget, it is still bigger than Defense. And that gap is due to get much wider in the coming years.

So why shouldn't you as a taxpayer learn to use this invaluable resource to solve some of your own health care problems? For example:

**Why pay for treatment at a local hospital...**
when some of the best doctors in the world get government money to perform procedures and operations for free?

**Why pay $200 to a doctor to answer a health question...**
when you can get better answers from a FREE medical researcher who spends a lifetime and millions of dollars studying just your disease? They can tell you what will be in the medical journals next year because they are financing the research today.

**Why pay the high cost of prescription drugs...**
when you might be able to get them for free?

**Why spend money on health books at the book store...**

when you can get FREE books, pamphlets and even videos that are more complete and more up-to-date?

**Why pay for a medical visit when you're unemployed or without insurance...**

when you can get free treatment at a local clinic?

**Why be harassed by a hospital for not paying a bill...**

when you can show that the hospital has to treat you for free if you can't afford to pay?

**Why trust a one-minute sound bite on the nightly news by a reporter who spends maybe one hour studying a recent health discovery...**

when you can call a government expert who spends a career studying the subject and will send you a free report showing you all the ifs, ands or buts of the discovery, and if this discovery really affects your life?

# The Art of Getting a Bureaucrat To Help You

Our greatest asset as information seekers is that we live in a society inhabited by people who are dying to talk about what they do for a living. However, in this world of big bureaucracies and impersonal organizations, it is rare that any of us get a chance to share what we know with someone who is truly interested. Perhaps that explains why psychiatrists are in such great demand.

This phenomenon can actually work to your advantage — almost anyone can find an expert on any topic if you are willing to make an average of seven telephone calls to eventually find that expert.

## The Value Of Experts In Today's Information Age

Using experts can be your answer to coping with the information explosion. Computers handle some problems of the information explosion because they are able to categorize and index vast amounts of data. However, many computerized databases fail to contain information that is generated by non-traditional sources, like documents that are buried in state and federal agencies.

Another problem is that many databases suffer from lack of timeliness because they offer indexes to articles and most publishers have long lead times for getting the material into print. And in our fast changing society, having the most current information is crucial, and these articles are often not as current in information as they should be.

Computers also contribute to a more serious problem. Because of their ability to store such large quantities of data, computers aggravate the information explosion by fueling the information overload. If you access one of the major databases on a subject such as Maine potatoes, most likely you will be confronted with a printout of 500 or more citations. Do you have the time to find and read all of them? How can you as a non-expert tell a good article from one that will just waste your valuable time retrieving and reading it?

The first step to cut through this volume of information is to find an expert specializing in Maine potatoes. Yes, such an individual exists! This person already will have read those 500 articles and will be able to identify the relevant ones that meet your information needs. This expert will also be able to tell you what will be in the literature next year on the subject of Maine potatoes, because he is probably in the midst of writing or reviewing forthcoming articles right now. And if you are in search of a fact or figure, this government bureaucrat might know the answer right off the top of his head. The best part of this research strategy is that all this valuable information can be accumulated for just the price of a telephone call.

## Case Study: How To Find Mr. Potato

The techniques for locating an expert can best be illustrated by a classic story from the days when I was struggling to start my first information brokerage company in 1975.

At the time the business amounted to just a desk and telephone crowded into the bedroom of my apartment. As so often happens in a fledgling enterprise, my first client was a friend. His problem was this: "I've got to have the latest information on the basic supply and demand of Maine potatoes within 24 hours."

My client represented a syndicate of commodity investors which invests millions of dollars in Maine potatoes. When he called, these potatoes were selling at double their normal price and he wanted to know why. I knew absolutely nothing about potatoes, but thought I knew where to find out. The agreement with my client was that I would be paid only if I succeeded in getting the information (no doubt you've guessed I no longer work that way).

## Luck With The First Telephone Call

The first call I made was to the general information office of the U.S. Department of Agriculture. I asked to speak to an expert on potatoes. The operator referred me to Mr. Charlie Porter. I wondered if this Mr. Porter was a department functionary with responsibility for handling crank calls, but the operator assured me that he was an agriculture economist specializing in potatoes. I called Mr. Porter and explained how I was a struggling entrepreneur who knew nothing about potatoes and needed his help to answer a client's urgent request. Charlie graciously gave me much of the information I needed, adding that he would be happy to talk at greater length either over the phone or in person at his office. I decided to go see him and meet a real expert face to face.

## Only Problem Was Getting Out Of Charlie Porter's Office

For 2 1/2 hours the next morning, the federal government's potato expert explained in minute detail the supply and demand of Maine potatoes. Charlie Porter showed me computer printouts that reflected how the price had doubled in recent weeks. For any subject that arose during our conversation, Charlie had immediate access to a reference source. Rows of books in his office covered every conceivable aspect of the potato market. A strip of ticker tape that tracked the daily price of potatoes from all over the country lay across his desk.

Here in Charlie's office was everything anyone might ever want to know about potatoes. The problem, it turned out, was not in getting enough information, but how to gracefully leave his office. Once Charlie started talking, it was hard for him to stop. It seemed that Charlie Porter had spent his lifetime studying the supply and demand of potatoes and finally someone with a genuine need sought his expertise on the subject closest to his heart.

## One Potato....Two Potato....

When I finally had to tell Charlie that I really had to leave, he pointed across the hall in the direction of a potato statistician whose primary responsibility was to produce a monthly report showing potato production and consumption in the United States. From this statistician I was to learn about all the categories of potatoes that are tallied. It turns out the U.S. Department of Agriculture counts all the potato chips sold every month, even how many Pringle potato chips are consumed in comparison to say, Lay's Potato Chips. The statistician offered to place me on the mailing list to receive all this free monthly data.

## The Art Of Getting An Expert To Talk

The information explosion requires greater reliance on experts in order to sift through this proliferation of enormous data. Cultivating an expert, however, demands an entirely different set of skills from using a library or a publication. You must know how to treat people so that they are ready, willing, and able to give you the information that you need. It is human nature for almost anyone to want to share their knowledge, but your approach will determine whether you ultimately get the expert to open up to your questions. So it is your job to create an environment that makes an individual want to share his expertise. Remember when dealing with both public and private sector experts, they will get the same paycheck whether they give you two weeks worth of free help or if they cut the conversation short after a minute or two.

## Expectations: The 7-Phone Call Rule

There is no magic to finding an expert. It is simply a numbers game which seems to take an average of seven telephone calls to find the answer you're looking for. Telephone enough people and keep asking each for a lead. The magic lies in how much information the expert will share once you find that individual. This is why it is essential to remember "the 7-phone call rule," and never stop at the second or third lead that seems to be going nowhere.

If you make several calls and begin to get upset because you are being transferred from one person to another, you will be setting yourself up to fail once you locate the right expert. What is likely to happen is that when your "Charlie Porter" picks up his telephone he is going to hear you complaining about how sick and tired you are of getting the runaround from his organization and colleagues. If you don't sound like you are going to be the highlight of Charlie's day, he will instantly figure out how to get rid of you fast.

This explains why some people are able to get information and others fail. Seasoned researchers know it is going to take a number of telephone calls and they will not allow themselves to get impatient. After all, the runaround is an unavoidable part of the information gathering process. Consequently, the first words that come out of your mouth are extremely important because they set the stage for letting the expert want to help you.

## Ten Basic Telephone Tips

Here are a few pointers to keep in mind when you are casting about for an expert. These guidelines amount to basic common sense but are very easy to forget by the time you get to that sixth or seventh phone call.

**1) Introduce Yourself Cheerfully**

The way you open the conversation will set the tone for the entire interview. Your greeting and initial comment should be cordial and cheerful. They should give the feeling that this is not going to be just another telephone call, but a pleasant interlude in his or her day.

**2) Be Open And Candid**

You should be as candid as possible with your source since you are asking the same of him. If you are evasive or deceitful in explaining your needs or motives, your source will be reluctant to provide you with information. If there are certain facts you cannot reveal such as client confidentiality, explain just that. Most people will understand.

**3) Be Optimistic**

Throughout the entire conversation you should exude a sense of confidence. If you call and say "You probably aren't the right person" or "You don't have any information, do you?" it makes it easy for the person to say "You're right, I can't help you." A positive attitude will encourage your source to stretch his mind to see what information he might have that could possibly help you.

**4) Be Humble And Courteous**

You can be optimistic and still be humble. Remember the old adage that you can catch more flies with honey than you can with vinegar. People in general, and experts in particular, love to tell others what they know, as long as their position of authority is not questioned or threatened. In fact, if they are made to feel like an expert by the way you treat them, chances are that they will give you more information than they originally intended.

**5) Be Concise**

State your problem simply. A long-winded explanation may bore your contact and reduce your chances for getting a thorough response.

**6) Don't Be A "Gimme"**

A "gimme" is someone who says "give me this" or "give me that," and has little consideration for the other person's time or feelings. Remember to "ask" for information or a particular document that you're interested in.

**7) Be Complimentary**

This goes hand in hand with being humble. A well placed compliment about your source's expertise or insight about a particular topic will serve you well. In searching for information in large organizations, you are apt to talk to many colleagues of your source, so it wouldn't hurt to convey the respect that your "Charlie Porter" commands, for example, "Everyone I spoke to said you are the person I must talk with." It is reassuring for anyone to know that they have the respect of their peers.

**8) Be Conversational**

Avoid spending the entire time talking about the information you need. Briefly mention a few irrelevant topics such as the weather, the Washington Redskins, or the latest political campaign. The more social you are without being too chatty, the more likely that your source will open up to you.

**9) Return The Favor**

You might share with your source information or even gossip you have picked up elsewhere. However, be certain not to betray the trust of either your client or another source. If you do not have any relevant information to share at the moment, it would still be a good idea to call back when you are further along in your research when you might have information of value to offer.

**10) Send Thank You Notes**

A short note, typed or handwritten, will help ensure that your source will be just as cooperative in the future.

# Sample Success Stories

Ok, all you skeptics. So, you really don't believe that if you call a government office they will actually do something good for you. I hope these case stories have the power to turn you around and make a believer out of you. Whether you are sick or well, rich or poor, or in or out of the medical profession, government resources can put you onto the fastest road to recovery, if you learn how to use them. Most of these stories were provided by the experts who work at the sources listed in this book. Others were taken from submissions to Information USA's recent "My Favorite Bureaucrat Contest."

## Elderly Women With Burning Mouth Condition Finds Relief

Two sisters were concerned about the health of their elderly mother who complained of a persistent burning sensation in her mouth. They took their mother to many doctors, dentists, clinics, and even to specialists, yet none of them could find anything wrong with her. They eventually contacted the National Institute of Dental Research who told her about a rare condition called, in fact, Burning Mouth, which most often affects post-menopausal, elderly women. The Institute was then able to send the sisters information that helped them take the necessary steps toward helping their mother.

## Woman With Eye Disease Gets Line On Free Treatment

A young woman diagnosed with Pseudotumor Cerebri needed help finding a local support group. The National Eye Institute referred her to the National Self Help Center and to the Self Help Clearinghouse of Greater Washington. In addition, the Institute told her about a clinical study on Idiopathic Intracranial

Hypertension (another term for pseudotumor) that she might qualify for being conducted by a university medical center.

## Florida Hospital Buys Patient Her Own Wheelchair

The Easter Seals Hospital in Tallahassee, Florida, gives all kinds of free health services to those who can't afford it. They offer free adult day health care for the elderly, and even bought an electric wheelchair for a woman who was a paraplegic. They've also bought insulin level monitors for diabetics, respiratory equipment for asthmatics, as well as crutches, leg braces, and walkers. They even pay for speech and physical therapy.

## Alzheimer's Patient Gets Free Care At Clinical Trial

A woman whose father is an Alzheimer's patient called the Alzheimer's Disease Education and Referral Center for information on drugs being tested for the disease. An information specialist discussed with her the types of drug trials that are going on across the country, then referred her to the nearest federally-sponsored Alzheimer's disease research center where her father could possibly receive free treatment.

## State Insurance Commissioner Shows How A Cancerous Mole Is More Serious Than Breast Enlargements

A woman in North Carolina got a notice from her insurance company stating that they were not going to pay for her claim to have a cancerous mole removed from her back. She knew of a fellow worker who had just been paid by the same insurance company to have her breasts enlarged and thought she was being treated unfairly. She contacted her state insurance commissioner and within the month received payment for her medical care.

## Medical Society Arranges Free Care For Ohio Woman

A 19-year-old called the Columbus, Ohio, Medical Society for help: she did not qualify for Medicaid, but she needed to see a doctor. The Medical Society called a local hospital for her and got them to agree to see her for free and to provide her with all her medications.

## Woman Gets Information On Newest Breast Cancer Treatment

A newly diagnosed breast cancer patient called the National Cancer Institute for information on treatment options. The Institute provided her with the most recent and up-to-date information on the available treatment options and identified clinical trials that investigate new treatments for early stage breast cancer.

## Center Locates Poem For Grieving SIDS Parent

A SIDS parent who had heard of a poem written by another SIDS parent in memory of her baby called the National Sudden Infant Death Syndrome Resource Center to get help locating it. The mother wanted to use the poem at her baby's memorial service. The staff was able to identify the poem, fax her a copy and give her contact information so she could get in touch with the author of the poem, and obtain permission to use it at her baby's funeral.

## Brother of Cancer Victim Learns How to Cope

The brother of a terminally ill patient called the National Cancer Institute for information on how to care for him. They referred the man to the nearest hospice program and provided him with information and materials to assist the family in coping with the illness.

## Parents Use Government To Track Down Daughter's Rare Disease Themselves And Out-Do The Doctors

A Florida couple became frustrated with the seeming lack of effort put forth by the medical community when it came to diagnosing just what was wrong with their 2-year-old daughter. Much of the advice was along the lines of, "Don't compare her to her older sister. All children mature and progress differently," or "Bring her back in 3 months and we'll take another look at her." The couple was not satisfied with the "wait and see" approach and began doing their own research. Along the way, they came upon a brochure from the National Organization of Rare Diseases (NORD). This and subsequent information helped them rule out erroneous diagnoses made by previous specialists and helped them identify some of the other complications that accompany their child's rare ailment. The parents credit NORD's networking program with connecting them with parents of other children with the same disease.

## Man Thinking About Eye Surgery Finds Out About Risks Involved

A man who was thinking about having corneal refractive surgery contacted the National Eye Institute. To help him make a more informed decision, they sent him results from the Prospective Evaluation of Radial Keratotomy (PERK), a National Eye Institute-sponsored clinical study of the procedure.

## Clearinghouse Helps Woman With Bladder Problem

A woman called the National Kidney and Urologic Diseases Information Clearinghouse. She was having recurrent bladder problems and wanted to know more about her doctor's tentative diagnosis of Interstitial Cystitis (IC), which he said was a difficult disorder to diagnose and treat. She asked the clearinghouse if this was true and if they had any information regarding treatment. The clearinghouse agreed with her doctor and told her that, at present, no treatment relieves the symptoms for IC patients. The clearinghouse enclosed a list of centers they support engaged in research related to Interstitial Cystitis. They also enclosed a literature search that listed materials about IC, and a list of organizations dealing with IC.

## Free Nursing Home Money After Medicaid Says No

A Worthington, Ohio, woman couldn't make it living independently any longer, but was disqualified for Medicaid coverage for a nursing home because of her savings. Through the federal Hill-Burton program she was able to receive money to cover her nursing home costs.

## Woman Tracks Down Information on Cushing's Syndrome

A woman called the National Kidney and Urologic Diseases Information Clearinghouse because she needed information on a rare disorder called Cushing's Syndrome. Although they do not have publications about this syndrome, they were able to refer her to the National Organization for Rare Disorders, as well as two other organizations that deal with rare kidney conditions.

## Man Gets Information on Lactose Intolerance

A man called the National Digestive Diseases Information Clearinghouse for information about his diet and lactose intolerance. They were able to provide him with publications that included general dietary guidelines. When the man asked for specific dietary advice, they referred him to a dietitian from the American Dietetic Association.

## Woman With Irritable Bowel Syndrome Finds Support Network

A woman called the National Digestive Diseases Information Clearinghouse for information on Irritable Bowel Syndrome (IBS). They were able to provide her with publications and information regarding a national intestinal disease foundation. The woman also expressed some concerns about dealing with the disease and her own feelings of isolation. To help out, the clearinghouse gave her the name of a person who coordinates a telephone network support system for people with IBS.

## Lead Poisoning Expert Provides Worried Mother With Expert Advice

A woman in Maryland was frightened and confused when she learned that her daughter tested positive for lead poisoning. She called a number of different agencies in an attempt to discover the causes, treatments, and effects of lead poisoning. Although she found a number of offices that she thought might be able of help, no one could give her any clear answers until she spoke with Dr. Susan Binder at the Centers For Disease Control in Atlanta. Dr. Binder listened to her story in detail and outlined the possible causes of the poisoning. Together they arrived at the conclusion that the recent house renovation was the likely culprit. Dr. Binder then discussed the potential long-term effects, some of the basic steps she could take to help her daughter, current research and controversies on the subject, and sent current literature. But most importantly, Dr. Binder referred her to local experts and resources in her area where she could turn for further assistance.

## Car Accident Victim Gets Free Overnight Hospital Stay

The Monroe Regional Medical Center in Ocala, Florida, provided free overnight care to an emergency car accident victim with a viral illness.

## Diabetic Gets New Information On Foot Problems

A man called the National Diabetes Information Clearinghouse for information on foot problems he was having related to diabetes. His doctor had told him that he may eventually lose his feet. The clearinghouse was able to send him information, fact sheets, and medical articles about foot problems, wound healing and infections, as well as peripheral vascular disease.

## Diabetic Woman Learns About Health And Pregnancy

A woman who had gestational diabetes with her first pregnancy called the National Diabetes Information Clearinghouse for information. She was trying to get pregnant again and wanted to avoid the same problems she'd had the first time. The clearinghouse provided her with a booklet, *Understanding Gestational Diabetes*, as well as several articles from a literature search. They also referred her to the American Diabetes Association, which has a booklet explaining meal planning and exchange lists of food.

## Single Mother Finishes College With Financial Assistance from State Pregnant Women's Program

A woman in Michigan found herself in her senior year of college, unmarried and pregnant. Her due date was shortly after the end of the semester in which she would receive her degree. As the due date approached, she felt great pressures: emotional, physical, academic, and most definitely financial. At that point, she heard about the Pregnant Women's Program at the State Department of Social Services, which provides financial assistance to pregnant women in need. Her case worker guided her step-by-step through the application process and made sure she got the financial help she needed to finish college and have her baby with as little stress as possible.

## Alzheimer's Center Gets Free Training Materials

The administrator of an adult day care center for Alzheimer's patients contacted the Alzheimer's Disease Education and Referral Center for help in training staff and developing activities for patients. The Center sent her a catalog of training materials it has available and a listing of other resources for training and activities planning from its computerized database.

## Stroke Victim Gets Help Finding Rehab Services

The family of a man who had recently suffered a stroke and was due to be released from the hospital needed help finding a rehabilitation facility that would accept him for speech and physical therapy. The National Rehabilitation Information Center referred them to a center in their area and also gave them information on support groups and equipment for stroke victims.

## State Health Care Official Gets Money And Private Bill To Help Terminally Ill Boy

A Wisconsin couple's insurance company would not cover the medical expenses for their terminally ill son. They turned to a state counselor for help. An attorney who works for the service was able to get an insurance company to pay the $17,000 disputed bill. He also got the Governor to pass a new law. As a result, their son is now included in a program that provides special funds that allow him to come home from the hospital for visits three times a week when he is stable.

## Paraplegic Gets Help Making His Home More Accessible

A recently disabled paraplegic needed to know how to make his home more accessible for his wheelchair. The National Rehabilitation Information Center sent him information and catalogs about products designed for disabled people, such as kitchen and bathroom equipment.

## Child With Learning Disability Gets Much-Needed Support

A woman whose ten-year-old son was just diagnosed with a learning disability needed help locating support groups for her son and herself. The National Institute on Deafness and Other Communication Disorders directed them to national and local organizations for more information, as well as providing them with publications and a literature search on the topic.

## Student Gets Free Help Writing Master's Thesis

A Master's student in Public Health contacted the National Maternal and Child Health Clearinghouse for materials on prenatal care among poor women. The clearinghouse provided a wide range of information, including current publications, resource guides listing other important titles/information sources in her area of interest, and referrals to several other government agencies and private organizations active in the area of prenatal care promotion and services.

## Business Gets Help Making Changes For Handicapped Access

A company interested in complying with the new Americans with Disabilities Act needed advice on building modifications they might have to make. The National Rehabilitation Information Center sent them precise information related to accessibility and equipment requirements under this new law.

## Health Fair Gets Free Help Organizing Event

A hospital health educator planning an annual health promotion fair for patients, staff, and the local community contacted the National Maternal and Child Health Clearinghouse for any relevant materials to help make the event a success. The clearinghouse supplied the hospital with bulk quantities of consumer-oriented publications appropriate for the general public, as well as posters and video tapes suitable for display during the event. The clearinghouse also referred them to other organizations that could provide free help in planning the event.

## Down and Out, Mother of Five Gets Last Chance From Congressman

A divorced mother of five, working full-time and living on $8,000 a year with no child support, could not even afford medical service for her children. One night in desperation and on the verge of a nervous breakdown, she wrote to her Congressman, Frank Thompson of New Jersey, about her story. Within one week she received a Medicaid identification card for each of her five children which would ensure them proper medical treatment.

## Pregnant Woman Gets Bilingual Information On Prenatal Care

A pregnant woman called the National Maternal and Child Health Clearinghouse for information materials that might help her properly care for her baby, both before and after birth, as well as similar materials in Spanish for her husband. The clearinghouse responded with literature on maternal nutrition, prenatal and newborn care, as well as addresses and phone numbers of sources for appropriate titles in Spanish. Since there was a history of genetic disorders in her family and she wanted to prepare for the eventual testing of her child, the clearinghouse also referred her to another office that gave her a reading list of the latest publications in print on the subject of genetic testing.

## Mother With Premature Baby Gets Help From State Nurse

A woman in Delaware learned that her baby would be born fourteen weeks early, and she began working with a nurse from her state's Early Intervention Program. After the birth of her son, the nurse visited him frequently throughout his four-month hospital stay, and after the baby had returned to his home, she visited him many times to thoroughly evaluate his developmental progress. She was the first to spot his hearing loss and helped the couple obtain a state-funded hearing aid for him. She diagnosed his need for speech, physical, and occupational therapy, and helped enroll him in an excellent school. At this time the nurse was experiencing severe difficulties of her own at home. Her husband was dying of cancer. Despite this, she continued to be an extremely dedicated and compassionate person.

## Woman With Endometriosis Gets Line On Free Treatment

A woman in her 30's had a terrible case of endometriosis and underwent a hysterectomy. But her problems continued to worsen and the endometriosis may have invaded her lungs and colon. On top of this, she was experiencing surgical menopause and needed estrogen. The National Institute of Child Health and Human Development was able to send her information on endometriosis and referred her to a national endometriosis organization that could, in turn, refer her to possible clinical studies for free treatment.

## Singer Finds Out How Not To Lose Her Voice

A woman feared that the amount of singing she does would put a strain on her vocal cords. The National Institute on Deafness and Other Communication Disorders sent her information on programs to prevent voice disorders. They also directed her to researchers on this topic, and sent her relevant publications.

## Center Helps Set Up New SIDS Program

A nurse with a State Maternal and Child Health Program was setting up a support group for SIDS parents, which had never been done before in her state. She called the National Sudden Infant Death Syndrome Resource Center for information, materials, publications, and examples of similar programs in other states. The staff was able to do a database search, as well as give her referrals and samples of program guidelines and publications from other states.

## National Institutes of Health Helps Woman With Brain Surgery and Diabetes

A 37-year-old woman began to quickly lose her eyesight, and within two months time was told she had a pituitary tumor and would need brain surgery. An information specialist at the National Institutes of Health (NIH) directed her to a brain surgeon who was located only 45 minutes away from her home in Arkansas. Unfortunately, as a result of the surgery she now suffers from Diabetes Insipidus, which is manifested by an uncontrollable urge to drink water. At times she drinks as much as five gallons in an hour. Again, NIH directed her to the National Organization of Rare Diseases. From there, she learned all about her condition, including facts that the doctors treating her didn't know. The organization also linked her up with other people who suffer from the same condition, one whom has even started a newsletter on the disease. NORD's newsletter keeps her updated on other people, as well as current legislation dealing with Orphan drugs.

## Parents of Deaf Child Get State Help

A couple in Pennsylvania decided they were ready for children after five years of marriage. When their first child was born, they were crushed to learn that the child was deaf. The woman quit her job to take care of the child's special needs. Shortly after this, the husband lost his job because of a plant closing. The woman turned to the state government for assistance and was happy to find Mr. Tornbloom who gave them a considerable amount of time, a wealth of information about programs and possibilities, and approved payment by the state for the child's hearing aid.

## Worried Mom Gets Bottom Line On Daughter's Acne Treatment

A mother called the National Institute of Arthritis and Musculoskeletal and Skin Diseases because her daughter had severe acne. Their dermatologist had tried many different treatments with little success. The mother wanted help understanding additional treatments the dermatologist was considering, such as putting the teenager on Acutane or birth control pills. The Institute sent the mother several articles on acne treatments, and referred her to the Acutane Hotline established by Roche Laboratories to answer consumers' questions. They also referred the mother to the American Academy of Dermatology for more information.

## State Consumer Office Saves Employee Thousands by Getting Insurance Company To Reverse Its Policy for Covering A Pre-Existing Case of Endometriosis

Mr. Gene Hackworth of the Insurance Department of the Consumer Protection Agency in West Virginia worked for close to a year to get an insurance company to reverse an unfair decision for a woman who was being stuck for thousands of dollars as a result of exploratory surgery for endometritis. Due to his efforts, the company paid the claim.

## Man Gets Line on Hip Replacement

A man called the National Institute of Arthritis and Musculoskeletal and Skin Diseases to find out where he could get a free hip replacement. Although the institute itself does not do this operation, they were able to refer him to a hotline established in his state that could explain some options or direct him to the appropriate place in his state for more information.

## State Worker Helps Couple Identify Little-Known Program To Pay For Baby's Skull Surgery

A couple in Illinois felt the financial pinch when they learned that their insurance did not cover the C-section birth of their new daughter. They were then devastated to learn that the skull surgery that was needed immediately for their new baby was also not covered. A case worker for the state Office of Crippled Children solved their problem. With his help, they sorted through the maze of forms and questions, and qualified for a program that paid for their baby's operation.

## Vet Gets Help From State Counselor When Congressman Fails

When a man from upstate New York received his military discharge, he had a service-connected disability. Yet he was turned away by the Veterans Administration which refused him financial compensation. He contacted his Congressman, but even he couldn't help. Years later when a co-worker asked about his limping, he told him his military disability story. The co-worker suggested that he see his brother-in-law who was a veteran's counselor for New York state. After a thorough medical exam, a review of the paperwork, and a hearing in front of the appeal board, the Veterans Administration approved him for compensation.

## Doctor Gets The Latest SIDS Information Faxed To Him

Recently, a physician from an intensive care unit in California called the National Sudden Infant Death Syndrome Resource Center for information on SIDS and other types of infant deaths. The doctor said that twins had just died in his section and he wanted information on other simultaneous deaths of twins from SIDS. The center performed a database search, and then faxed citations of articles dealing with the subject to the doctor.

## Illinois Woman Sees Again

As a result of a spinal tap, a woman in Illinois contracted Multiple Sclerosis. The effects of her disease caused her to lose her eyesight, lose her job, and have a car accident. In addition to the financial strains she already faced, the roof on her house also had to be replaced. She went to the state's Office of Rehabilitation to see if they could help her find employment. The counselor questioned the diagnosis of her eye condition and paid for another eye test. As a result of the test, she had eye surgery and regained her eyesight.

## Center Helps Out At A SIDS Funeral

A grandmother of a SIDS infant contacted the National Sudden Infant Death Syndrome Resource Center immediately after her grandchild's death. She wanted information sheets or other publications explaining what SIDS is so that they could be given to those attending the funeral. This way the family would be spared the painful process of explaining the condition. The staff prepared the publications and delivered them in person to the grandmother's home the night before the funeral.

## Woman With Rare Disease Gets Help In Treatment And Support

A woman in her late 40's who was diagnosed with a very rare and incurable disease contacted the National Organization of Rare Diseases to find out all she could and where the latest testing was being done. NORD sent her brochures and also the names of others across North America that had the same disease. The woman has managed to travel to visit some of these people and attend several organized support groups. She found these meetings, both group and individual, to be central to her ability to cope with her diagnosis and lead as full and productive a life as she can.

## Head Injury Victim Gets Help With Loss of Taste

A woman's husband had a serious fall that created trauma to his head, and as a result was unable to taste his food. The National Institute on Deafness and Other Communication Disorders sent her all kinds of publications related to such head injuries and also referred her to other organizations that could help them understand taste disorders.

## Student Gets Free Help Writing Paper On Leukemia

A high school student preparing a paper for a science class called the National Cancer Institute for background information on leukemia and the use of bone marrow transplants. They provided her with booklets and research reports to help develop the paper.

## Disabled Woman Gets The Gift Of Life From Vocational Rehabilitation Counselor

In 1986, a woman was diagnosed with Multiple Sclerosis. She met up with Dorothy Winegrad of the Maryland State Department of Education's Division of Vocational Rehabilitation. Mrs. Winegrad assessed her situation, and recommended that she obtain a scooter and an elevator to lower her stair glide and her wheelchair to street level from her front porch. Unfortunately, the woman was unemployed and didn't have the thousands of dollars needed to purchase the items. Through the state program, Mrs. Winegrad arranged for her to obtain all the items at no cost.

## Perfume Man Who Loses Sense of Smell Gets Help

For no apparent reason, a man who worked in the perfume industry lost his sense of smell. The National Institute on Deafness and Other Communication Disorders directed him to organizations that study this disorder and could inform him about current research being done on this topic.

## T.V. Station Gets Help With Breast Cancer Awareness Program

The Public Service Director of a local television station called the National Cancer Institute for information on breast cancer screening. The Institute's Outreach Coordinator provided Public Service Announcements and a 30-minute video program on mammography and provided suggestions for developing a local program on breast cancer screening.

## High-Risk Woman Gets Line On Free Breast Cancer Prevention

A 50-year-old woman with a family history of breast cancer called the National Cancer Institute for information on a prevention trial for women at high risk for breast cancer. They referred her to the researchers in her area conducting the study for information on free enrollment.

# Free
# Health Care

For many years I was aware that hundreds of thousands of patients, both rich and poor, can receive free medical treatment from various government programs. And for many years I also believed that most people, especially those within the health care community, knew of these programs and opportunities. But my perceptions changed when I recently helped a woman in my neighborhood who needed a simple examination by a cardiologist.

The woman was unemployed, had no money, and of course, no health insurance coverage. A doctor at a local clinic prescribed an anti-depressant drug but said that before he could give it to her, she needed to be examined by a cardiologist. He said she had to get the cardiologist examination on her own. I had to make over *thirty* telephone calls to get her a free examination.

What I learned by making all those telephone calls was that most people in the health care community did not even know what free services were available to the public. I even called a number of local cardiologists, and they seemed to be the least helpful of all. Not only were they not set up to handle patients for free, they had no suggestions as to how this woman could get the care she needed. They didn't even know that their own medical association provided a referral service to provide aid to those who can't afford to pay.

## Our Survey Of 100 Doctors

After this experience, my staff performed an undercover investigation in which we approached one hundred cardiologists around the country with the same problem. Here is what we found:

- *4% said they would examine her even if she did not have money or insurance.*

- *5% said they would not examine her but had other suggestions that proved to be helpful.*
- *25% said they would not examine her, and suggested other solutions that proved of no value.*
- *66% said that they would not see her and had no idea where to turn.*

## 83% of Congress Unaware of Current Federal Health Care Programs

Maybe you're thinking that it's OK for doctors not to be aware of the free medical help that's available because most of this help is from the government and you can't expect doctors to know a lot about the government. That's what we thought too, so we decided to go undercover again and contact 100 members of the U.S. Congress to see what they knew.

We called their offices and said that our mother lived in their voting district, made very little money, had no insurance, did not qualify for Medicare or Medicaid, and needed a heart operation. We also said that mom had to take drugs costing $100 per month and couldn't afford it. It's also important to note that at each office we asked to speak to the health care expert on the staff. Seventy one percent of them did not know about the free drug programs offered by pharmaceutical companies, and 83% of them had no idea about the same federal programs that they as federal legislators are responsible for funding.

| Percent of Congress Who Know About Free Health Care Programs | | | |
|---|---|---|---|
| | **Senate** | **House** | **Total** |
| Knew More than Medicare/Medicaid | 18% | 16% | 17% |
| Knew of Free Hospitalization Program | 16% | 16% | 16% |
| Knew about Physicians Who Get Grants | 2% | 2% | 2% |
| Knew of Free Drug Program | 34% | 24% | 29% |
| Offered Other Suggestions | 12% | 8% | 10% |

If you would like more details on either of these studies, you can contact the office of Information USA, Inc. in Kensington, Maryland.

What follows in this section is a listing of those places, both nationally and locally, you can turn to for free health care and treatment. Some programs will take you only if you can't afford treatment or have no health insurance coverage, while other programs will take you no matter who you are, rich or poor.

## Free Medical Care for Rich and Poor By the Best Doctors in the World

Each year hundreds of thousands of patients receive free medical care by some of the best doctors in the world. Medical research professionals receive millions of dollars each year to study the latest causes, cures and treatments to various diseases or illnesses. If your health condition is being studied somewhere, you may qualify for what is called a "clinical trial" and get treatment for free. These clinical trials can also be used when your doctor recommends an experimental new treatment.

There are several ways to find out about ongoing clinical trials across the nation. Your first call should be to the National Institutes of Health (NIH) Clinical Center. NIH is the federal government's focal point for health research and is one of the world's foremost biomedical research centers. The Clinical Center is a 540-bed hospital that has facilities and services to support research at NIH. They also have an adjacent Ambulatory Care Research Facility that provides additional space and facilities for outpatient research. Your doctor should contact

The Patient Referral Line
(301) 496-4891

to find out if your diagnosis is being studied, and to be put in contact with the primary investigator who can then tell if you meet the requirements for the study. An information brochure is available describing the Clinical Center programs.

☎ Contact:
Clinical Center
National Institutes of Health

Bethesda, MD 20892
(301) 496-2563

If your doctor diagnoses you for a disease but you can't afford treatment, you should check to see whether the National Institutes of Health is studying the disease and looking for patients to be treated at no cost.

In 1994, the Clinical Center at NIH in Bethesda, Maryland, treated 82,500 patients--so it's not as if only the lucky or the rich get to take part in the clinical studies. Keep in mind, though, that most doctors aren't even aware of what is being studied at NIH and probably won't think of a clinical study as an option for you--so *you* may very well have to tell your doctor that NIH is looking for patients with your diagnosis. The list of diseases studied at NIH includes almost everything from writers' cramp and lupus, to AIDS and PMS.

Referring doctors and dentists are welcome to visit their patients at the Clinical Center. When a patient is discharged, the referring doctor or dentist receives a full report on the results of studies and the treatment given. Cooperation of doctors, dentists and patients is appreciated for follow-up observation of patients after they have been discharged.

## Patient Referrals

Again, patients are admitted to the Clinical Center *only* on referral by a doctor or dentist. Your complete diagnosis and medical history is necessary for admission.

Your doctor should make preliminary inquiries by telephone to determine if your diagnosis may be of interest to investigators. If your disease is under active investigation, your doctor may be asked to submit the diagnosis and medical history in writing to the principal investigator.

Your doctor may call the institute contact listed or the patient referral number at (301) 496-4891. To obtain telephone numbers of principal investigators or other staff, call (301) 496-2351.

## Financial Assistance

If necessary, the Clinical Center Social Work Department will help prospective patients with personal problems concerning their admission. This department *cannot* provide financial assistance to individuals and their families except in certain emergency situations. For more information, contact the Social Work Department at (301) 496-2381.

Patients are not financially responsible for medical, surgical or other hospital services performed at the Clinical Center; however, the patient's transportation costs *usually* cannot be paid.

## Eligibility Requirements

1. You must be referred by a physician or dentist in private practice, hospital, clinic or other medical organization.

2. Your specific disease or condition must be under active investigation by NIH physicians at the time of admission.

3. Each Institute considers your age, weight, sex, general health the and length of their waiting list to qualify you as a patient for admission. Possibilities for long-term inpatient status and extended follow-up observations may also be

considered. Apart from the medical considerations listed above, there are no other restrictions based on race, creed, age, sex or color.

4. You must have a reasonable understanding of your role in a research study.

## Length of Stay

You will be returned to the care of your referring doctors or institutions, or to your family, when your participation in a study has been completed and your medical condition permits. The clinical director of the Institute in which you are under study is responsible for making these determinations.

## Accuracy of Information

The information in this section is the most up-to-date possible at the time of publication of this book. However, each year the Clinical Center publishes a new directory of clinical studies that includes the most recently-funded studies, along with those that continue to be funded. So to ensure that the following studies are still underway and looking for patients, you'll have to contact the Center. Also, an up-to-date index of the current clinical studies is carried on the AMA/GTE Telenet Medical Information Network. Quarterly index updates are available on the information network to Telenet subscribers.

# NIH Clinical Studies

What follows is a listing of 1995 Clinical Studies being conducted at the National Institutes of Health. For more information on how to become a clinical trials patient, see the "Free Medical Care for Rich and Poor by the Best Doctors in the World" Section in the first chapter of this book.

## National Institute on Aging

Mark B. Schapiro, M.D., Deputy Clinical Director
Telephone referrals of patients should be directed to:
Carol J. Fuchs-Kinslow, MSSW
Social Worker . . . . . . . . . . . . . . . . . . . . . . (301) 496-4754

**Laboratory of Neurosciences**
*Section on Brain Aging and Dementias*

## National Institute on Alcohol Abuse and Alcoholism

Gerald L. Brown, M.D., Clinical Director
Telephone referrals of patients should be directed to:
Irene Culver . . . . . . . . . . . . . . . . . . . . . . (301) 496-1993

**Laboratory of Clinical Studies**
*Brain Imaging in Alcoholism and Individuals at Risk for Alcoholism*
*Chronic Organic Brain Syndromes of Alcoholism*
*Clinical and Family Studies*
*Cognitive Neuroscience Studies in Alcoholism*
*Pharmacologic Reduction of Alcohol Consumption*
*Treatment of Alcohol Withdrawal*
*Neuropharmacology of Alcoholism*

*Characterization of Abusive Behavior Patterns*
*Characterization of Smoking Withdrawal in Alcoholics*

## National Institute of Allergy and Infectious Diseases

H. Clifford Lane, M.D., Clinical Director
AIDS Studies . . . . . . . . . . . . . . . . . . . . . . . . (800) 243-7644

*Acquired Immunodeficiency Syndrome (AIDS) and Other Syndromes Associated with Human Immunodeficiency Virus (HIV) Infection*
*Anti-retrovirals:*
Candace Kurtz, AIDS Protocol Office, (800) 243-7644
*Anti-infectives:*
Candace Kurtz, AIDS Protocol Office, (800) 243-7644
*Candidiasis* John Bennett, M.D., (301) 496-3461
*Immune-based Therapies for HIV*
Candace Kurtz, AIDS Protocol Office, (800) 243-7644
*Immunopathogenic Mechanisms of HIV Infection*
("Long-term non-progressors")
Barbara Baird, R.N., (301) 402-0980, ext. 420
or (others) Oren Cohen, M.D., (301) 496-5508
*Asthma* Dean Metcalfe, M.D., (301) 496-2165
*Chediak-Higashi Syndrome* John I. Gallin, M.D., (301) 496-4114
*Cryptococcosis* John Bennett, M.D., (301) 496-3461
*Epstein-Barr Virus* Stephen Straus, M.D., (301) 496-5221
*Gluten-Sensitive Enteropathy (Coeliac Sprue)*
Warren Strober, M.D., (301) 496-9662
*Granulomatous Diseases* John I. Gallin, M.D., (301) 496-4114
*Chronic Granulomatous Diseases of Childhood*
John I. Gallin, M.D., (301) 496-4114
or Harry Malech, M.D., (301) 496-1344
*Herpes Simplex Virus Infections*
Stephen Straus, M.D., (301) 496-5221
*Hyperimmunoglobulin and Recurrent Infection (Job's Syndrome)*
John I. Gallin, M.D., (301) 496-4114

*Immunodeficiency Diseases* Warren Strober, M.D., (301) 496-9662
*Inflammatory Bowel Disease* Warren Strober, M.D., (301) 496-9662
*Mastocytosis and Urticaria Pigmentosa*
Dean Metcalfe, M.D., (301) 496-2165

*Mycobacterial Infections*
*Treatment with Interleukin-2*
Michael Sneller, M.D., (301) 496-1124
*Evaluation of Underlying Host Immune Abnormalities and for Treatment with Interferon Gamma and other Cytokines*
Steven M. Holland, M.D., (301) 402-7684
*Neutropenia* Harry Malech, M.D., (301) 496-1344
or John I. Gallin, M.D., (301) 496-4114
*Parasitic Diseases: Amebiasis, Chagas' Disease, Cryptosporidiosis, Cysticercosis, Echinococcosis, Filariasis, Giardiasis, Leishmaniasis, Malaria, Onchocerciasis, Schistosomiasis, Strongyloidiasis and Toxoplasmosis*
Theodore Nash, M.D., (301) 496-6920
Franklin Neva, M.D., (301) 496-2486
or Thomas Nutman, M.D., (301) 496-5398
*Recurrent Pyogenic Infections* John I. Gallin, M.D., (301) 496-4114
*Varicella-Zoster Infections* Stephen Straus, M.D., (301) 496-5221
*Vasculitis* Michael Sneller, M.D., (301) 496-1124
or Carol Langford, M.D., (301) 496-1124

## National Institute of Arthritis and Musculoskeletal and Skin Diseases

John H. Klippel, M.D., Clinical Director
Telephone referrals should be directed to individuals listed under each subject area.

**Arthritis and Rheumatism Branch**
*Polymyositis and Dermatomyositis and Related Myopathies*
Paul H. Plotz, M.D., (301) 496-1474
*Juvenile Dermatomyositis and Other Idiopathic Inflammatory Myopathies of Childhood* Lisa G. Rider, M.D., (301) 496-6913

*Rheumatoid Arthritis* Ronald L. Wilder, M.D., Ph.D., Arthritis and Rheumatism Branch, (301) 496-3373
*Systemic Lupus Erythematosus*
Mark F. Gourley, M.D., (301) 496-5236
*Antiphospholipid Antibody Syndrome*
Michael D. Lockshin, M.D., (301) 496-0802
*Environmentally-Associated Connective Tissue Diseases*
Frederick W. Miller, M.D., Ph.D., (301) 496-6913
*Cystinuria*
Daniel L. Kastner, M.D., Ph.D., (301) 496-3374
*Familial Mediterranean Fever*
Daniel L. Kastner, M.D., Ph.D., (301) 496-3374

**Dermatology Clinical Research Unit**
*Skin Cancer, Disorders of Cornification*
John Di Giovanna, M.D., (301) 402-1607
*Genodermatoses* Sherri J. Bale, Ph.D., (301) 402-2679

## National Cancer Institute

Gregory A. Curt, M.D., Clinical Director
Telephone referrals should be directed to physicians listed under each study.

**Biological Response Modifiers Program**
Dan L. Longo, M.D., Acting Chief
Clinical Research Branch . . . . . . . . . . . . . . . (301) 846-1520

**Dermatology Branch**
Chief: Stephen I. Katz, M.D., Ph.D. . . . . . . . . . . (301) 496-2481
*Basal Cell Carcinoma* (especially nevoid basal cell carcinoma)
*Benign Mucosal Pemphigoid* (ocular pemphigoid)
*Bullous Pemphigoid*
*Dermatitis Herpetiformis*
*Disorders of Keratinization* (Ichthyoses, Darier's Disease)

*Epidermodysplasia Verruciformis* (Genetic predisposition for flat warts and squamous cell carcinoma)
*Epidermolysis Bullosa Acquisita*
*Erythema Elevatum Diutinum*
*Granuloma Faciale*
*Erythema Multiforme*
*Herpes Gestationis*
*Multiple Warts*
*Pemphigus Foliaceus*
*Pemphigus Vulgaris*
*Psoriasis*
*Sezary Syndrome*
*Vasculitis*
*Vulvodynia*
*Xeroderma Pigmentosum*

**Epidemiology Program**
Chief: Joseph F. Fraumeni, Jr., M.D. . . . . . . . . . . (301) 496-1611

**Experimental Immunology Branch**
Chief: Ronald E. Gress, M.D. . . . . . . . . . . . . . . (301) 496-1791
*Malignant Disease*

**Medicine Branch**
Chief: Robert E. Wittes, M.D. . . . . . . . . . . . . . . (301) 496-4916
*Hodgkin's Disease and Non-Hodgkin's Lymphoma*
*Ovarian Carcinoma*
*Breast Carcinoma*
*AIDS/Kaposi's Sarcoma*
*Colon Cancer*

**Clinical Pharmacology Branch**
Acting Chief: Eddie Reed, M.D. . . . . . . . . . . . . . (301) 402-1357
*Prostate Cancer*

**Metabolism Branch**
Chief: Thomas A. Waldmann, M.D. . . . . . . . . . . (301) 496-6653

*Agammaglobulinemia*
*Ataxia-Telangiectasia*
*Growth Hormone Deficiency*
*Hypogammaglobulinemia*
*Cutaneous T-Cell Lymphomas (Sezary Syndrome)*
*Adult T-Cell Leukemia*
*T-Cell Type Large Granular Lymphocytic Leukemia*
*Tropical Spastic Paraparesis*

**NCI-Navy Medical Oncology Branch**
Chief: Carmen Allegra, M.D. . . . . . . . . . . . . . . . . (301) 496-0901

**Pediatric Branch**
Chief: Philip A. Pizzo, M.D. . . . . . . . . . . . . . . . . (301) 496-4256
*Acute Leukemia*
*Ewing's Sarcoma*
*Brain Tumors*
*Non-Hodgkin's Malignant Lymphoma (especially Burkitt's Lymphoma)*
*Osteogenic Sarcoma*
*Rhabdomyosarcoma and Undifferentiated Sarcomas*
*Acquired Immunodeficiency Syndrome (AIDS)*

**Radiation Oncology Branch**
Chief: Paul Okunieff, M.D. . . . . . . . . . . . . . . . . . (301) 496-5457
*Breast Cancer*
*Unresectable Sarcomas*
*Gliomas*
*Hodgkin's Disease*
*Non-Hodgkin's Malignant Lymphomas*
*Oat Cell Cancer*
*Gastric Cancer*
*Carcinoma of the Bladder*
*Abdominal Sarcomas*
*Ovarian Cancer*
*Cervix Cancer*

**Surgery Branch**
Chief: Steven A. Rosenberg, M.D., Ph.D. . . . . . . (301) 496-4164
Admitting Officer: David N. Danforth, Jr., M.D. . . (301) 496-1534
*Sarcomas of Bone and Soft Tissues*
*Breast Cancer*
*Melanoma*
*Lung Cancer*
*Renal Cancer*
*Bladder Cancer*
*Metastatic Colorectal Cancer*
*Cancer of the Pancreas*
*Cancer of the Stomach*

## National Institute of Child Health and Human Development

Lynnette K. Nieman, M.D., Clinical Director
Telephone referrals of patients should be directed to physicians listed under each branch. General inquiries should be directed to:
Lynnette K. Nieman, M.D., Clinical Director . (301) 496-1068

**Human Genetics Branch**
Acting Chief: Joan C. Marini, M.D., Ph.D. . . . . . (301) 496-6683
*Carbohydrate-Deficient Glycoprotein Syndrome*
*Cystinosis*
*Lysosomal Storage Disorders*
*Amino Acid Disorders*
$\alpha_1$*-Antitrypsin Deficiency*
*Hermansky-Pudlak Syndrome*
*Menkes Disease*
*Osteogenesis Imperfecta*
*Sialic Acid Disorders*

**Perinatology Research Branch**
Chief: Roberto Romero, M.D. . . . . . . . . . . . . . . (202) 687-2329
*Current Pregnancy*
*Past Pregnancy History, with Another Pregnancy Anticipated*

**Developmental Endocrinology Branch**
Acting Chief: Carolyn A. Bondy, M.D. . . . . . . . . . (301) 496-4686
*Cushing's Syndrome*
*Nelson's Syndrome*
*Congenital Adrenal Hyperplasia*
*Adrenal Insufficiency*
*Short Stature*
*Premature Ovarian Failure*
*Congenital or Acquired Hypothyroidism*
*Turner Syndrome*
*Hypophosphatemic Rickets*
*Precocious Puberty*
*Delayed Puberty and Kallmann's Syndrome*
*Hirsutism and Virilism*
*Multiple Miscarriages*
*Infertility*
*Pituitary Tumors*
*Ambiguous Genitalia*
*Autoimmune Polyglandular Disorders*
*Hypoparathyroidism*

**Cell Biology and Metabolism Branch**
Chief: Richard D. Klausner, M.D. . . . . . . . . . . . . . (301) 496-6368

**Laboratory of Comparative Ethology**
Chief: Stephen J. Suomi, Ph.D. . . . . . . . . . . . . . . (301) 496-6832
*Developmental Psychology*

## National Institute on Deafness and Other Communication Disorders

Ralph Naunton, M.D., Acting Clinical Director
Telephone referrals should be directed to:
Suzanne Lischynsky . . . . . . . . . . . . . . . . . . (301) 496-7491
(301) 496-0771 (TDD)

*Voice or Laryngeal Disorders*
Christy Ludlow, Ph.D., (301) 496-9365
(301) 496-0771 (TDD)
*Speech Disorders* Christy Ludlow, Ph.D., (301) 496-9365
(301) 496-0771 (TDD)
*Hereditary Hearing Impairments*
Marci Lesperance, M.D., (301) 496-7491
(301) 496-0771 (TDD)

## National Institute of Dental Research

Bruce J. Baum, D.M.D., Ph.D., Clinical Director
Telephone referrals should be directed to the investigators listed after each study description.

*Salivary Gland Function and Dysfunction*
Philip C. Fox, D.D.S., (301) 496-4278
*Taste and Related Oral Sensory Disorders*
James M. Weiffenbach, Ph.D., (301) 496-4278
*Oral Motor Dysfunction*
Bruce J. Baum, D.M.D., Ph.D., (301) 496-1363
*Oral Surgery*
Raymond Dionne, D.D.S., Ph.D., (301) 496-5483
*Chronic Facial Pain* Donald J. DeNucci, D.D.S., M.S.,
or Raymond Dionne, D.D.S., Ph.D. (301) 496-5483
*Painful Diabetic Neuropathy* Mitchell Max, M.D., (301) 496-6695
*Reflex Sympathetic Dystrophy or Causalgia*
Mitchell Max, M.D., (301) 496-6695
*Post-herpetic Neuralgia* Mitchell Max, M.D., (301) 496-6695

## National Institute of Diabetes and Digestive and Kidney Diseases

James E. Balow, M.D., Clinical Director
Telephone referral should be directed to physicians listed under each study:

*Blood Diseases* N. Raphael Shulman, M.D., Clinical Hematology Branch, (301) 496-4787
*Chronic Viral Hepatitis* Jay H. Hoofnagle, M.D., Liver Diseases Section, (301) 402-3236
*Diabetes Mellinus* Monica Skarulis, M.D., Derek LeRoith, and Simeon Taylor, M.D., Diabetes Branch, (301) 496-4658
*Gastrointestinal Diseases* Robert T. Jensen, M.D., Gastroenterology Section, (301) 496-4201
*Hypoglycemia* Monica Skarulis, M.D. and Simeon Taylor, M.D., Diabetes Branch, (301) 496-4658
*Parathyroid Disorders and Metabolic Bone Diseases*
S.J. Marx, M.D., (301) 496-5051 and A.M. Spiegel, Metabolic Diseases Branch, (301) 496-4128
*Pituitary Tumors and Hypopituitarism*
Richard C. Eastman, M.D., Derek LeRoith, M.D., and Monica Skarulis, M.D., Diabetes Branch, (301) 496-4658
*Primary Biliary Cirrhosis*
Jay H. Hoofnagle, M.D., Liver Diseases Section, (301) 402-3236
*Kidney Diseases* Howard A. Austin III, M.D., James E. Balow, M.D., and Dimitrios T. Boumpas, M.D., Kidney Disease Section, (301) 496-3092
*Thyroid Neoplasms* Bruce D. Weintraub, M.D., (301) 496-3405 or Jacob Robbins, M.D., Molecular and Cellular Endocrinology Branch, (301) 496-5761
*Inappropriate Secretion of TSH, Hypothyroidism*
Bruce D. Weintraub, M.D., Molecular and Cellular Endocrinology Branch, (301) 496-3405
*Zollinger-Ellison Syndrome* Robert T. Jensen, M.D., Gastroenterology Section, (301) 496-4201
*Hemoglobinopathies* Griffin P. Rodgers, M.D., Laboratory of Chemical Biology, (301) 496-5408

## National Institute on Drug Abuse

Jean-Lud Cadet, M.D., Carol Contoreggi, M.D., Annie Umbricht, M.D., Acting Clinical Directors

Telephone referrals should be directed to:
Recruitment Unit . . . . . . . . . . . . . . . . . . . . (410) 550-1502

*Biopsychosocial Components of Drug Abuse Studies*
*Etiology of Drug Abuse Studies*
*Twin Studies*
*Treatment of Drug Withdrawal*
*Treatment of Drug Abuse*

## National Eye Institute

Scott Whitcup, M.D., Clinical Director
Telephone referral of patients should be directed to:
Scott Whitcup, M.D., Clinical Director . . . . . (301) 496-3123

**Clinical Branch**
*Glaucoma: Studies of the Factors Controlling Intraocular Pressure*
Carl Kupfer, M.D., Clinical Branch, (301) 496-2234
*Neuro-Ophthalmology* Ed Fitzgibbons, M.D.,
Laboratory of Sensorimotor Research, (301) 496-7144
*Vitreo-Retinal Disease* Frederick Ferris, M.D.,
Clinical Trials Branch, (301) 496-6583
*Congenital and Acquired Deficiencies of Visual Function*
Rafael C. Caruso, M.D.,
Ophthalmic Genetics and Clinical Services Branch, (301) 496-3577
*Retinal Degeneration* Muriel Kaiser, M.D.,
Ophthalmic Genetics and Clinical Services Branch, (301) 496-3577
*CMV Retinitis* Scott Whitcup, M.D.,
Clinical Branch, (301) 496-3123
*Uveitis* Robert Nussenblatt, M.D., Laboratory of Immunology
or Scott Whitcup, M.D., Clinical Branch, (301) 496-3123
*Cataracts* Muriel Kaiser, M.D., or Manuel Datiles, M.D.,
Ophthalmic Genetics and Clinical Services Branch, (301) 496-3577
*Ophthalmic Congenital and Genetic Disease*
Muriel Kaiser, M.D., or Manuel Datiles, M.D.,
Ophthalmic Genetics and Clinical Services Branch, (301) 496-3577

## National Heart, Lung, and Blood Institute

Harry R. Keiser, M.D., Clinical Director
Telephone referrals should be directed to the physicians listed under each study.

**Cardiology Branch**
Chief: Stephen E. Epstein, M.D. . . . . . . . . . . . . . . (301) 496-5817
*Coronary Artery Disease* Arshed Quyyumi, M.D., (301) 496-0022
*Microvascular Angina* Richard Cannon, M.D., (301) 496-9895
*Inherited Cardiac Diseases* Lameh Fananapazir, M.D. and Neal Epstein, M.D., Inherited Cardiac Diseases Section, (301) 496-5202
*Valvular Heart Disease* Julio Panza, M.D., (301) 496-2634

**Hypertension-Endocrine Branch**
Chief: Harry R. Keiser, M.D. . . . . . . . . . . . . . . . . (301) 496-1518
*Essential Hypertension*
*Familial Hypertension*
*Pheochromocytoma*
*Steroid Hypertension*
*Hypokalemia*

**Molecular Disease Branch**
Chief: H. Bryan Brewer, Jr., M.D. . . . . . . . . . . . (301) 496-5095
*Hyperlipidemia (Hyperlipoproteinemia)*
*Hypolipidemia (Hypolipoproteinemia)*

**Hematology Branch**
Chief: Neal S. Young, M.D. . . . . . . . . . . . . . . . (301) 496-5093
*Aplastic Anemia and Myelodysplasia*
*Multiple Myeloma and Chronic Myelogenous Leukemia*
*Sickle Cell Anemia*

**Pulmonary-Critical Care Medicine Branch**
Chief: Joel Moss, M.D., Ph.D. . . . . . . . . . . . . . . (301) 496-3632
*Interstitial Lung Disease*

*Asthma (Reactive Airways)*
*Chronic Bronchitis*
*$\alpha_1$-Antitrypsin*

## National Institute of Mental Health

David R. Rubinow, M.D., Clinical Director
Telephone referrals of patients should be directed to:
Nazli Haq, M.A. . . . . . . . . . . . . . . . . . . . . . (301) 496-1337

*Depression and Mania (Bipolar)* Nazli Haq, M.A., Office of the Clinical Director, (301) 496-1337

*Bipolar Disorder Genetic Study* Liz Maxwell, M.S.W., Clinical Neurogenetics Branch, (301) 496-8977

*Unipolar Disorder* David Michelson, M.D., Clinical Neuroendocrinology Branch, (301) 496-0083 or Debbie Hu, (301) 496-6979

*Depression in Women* David Michelson, M.D., Clinical Neuroendocrinology Branch, (301) 496-0083 or Lauren Hill, M.A., (301) 496-6978

*Menstrual and Menopausal Mood and Behavioral Disorders* Anne Bowles, Consultation-Liaison Service, (301) 496-9675

*Seasonal Affective Disorder (SAD)* Holly Clark, L.C.S.W., Clinical Psychobiology Branch, (301) 496-7427
Ron Barnett, Ph.D., (301) 496-0500
or Fran Myers, R.N., (301) 496-6565, ext. 209

*Anxiety Disorders* Barbara Scupi, L.C.S.W., Biological Psychiatry Branch, (301) 496-7141

*Panic Disorder Genetic Study* Liz Maxwell, M.S.W., Clinical Neurogenetics Branch, (301) 496-8977

*Anxiety Disorders and Pregnancy* Margaret Altemus, M.D., Laboratory of Clinical Science, (301) 496-3421

*Obsessive-Compulsive and Anxiety Disorders* David Keuler, M.A., Laboratory of Clinical Science, (301) 496-3421

*Borderline Personality Disorder* Kathleen O'Leary, M.S.W., Neuroscience Center at St. Elizabeths, (202) 373-6068

*Schizophrenia* Judy Schreiber, M.S.W., Experimental Therapeutics Branch, Clinical Center, (301) 496-7128; Admissions Office, Llewellyn Bigelow, M.D., Neuroscience Center at St. Elizabeths, (202) 373-6100; or Kayleen Hadd, R.N., Experimental Therapeutics Branch, (301) 496-2082

*Schizophrenia Disorder Genetic Study* Liz Maxwell, M.S.W., Clinical Neurogenetics Branch, (301) 496-8977

*Tardive Dyskinesia and Other Movement Disorder*
Admissions Office, Neuroscience Center at St. Elizabeths, (202) 373-6100

*Disorders of Attention and Cognition* Alan F. Mirsky, M.D., Laboratory of Psychology and Psychopathology, (301) 496-2551

*Rapid Cycling Mood Disorders*
Amy Iwan, B.A., Clinical Psychobiology Branch, (301) 496-6981 or Ellen Leibenluft, M.D., (301) 496-2141

*Childhood Mental Illness*
Gail Ritchie, M.S.W., Child Psychiatry Branch, (301) 496-0851 or (301) 496-6080
Marge Lenane, M.S.W., Child Psychiatry Branch, (301) 496-7962 or Susan Swedo, M.D., Child Psychiatry Branch, (301) 496-6081

*Attention-Deficit Hyperactivity Disorder in Children and Adults*
Peter Jons, B.A., Child Psychiatry Branch, (301) 496-4707

*Attention-Deficit Hyperactivity Disorder (ADHD) in Adults*
Peter Jons, B.A., Child Psychiatry Branch, (301) 496-4707

*Autism, Lesch-Nyhan Disorder and Tourette's Syndrome in Children and Adults* Monique Ernst, M.D., Ph.D., Child Psychiatry Branch, (301) 496-4707

*Eating Disorders in Adults* Harry Gwirtsman, M.D., Clinical Neuroendocrinology Branch, (301) 496-6884

*Developmental Psychology* Marian Radke Yarrow, Ph.D., Laboratory of Developmental Psychology, (301) 496-1091

*Alzheimer's Disease* Sue Bell, M.S.W., Laboratory of Clinical Science, (301) 496-3421

*Genetic Studies* Liz Maxwell, Clinical Neurogenetics Branch, (301) 496-8977

*Genetic Disorders* Edward Ginns, M.D., Ph.D., or Ellen Sidransky, M.D., Clinical Neuroscience Branch, (301) 496-0373

## National Institute of Neurological Disorders and Stroke

Mark Hallett, M.D., Clinical Director
Telephone referrals should be directed to the individuals listed under each study.

**Developmental and Metabolic Neurology Branch**
Chief: Roscoe O. Brady, M.D. . . . . . . . . . . . . . . . (301) 496-3285
Chief: Section on Clinical Investigations and Therapeutics,
Norman W. Barton, M.D., Ph.D. . . . . . . . . . (301) 496-1465
*Sphingolipidoses, Mucopolysaccharidoses and other Metabolic Storage Disorders*
*Neurogenetic Diseases*
*Progressive Dementia in Children*

**Neuroimmunology Branch**
Acting Chief: Henry F. McFarland, M.D. . . . . . . . (301) 496-1801

*Multiple Sclerosis*
*Familial Multiple Sclerosis*
*Subacute Sclerosing Panencephalitis*
*Neurological Diseases Related to HTLV-I*

**Experimental Therapeutics Branch**
Chief: Thomas N. Chase, M.D. . . . . . . . . . . . . . (301) 496-7993
*Extrapyramidal Disorders*
*Dementing Disorders*

**Surgical Neurology Branch**
Chief: Edward H. Oldfield, M.D. . . . . . . . . . . . . (301) 496-5728
*Brain Tumors*

*Spinal Arteriovenous Malformations*
*Pituitary Tumors*
*Syringomyelia*

**Medical Neurology Branch**
Chief: Mark Hallett, M.D. . . . . . . . . . . . . . . . . . . (301) 496-1561

***Human Motor Control Section***
Chief: Mark Hallett, M.D. . . . . . . . . . . . . . . . . . . (301) 496-1561
*Voluntary Movement Disorders*
*Involuntary Movement Disorders*

***Neuromuscular Diseases Section***
Chief: Marinos Dalakas, M.D. . . . . . . . . . . . . . . . (301) 496-9979
*Post-Polio Syndrome and Other Related Motor Neuron Diseases*
*Chronic Demyelinating Polyneuropathies*
*Inflammatory Myopathies*
*Neuromuscular Diseases*
*HIV-related Neuromuscular Disorders*
*Metabolic Myopathies, Periodic Paralysis and Channel Disorders*

***Cognitive Neuroscience Section***
Chief: Jordan Grafman, Ph.D. . . . . . . . . . . . . . . . (301) 496-0220
*Brain Behavior Studies*

**Clinical Neuroscience Branch**
Chief: Irwin Kopin, M.D. . . . . . . . . . . . . . . . . . . (301) 496-4297
*Autonomic Nervous System Disorders*
*Familial Alzheimer's Disease*

**Epilepsy Research Branch**
Acting Chief: William H. Theodore, M.D. . . . . . . (301) 496-1505

***Clinical Epilepsy Section***
Chief: William H. Theodore, M.D. . . . . . . . . . . . (301) 496-1505
*Epilepsy*

**Neuroimaging Branch**
Chief: Giovanni Di Chiro, M.D. . . . . . . . . . . . . . (301) 496-6801
*Brain Tumors*
*Cerebral Ischemia*
*Movement Disorders*

**Stroke Branch**
Chief: John M. Hallenbeck, M.D. . . . . . . . . . . . . (301) 496-6579
*Stroke*
*At-Risk-For-Stroke*

## Clinical Center

John I. Gallin, M.D., Director

**Critical Care Medicine Department**
Telephone referrals should be directed to:
AIDS Protocol Office . . . . . . . . 1-800-243-7644 (AIDS-NIH)
*HIV and Acquired Immune Deficiency Syndrome*

**Medical Genetics Program**
Telephone referrals should be directed to:
Sandra Schlesinger, M.S., Clinical Coordinator (301) 496-1380

William A. Gahl, M.D., Ph.D., Dilys Parry, Ph.D., Program Directors
(301) 496-6683 or (301) 496-4947
*The Interinstitute Medical Genetics Program*

## Doctors Who Get Grants To Study Your Illness

In addition to the free clinical studies at NIH described in the preceding section, there are thousands of other doctors who get research money and may be able to treat your condition for free. You can locate these doctors through the Division of Research Grants at NIH. This office can conduct a CRISP (Computer Retrieval for Information on Scientific Projects) search for you at no charge. The search can provide you with information on grants awarded to the National Institutes of Health, Food and Drug Administration, and other government research institutions, universities, or hospitals that deal with the topic in which you are interested. They have a free brochure available that describes their services.

☎ Contact:
Division of Research Grants
5333 Westbard Ave., Room 148
Bethesda, MD 20895
(301) 496-7543

What follows is an example of a CRISP search done on Headaches/Migraines. The information you receive includes the title of the study, the investigator, the research facility, the amount of the grant, as well as a detailed description of the purpose of the study.

# CRISP Search Request
# Topic: Headache Research

Title: *Psychophysiological Assessment of Stress in Chronic Pain*
Investigator: Ohrbach, Richard, SUNY At Buffalo,
355 Squire Hall Med.
Buffalo, NY 14214
Organization: State University of New York at Buffalo
Award Amount: $67,303

Title: *Neural and Endothelial Regulators of Cerebrovascular Tone*
Investigator: Brayden, Joseph E.
University of Vermont, Dept. of Pharmacology
Burlington, VT 05405
Organization: University of Vermont & State Agricultural College
Award Amount: $52,432

Title: *Medical Care and Risks of Dysfunctional Chronic Pain*
Investigator: Von Korff, Michael R.
Center for Health Studies
1730 Minor Ave., Suite 1600
Seattle, WA 98101-1448
Organization: Group Health Cooperative of Puget Sound
Award Amount: $73,600

Title: *Explanation in the Clinical Setting*
Investigator: Buchanan, Bruce G., Intelligent Systems Laboratory
Pittsburgh, PA 15260
Organization: University of Pittsburgh at Pittsburgh
Award Amount: $499,187

Title: *Genetic Epidemiology of Psychiatric Disorders*
Investigator: Merikangas, Kathleen R.

40 Temple St., Lower Level
New Haven, CT 06510-3223
Organization: Yale University
Award Amount: $65,433

Title: *Psychological Treatment of Headache*
Investigator: Blanchard, Edward B.
1535 Western Ave.
Albany, NY 12203
Organization: State University of New York at Albany
Award Amount: $116,890

Title: *Trigeminal Nerve--Control of the Brain Vasculature*
Investigator: Moskowitz, Michael A.
Massachusetts General Hospital
Fruit St., Boston, MA 02114
Organization: Massachusetts General Hospital
Award Amount: $282,399

Title: *Drug and Non-drug Treatment for Adult and Pediatric Migraine*
Investigator: Andrasik, Frank
University of West Florida
11000 University Parkway
Pensacola, FL 32514-5751
Organization: University of West Florida
Award Amount: $251,602

Title: *Pentosan Polysulfate as Prophylaxis for Migraine*
Investigator: Bigelow, L.B.
National Institute of Mental Health
Bethesda, MD
Organization: National Institute of Mental Health

Title: *Collaborative Studies of Less Common or Less Debilitating Neurologic Disorders*
Investigator: Roman, G.C., National Institute of Neurological

Disorders and Stroke
National Institutes of Health
Organization: NINDS

Title: *Erythema Multiforme--A Clinical Pathogenetic Study*
Investigator: Weston, William L., University of Colorado
School of Medicine
4200 West Ninth Ave., Box B153
Denver, CO 80262
Organization: University of Colorado Health Sciences Center
Award Amount: $167,349

Title: *Drug Dependence Clinical Research Program: Neurologic Sequelae of Cocaine Use*
Investigator: Rowbotham, Michael C.
University of California
401 Parnassus Ave.
San Francisco, CA 94143
Organization: University of California, San Francisco
Award Amount: $74,240

Title: *TMD Longitudinal Studies--Clinical/Chronic Pain Syndrome: Longitudinal Studies of Tempor-mandibular Disorders*
Investigator: Dworkin, S.F., University of Washington
School of Dentistry
Seattle, WA 98195
Organization: University of Washington
Award Amount: $196,489

Title: *TMD Longitudinal Studies--Clinical/Chronic Pain Syndrome: Longitudinal Studies of Chronic Pain Syndrome in TMD*
Investigator: Von Korff, M., University of Washington
School of Dentistry
Seattle, WA 98195
Organization: University of Washington
Award Amount: $196,489

Title: *Compliance in the Physicians' Health Study*
Investigator: Glynn, Robert J.
Brigham and Women's Hospital
55 Pond Ave.
Organization: Brigham and Women's Hospital
Award Amount: $38,563

Title: *Cost-Effective Management of HIV-related Illnesses*
Investigator: Tosteson, Anna, Dartmouth Medical School
1 Medical Center Dr.
Lebanon, NH 03756
Organization: Dartmouth College
Award Amount: $196,911

Title: *The Classification of Anxiety Disorders*
Investigator: Barlow, David H.
State University of New York at Albany
1400 Washington, Ave.
Albany, NY 12222
Organization: State University of New York at Albany
Award Amount: $233,953

Title: *Clinical Stroke Research Center: Stroke Prevention in Young Women*
Investigator: Kettner, Steven J.
University of Maryland Hospital
22 S. Greene St.
Baltimore, MD 21201
Organization: University of Maryland, Baltimore Professional School
Award Amount: $312,859

Title: *General Clinical Research Center: Marijuana-- Repeated Smoking in Humans (Marijuana-Alcohol Hangover)*
Investigator: Chait, Larry D.
University of Chicago
5841 S. Maryland Ave.

Chicago, IL 60637
Organization: University of Chicago
Award Amount: $34,508

Title: *General Clinical Research Center: Humoral and Cellular Mediated Immunity*
Investigator: Fireman, Philip A.
Children's Hospital of Pittsburgh
3705 Fifth Ave. at Desoto
St., Pittsburgh, PA 15213
Organization: Children's Hospital of Pittsburgh
Award Amount: $16,051

Title: *Antibody-toxin Conjugates for the Treatment of Human Brain Tumors*
Investigator: Youle, R.J.
National Institute of Neurological Disorders and Stroke, NIH
Bethesda, MD
Organization: NINDS

A second place to look is at the National Library of Medicine where you can conduct a search on their MEDLINE database (part of their MEDLARS databases). This search can provide you with citations and abstracts on your diagnosis and clinical trials from 6.6 million articles from approximately 3,600 biomedical journals published in the United States and abroad. You can access this system through a computer and modem. They also sell a GRATEFUL Med software program for $29.95 which is Macintosh and IBM-compatible, and makes it easier to access the library's collection. Libraries in your area, as well as medical schools may have access to the MEDLARS databases, and you may be able to have someone conduct a search for you for a small fee. Your regional medical library can also direct you to libraries near you that have access, or they may be able to provide the search for you. They can be reached at (800) 338-7657. For more information about accessing MEDLARS or buying the GRATEFUL Med software:

☎ Contact:

MEDLARS Management Section
National Library of Medicine
Bldg. 38A, Room 4N421
8600 Rockville Pike
Bethesda, MD 20894
(800) 638-8480

## Free Health Care At Your Hospital

Do you need an operation? Has an unexpected health crisis occurred? Are you worried about paying your hospital bills? Many hospitals, nursing homes, and clinics offer free or low-cost health care under the Hill-Burton free care program. You are eligible if your income falls within the Poverty Income Guidelines. You must request and apply for Hill-Burton assistance (you can even apply after you have been discharged). Each Hill-Burton facility can choose which types of services to provide at no charge or reduced charge, and must give you a written individual notice that will tell you what types of services are covered. They also must provide a specific amount of free care each year, but can stop once they have given that amount. A special hotline has been established that distributes information on applying for Hill-Burton assistance, and can answer questions regarding eligibility guidelines, facilities obligated to provide services, and help with filing a complaint. If you do not qualify for Hill-Burton assistance, don't worry: many hospitals have special funds to provide care for the poor. The hospital business offices can help you apply for various forms of government assistance, as well as set up payment plans you can afford. They can't help you if they don't know you have a problem. For more information on Hill-Burton:

☎ Contact:

Office of Health Facilities
Health Resources and Services Administration
Department of Health and Human Services
5600 Fishers Lane, Room 11-03
Rockville, MD 20857
(800) 638-0742
(800) 492-0359 (in MD).

## Local Free Health Clinics

Your local health department (found in the blue pages of your phone book) often operates free or sliding-fee-scale clinics and screening centers to handle non-emergency health problems. Many operate prenatal and well-baby clinics as well. The services and fees vary from place to place, so contact the health department to find out about eligibility, hours of service, and services provided. According to the National Association of Community Health Centers, federally sponsored community health centers serve six million people, and four to six million people are served at other-sponsored health centers. However, some problems exist. Because of the increase demand for low-cost health care, many centers are closing off registration and are carrying waiting lists of 15 to 20 percent of their current case load. The demand and availability of local health centers do vary, so don't overlook this resource. To find out about local clinics:

☎ Contact:
Your State Department of Public Health
(See listing below)

### Public Health Hotlines

**Alabama**
Department of Public Health
434 Monroe St.
Montgomery, AL 36130
(205) 613-5300

**Alaska**
Department of Health and Social Services
P.O. Box 110640
Juneau, AK 99811
(907) 465-3347

**Arizona**
Department of Health Services
1740 W. Adams St.
Phoenix, AZ 85007
(602) 542-1000

**Arkansas**
Department of Health
4815 W. Markham St.
Little Rock, AR 72205
(501) 661-2000

**California**
Department of Health Services
714 P St.
Sacramento, CA 95814
(916) 445-4171

**Colorado**
Department of Health
4210 E. 11th Ave.
Denver, CO 80220
(303) 692-2000

**Connecticut**
Department of Health Services
150 Washington St.
Hartford, CT 06106
(203) 566-4800

**Delaware**
Division of Public Health
P.O. Box 637
Dover, DE 19901
(302) 739-4701

**District of Columbia**
Commission of Public Health
613 G St NW
Washington, DC 20001
(202) 727-0014

**Florida**
Health and Rehabilitative Services Department
1323 Winewood Blvd.
Tallahassee, FL 32399
(904) 487-2705

**Georgia**
Public Health Division
Department of Human Resources
2 Peachtree St., NW
Atlanta, GA 30309
(404) 657-2700

**Hawaii**
Department of Health
P.O. Box 3378
Honolulu, HI 96801
(808) 586-4410

**Idaho**
Division of Health
Department of Health and Welfare
Towers Building
4th Floor
P.O. Box 83720
Boise, ID 83720
(208) 334-5945

**Illinois**
Maternal and Child Health
Department of Public Health
535 W. Jefferson St.
Springfield, IL 62761
(217) 524-5989
Beautiful Babies
(800) 545-2200

**Indiana**
State Board of Health
1330 W. Michigan St.
Indianapolis, IN 46206
(317) 383-6100

**Iowa**
Department of Public Health
Lucas State Office Building
Des Moines, IA 50319
(515) 281-5605

**Kansas**
Department of Health and Environment
Landon Office Building
Topeka, KS 66620
(913) 296-1343

**Kentucky**
Department for Health Services
275 E. Main St.
Frankfort, KY 40601
(502) 564-3970

**Louisiana**
Dept. of Health and Hospitals
325 Loyola Ave.
New Orleans, LA 70112
(504) 568-5050

**Maine**
Department of Human Services
State House Station #11
Augusta, ME 04333
(207) 289-3707

**Maryland**
Department of Health and Mental Hygiene
201 W. Preston St.
Baltimore, MD 21201
(410) 225-6500

**Massachusetts**
Department of Public Health
150 Tremont St.
Boston, MA 02111
(617) 727-0201

**Michigan**
Department of Public Health
3423 N Martin Luther King Blvd.
Lansing, MI 48909
(517) 335-8000

**Minnesota**
Department of Health
717 Delaware St., SE
Minneapolis, MN 55440
(612) 623-5000

**Mississippi**
Department of Health
2423 N. State St.
Jackson, MS 39216
(601) 960-7635

**Missouri**
Department of Health
P.O. Box 570
Jefferson City, MO 65102
(314) 751-6062

**Montana**
Health Services Division
Health and Environment Sciences
Cogswell Building
Helena, MT 59620
(406) 444-4473

**Nebraska**
Department of Health
301 Centennial Mall S.

P.O. Box 95007
Lincoln, NE 68509
(402) 471-2133

**Nevada**
Department of Human Resources
505 E. King St.
Carson City, NV 89710
(703) 687-4740

**New Hampshire**
Department of Health and Welfare
Hazen Dr.
Concord, NH 03301
(603) 271-4501

**New Jersey**
Department of Health
CN 360
Trenton, NJ 08625
(609) 292-7837

**New Mexico**
Department of Health
1190 St. Francis Dr.
Santa Fe, NM 87502
(505) 827-2613

**New York**
Department of Health
Empire State Plaza
Albany, NY 12237
(518) 474-7354

**North Carolina**
Department of Health
P.O. Box 27687
Raleigh, NC 27611
(919) 715-4125

**North Dakota**
Department of Health
State Capitol
600 E. Boulevard
Bismarck, ND 58505
(701) 328-2372

**Ohio**
Department of Health
246 N. High St.
P.O. Box 118
Columbus, OH 43266
(614) 466-3543

**Oklahoma**
Department of Health
1000 NE 10th
P.O. Box 53551
Oklahoma City, OK 73152
(405) 271-4200

**Oregon**
Health Division
Department of Human Resources
800 NE Oregon St.
Portland, OR 97232
(503) 731-4000

**Pennsylvania**
Bureau of Community Health
P.O. Box 90
Harrisburg, PA 17120
(717) 787-4366

**Rhode Island**
Department of Health
3 Capitol Hill
Providence, RI 02908
(401) 277-2231

**South Carolina**
Health and Environmental Control
2600 Bull St.
Columbia, SC 29201
(803) 734-5000

**South Dakota**
Department of Health
Anderson Building
Pierre, SD 57501
(605) 773-3361

**Tennessee**
Department of Health
Tennessee Tower, 9th Floor
312 8th Ave. N
Nashville, TN 37247
(615) 741-3111

**Texas**
Department of Health
1100 W. 49th St.
Austin, TX 78756
(512) 458-7111

**Utah**
Department of Health
288 N. 1460 W
Salt Lake City, UT 84116
(801) 538-6101

**Vermont**
Department of Health
P.O. Box 70
Burlington, VT 05402
(802) 863-7200

**Virginia**
Department of Health
109 W Main St.
Richmond, VA 23219
(804) 786-3561

**Washington**
Department of Health
1112 SE Quince
P.O. Box 47890
Olympia, WA 98504
(206) 753-5871

**West Virginia**
Bureau of Public Health
Building 3, Room 518
Charleston, WV 25305
(304) 558-2971

**Wisconsin**
Bureau of Public Health
Health and Social Services Department
1414 E Washington Ave.
Madison, WI 53703
(608) 266-1251

**Wyoming**
Department of Health
Hathaway Building
Cheyenne, WY 82002
(307) 777-7656

# Federal Medical Programs For Elderly, Disabled And Low Income

How do you know if you qualify for Medicare or Medicaid? The Medicare Program is a federal health insurance program for persons over 65 years of age and certain disabled persons. It is funded through Social Security contributions, premiums, and general revenue. The Medicaid Program is a joint federal/state program which provides medical services to the needy and the medically needy. Eligibility and services for this program vary from state to state. To locate an office near you, look in the blue pages of your phone book under Human Services or:

☎ Contact:
Medicare Hotline
Health Care Financing Administration
330 Independence Ave., SW
Washington, DC 20201
(800) 638-6833
(800) 492-6603

This hotline can provide you with information regarding Medicare, Medicaid, and Medigap questions. They can refer you to the proper people to answer your questions, as well as provide you with publications on your topic of interest. This is also the number to call if you suspect abuse or fraud of Medicare or Medicaid, as well as if you suspect improper sales practices of Medigap policies.

## New Law Provides Free Health Care For Children

Are you pregnant or the parent of young children? Do you have a child with special needs? The federal government provides block grants, called Title V, to each state to provide maternal and child (including teens) health care services. Each state has some latitude as to how they spend the money, but 30% must go to providing services for children with special health care needs, and 30% for children and adolescents. The Maternal and Child Health Division of your state Department of Health is responsible for administering the funds. The states are required by Title V to start establishing 800 numbers to provide information regarding services available in the state (see state by state listing later in this chapter).

Federal law requires that all states provide Medicaid to pregnant women and children through the age of six whose income does not exceed 133% of the poverty line. Federal poverty thresholds in 1994 were $7,360 for one person, $9,840 for two, $12,320 for three, and $14,800 for four people. The government is going to raise the age level for Medicaid benefits one year at a time until all children are covered to age eighteen. Many states have additional benefits for children and programs for children with special needs. The following states have extended Medicaid coverage:

- *Minnesota*: covers everyone with income below 225% of the federal poverty line, or about $33,000 for a family of four.
- *Vermont*: all children under eighteen with family incomes below 225% of the federal poverty line, or about $33,000 for a family of four.
- *Washington*: all children to age eighteen with family incomes 100% of federal poverty line, or about $14,800 for

a family of four.

- *Wisconsin*: children one to six with family incomes below 155% of federal poverty line, or about $22,940 for a family of four.
- *Maine*: all children to age 18 with family incomes below 125% of poverty line, or about $8,500 for a family of four.
- 23 states have extended coverage for all pregnant women whose incomes are 100% of poverty line, or about $13,950.
- Several states, such as Ohio and West Virginia, have established special programs for children with special health care needs.

There are several ways to find out more about the programs available in your state. You can call the local department of health (found in the blue pages in your phone book), or the state Department of Health and the Maternal and Child Health Hotlines (listed below). Each year states enact new legislation to help provide health care for those in need. Your state representative can keep you updated regarding new legislation. To find out more about the programs available in your state:

☎ Contact:
Your State
Maternal and Child Health Hotline
(See listing below)

## Maternal and Infant Care Hotlines

**Alabama**
Maternal and Infant Care
434 Monroe St.
Montgomery, AL 36130
(205) 242-5766

Stork Line Referral Information
(800) 654-1385
This hotline can refer people to local maternal and infant health centers.

**Alaska**
Division of Public Assistance
Department of Health and Social Services
P.O. Box 110640
Juneau, AK 99811-0640
(907) 465-3347

**Arizona**
Information Referral Service
1515 East Osbourne at the Annex
Phoenix, AZ 85014
(602) 263-8856
Health Care Referral
(800) 352-3792

**Arkansas**
Section of Maternal and Child Health
Arkansas State Department of Health
4815 W. Markham
Little Rock, AR 72205
(501) 661-2251
Health Care Clearinghouse
(800) 336-4797
This hotline can refer you to local resources.

**California**
Maternal and Child Health
State Department of Health
714 P. St., Room 740
Sacramento, CA 95814
(916) 657-1347
(800) BABY-999
(222-9999)
This hotline can refer you to local maternal and child health resources.

**Colorado**
Family Health Services
Colorado Department of Health
4210 East 11th Ave.
Denver, CO 80220
(303) 331-8360
(800) 688-7777
This hotline can refer you to local maternal and child health resources.

**Connecticut**
Connecticut Association for Human Services
880 Asylum Ave.
Hartford, CT 06105
(203) 522-7762

INFOLINE- The following numbers can refer you to the appropriate resources in your area:
North West Region
(203) 759-2000
South Central Region
(203) 867-4150
East Region
(203) 886-0516
North Central Region
(203) 522-4636
South West Region
(203) 853-2525
To access your closest region
(800) 203-1234

**Delaware**
Division of Public Health
Health and Social Services Dept.
P.O. Box 637
Dover, DE 19903
(302) 739-4701

Help Line
(800) 464-HELP
The Helpline can refer you to local health services, as well as provide you with other state services and information.

### District of Columbia

Office of Maternal And Child Health
Commission of Public Health
613 G St NW
Suite 628
Washington, DC 20001
(800) MOM-BABY
(202) 727-0393

### Florida

Maternal and Child Health
Health and Rehabilitative Services Department
1317 Winewood Blvd.
Tallahassee, FL 32399
(904) 487-2705
(800) 451-BABY
This hotline can refer you to local maternal and child health resources.

### Georgia

Family Health Services Section
Division of Public Health
Department of Human Resources
2 Peachtree St., SW
8th Floor
Atlanta, GA 30303
(404) 657-2850
This hotline can refer you to local maternal and child health resources.

### Hawaii

Family Health Services Division
State of Hawaii
Department of Health
3652 Kilawea Ave.
Honolulu, HI 96816
(808) 733-9017
(808) 275-2000
This number can refer you to local maternal and child health resources.

### Idaho

Bureau of Maternal and Child Health
Idaho Department of Health and Welfare
450 W. State St.
Boise, ID 83720
(208) 334-5967
(800) 926-2588
This number can refer you to local maternal and child health resources.

### Illinois

Department of Public Health
535 W. Jefferson St.
Springfield, IL 62761
(217) 782-4977
Contact your local health department.

### Indiana

Division of Maternal and Child Health
Indiana State Board of Health
1330 W. Michigan St.
Suite 236N
Indianapolis, IN 46206
(317) 383-6478

Family Wellness Health Line
(800) 433-0746
This hotline can refer you to local resources for help.

**Iowa**
Family and Community Health
Department of Public Health
Lucas State Office Bldg.
Des Moines, IA 50319
(515) 281-3931
Healthy Families
(800) 369-2229
This hotline can refer you to local resources.

**Kansas**
Electronic Data Systems-Recipients Assistance
P.O. Box 4649
Topeka, KS 66604
(913) 273-8557
(800) 658-4690

SRS- Division of Medical Services
915 SW Harrison
Room 628 South
Docking State Office Building
Topeka, KS 66612
(913) 296-3981

**Kentucky**
Division of Maternal and Child Health
Department of Health Services
State Dept. of Human Resources
275 East Main St.
Frankfort, KY 40621
(502) 564-4830
(800) 372-2973
This hotline can refer you to local maternal and child health resources.

**Louisiana**
Department of Health and Hospitals
325 Loyola Ave.
New Orleans, LA 70112
(504) 568-5051
(800) 922-DIAL
This hotline can refer you to local resources.
(800) 251-BABY

**Maine**
Division of Maternal and Child Health
Department of Human Services
151 Capitol St.
State House- Station 11
Augusta, ME 04333
(207) 287-3311
(800) 698-3624
(800) 437-9300
(207) 775-7231
This hotline can answer your maternal and child health questions.

**Maryland**
Department of Health and Mental Hygiene
201 W. Preston St., 5th Fl.
Baltimore, MD 21201-2399
(410) 225-6538
(MAC- Maryland Access to Care Program)
(800) 492-5231
This 800 number can refer you to local services.

### Massachusetts

Bureau of Family & Community Health
Massachusetts Department of Public Health
150 Tremont St.
Boston, MA 02111
(617) 727-0940
The following numbers can refer you to the proper maternal and child health resources:

Boston Region
(800) 531-2229
Central Region
(800) 227-7748
North East Region
(800) 992-1895
South East Region
(800) 642-4250
West Region
(800) 992-6111

### Michigan

Bureau of Child & Family Services
Division of Family & Community Health
3423 N Martin Luther King Jr. Blvd.
P.O. Box 30035
Lansing, MI 38909
(517) 335-8945
(800) 26-BIRTH
This hotline can refer you to local resources for all your health and human services needs.

### Minnesota

Department of Human Services
444 Lafayette Rd.
St. Paul, MN 55155
(612) 296-6117
Maternal and Child Health Referrals
(800) 657-3672
Health and Human Services
(800) 652-9747

### Mississippi

Department of Health
2423 N. State St.
Jackson, MS 39215
(601) 960-7484
(800) 222-7622
This hotline can refer you to local health resources.

### Missouri

Division of Child and Family Health Care
Department of Health
P.O. Box 570
Jefferson City, MO 65102
(800) 835-5465
TELL-LINK

### Montana

Health Services and Medical Facilities Division
Department of Health and Environmental Sciences
Cogswell Building
1400 Broadway
Helena, MT 59620-0901
(406) 444-4740
(800) 762-9891
This hotline can refer you to local maternal and child health resources.

## Nebraska

Maternal and Child Health
State Department of Health
301 Centennial Mall South
P.O. Box 95007
Lincoln, NE 68509
(402) 471-2907
Healthy Mother/Healthy Baby Coalition
(800) 862-1889

## Nevada

Family Health Services
Nevada Health Division
Kinkhead Building
State Department of Human Resources
505 East King St., Room 205
Carson City, NV 89710
(702) 687-4885
(800) 992-0900 ext. 4885
This hotline can refer you to local maternal and child health resources.

## New Hampshire

Helpline
2 Industrial Park Dr.
Concord, NH 03301
(800) 852-3388
(603) 225-9000
This 24-hour helpline for social services answers questions regarding emergency health, spouse or child abuse, suicide, food, housing, clothing, alcohol and drug problems, and more.

## New Jersey

Maternal and Infant Health
New Jersey Dept. of Health
CN364
50 E State St.
Trenton, NJ 08625-0364
(609) 292-5616
(800) 328-3838
This office can answer questions regarding maternal and infant health, and can refer to clinics for prenatal, and child health programs. People looking for other health services should contact your local health department.

## New Mexico

Department Of Health
1190 St. Francis Dr.
Santa Fe, NM 87502
(505) 827-2613
The Department of Health can refer you to your local district for further information and help.

Information Center
DD Planning Council
435 St. Michael's Dr., Bldg. D
Santa Fe, NM 97501
(800) 552-8195
(505) 827-6260
This is an information center for New Mexicans with disabilities and BABYNET. They can refer people to clinics, and handle referrals for prenatal, postnatal and well-baby care. They have an information database to direct you to services in your area.

## New York

Growing Up Healthy
New York State Dept. of Health

8th Floor, Room 789
Empire State Plaza
Albany, NY 12237
(800) 522-5006
(518) 474-1964
This hotline can provide you with information on receiving low-cost pregnancy testing, prenatal and post natal care, as well as information on where to obtain well-baby care.

**North Carolina**
Care Line
Department of Human Resources
325 N. Salisbury St.
Raleigh, NC 27603
(800) 662-7030
(919) 733-4261
This hotline can answer your questions regarding where to obtain health care and other human services, such as welfare, food stamps, and other entitlement programs.

**North Dakota**
Division of Maternal and Child Health
State Department of Health and Consolidated Labs
600 E Boulevard Ave.
State Capitol Building
Bismarck, ND 58505
(701) 328-2493
(800) 472-2286
This hotline can provide you with information on family planning, health promotion and education, WIC, and other maternal and child health information.

Children With Special Health Care Needs
Department of Human Services
State Capitol Building
Bismarck, ND 58505
(701) 224-4814
(800) 472-2622 x2436
This hotline can provide answers to all your question regarding children with special health care needs. They have information on case management, special education, medical specialties, dental care, hospitalization, and much more.

**Ohio**
Healthy Babies Health Line
Bureau of Maternal and Child Health
Ohio Department of Health
P.O. Box 118
Columbus, OH 43266
(614) 466-5332
(800) 624-BABY
This hotline can direct you to prenatal, postnatal and well baby clinics, as well as your local WIC, Medicaid, and other human services offices.

**Oklahoma**
Health Line
1000 NE 10th St.
Department of Health
Oklahoma City, OK 73117-1299
(405) 271-4200
This health line can refer you to helpful clinics in the Oklahoma City area.

Community Council of Central Oklahoma
Information and Referral
P.O. Box 675
Oklahoma City, OK 73101
(405) 272-0049
This health line deals with all health concerns, referring people to health clinics in Oklahoma, Canadian and Cleveland counties.

### Oregon

Safe Net
Multnamah County
426 SW Stark
Portland, OR 97204
(800) SAFE-NET
This hotline handles maternal and child health care needs (including teens). They deal with such issues as primary care, family planning, and have a roster of private physicians and clinics.

### Pennsylvania

Health Hotline
Pennsylvania Department of Health
Division of Health Promotion
P.O. Box 90, Room 1003
Health and Welfare Building
Harrisburg, PA 17108
(800) 692-7254
(717) 787-5900
This hotline can provide you with community clinic information, immunizations, AIDS/STD testing, some prenatal and well-baby care, but no referrals to doctors, hospitals, or primary care.

### Rhode Island

Right Start
Rhode Island Department of Health
3 Capitol Hill, Room 302
Providence, RI 02908
(800) 346-1004
This hotline is designed to hook up uninsured Pregnant women with health clinics in their area. They can also direct you to early childhood well-baby centers.

### South Carolina

South Carolina Department of Health
1st Nine Care Line- MH
Robert Mills Complex
Box 101106
Columbia, SC 29211
(803) 734-3350
(800) 868-0404
This hotline serves pregnant women and women with children under the age of one. For other health care questions contact your local health department.

### South Dakota

Health Services
Department of Health
Anderson Bldg.
445 E Capitol Ave.
Pierre, SD 57501
(605) 773-3737
(800) 658-3080
This office can refer you to community health services, WIC,

emergency services, maternal and child health care, and health promotion.

**Tennessee**
Maternal and Child Health Section
Tennessee Department of Health and Environment
Bureau of Health Services
Tennessee Tower Bldg
10th Floor
312 8th Ave
Nashville, TN 37247-4701
(615) 741-7353
(800) 428-BABY (2229)
Although this hotline is set up to handle calls from pregnant women and mothers, they can direct all callers to local health services.

**Texas**
BABY LOVE
Maternal and Child Health
Texas Department of Health
1100 West 49th St.
Austin, TX 78756
(512) 458-7700
(800) 4-Baby Love (422-2956)
This office can refer you to local health centers, child health clinics, WIC and Medicaid offices, and other well baby resources.

**Utah**
Maternal & Infant Health
44 Medical Drive
Salt Lake City, UT 84114
(801) 584-8284
Pregnancy Risk Line
(800) 826-9662
Medicine, Drugs and Chemicals
(800) 822-2229
Baby Watch
(800) 839-8200

**Vermont**
Medical Services
Vermont Department of Health
P.O. Box 70
Burlington, VT 05402
(802) 863-7330
This hotline deals only with pregnancies, and can refer you to different agencies. For all other health concerns contact your local health department.

**Virginia**
Department of Health
1500 E Main, Room 136
Richmond, VA 23219
(804) 786-3561
Contact your local health department.

**Washington**
Department of Health
1112 SE Quince, M/S: 7890
Olympia, WA 98504-7890
(206) 753-5871
Contact your local health department.

**West Virginia**
Division of Maternal and Child Health
State Department of Health
1411 Virginia St., E

Charleston, WV 25301
(800) 642-8522
(304) 558-5388
This office handles women and children's services, referrals to local health centers, early intervention programs, WIC, family planning, high risk pregnancy programs, pediatricians, birthing centers, dental heal, cancer prevention, and adolescent pregnancy programs.

Client Services
Health and Human Resources Department
State Capitol Complex
Charleston, WV 25305
(304) 558-2400
(800) 642-8589
This hotline can answer questions regarding case eligibility for benefits, and can refer callers to local health centers.

**Wisconsin**
Division of Health
Health and Social Services Department
1 W. Wilson St.
Madison, WI 53703
(608) 266-1511
Contact your local health department.

**Wyoming**
Division of Public Health
Department of Health
Hathaway Bldg.
Cheyenne, WY 82002
(307) 777-6186
This office can refer you to local health care services.

## It's The Law: Care At Hospital Emergency Rooms

If you walk into an emergency room, do they have to treat you? Emergency rooms are now required by federal law to provide an initial screening to assess a patient's condition, which is designed to stop the automatic transfer of people unable to pay. Emergency rooms must also treat emergency situations until they are stabilized, then they can refer you to other hospitals or clinics for further treatment. Emergency medicine encompasses the immediate decision making and action necessary to prevent death or any further disability for patients in health crises. It also includes interventions necessary to stabilize the patient, as well as short-term assessment of the patient's condition beyond the immediate life, limb, and disability threats. If you feel you have been denied service, or received insufficient care, you should complain to your regional Health Care Financing Administration, who then will investigate your complaint. Because of the increase in the number of people who cannot afford or do not qualify for health insurance, many people wait to seek treatment until the situation becomes so terrible they end up in the emergency room. People are also using the emergency room as their primary care physician. By using some of your other options to receive health care, you can receive needed treatments sooner and from more appropriate sources.

## Regional Health Care Financing Administration Offices

*** Region 1**
JF Kennedy Federal Building
Government Center
Boston, MA 02203
(617) 565-1188

*** Region 2**
26 Federal Plaza
JK Javits Federal Building
New York, NY 10278
(212) 264-4488

*** Region 3**
3535 Market St., Gateway Building
P.O. Box 7760
Philadelphia, PA 19101
(215) 596-1351

*** Region 4**
101 Marietta Tower
Atlanta, GA 30323
(404) 331-2329

*** Region 5**
105 W. Adams St.
Chicago, IL 60603
(312) 886-6432

*** Region 6**
1200 Main Tower Building
Dallas, TX 75202
(214) 767-6427

*** Region 7**
601 E 12th St.
Federal Building
Kansas City, MO 64106
(816) 426-5233

*** Region 8**
1961 Stout St.
Federal Office Building
Denver, CO 80294
(303) 844-2111

*** Region 9**
75 Hawthorne St.
San Francisco, CA 94105
(415) 744-3502

*** Region 10**
2201 Sixth Ave.
Blanchard Plaza
Mail Stop RX-40
Seattle, WA 98121
(206) 553-0425

## Physicians Who Volunteer In Your Area

Where are the free clinics in your area? Do you have volunteer physician groups near you? Your local medical society can be a great resource to answer these questions. Although service varies from place to place, most medical societies know about the different county programs, groups of physicians who volunteer their services, free clinics, and other helpful information, and can refer you to the appropriate place for help. Several of the societies actually assist people in making appointments, while others direct you to an initial screening with the health department. According to a recent American Medical Association survey, physicians average 6.6 hours per week of free or reduced fee care. This amounts to $6.8 billion annually. To find out if there are local opportunities available for you:

☎ Contact:
Your State Medical Association
(See listing below)

### Medical Association Hotlines

**Alabama**
Medical Association of the State of Alabama
19 S. Jackson St.
Montgomery, AL 36102
(205) 263-6441

**Alaska**
Alaska State Medical Association
4107 Laurel St.
Anchorage, AK 99508
(907) 562-2662

**Arizona**
Arizona Medical Association
810 W. Bethany Home Rd.
Phoenix, AZ 85103
(602) 246-8901

**Arkansas**
Arkansas Medical Society
P.O. Box 5776
Little Rock, AR 72205
(501) 224-8967

**California**
California Medical Association
P.O. Box 7690
San Francisco, CA 94120
(415) 541-0900

**Colorado**
Colorado Medical Society
P.O. Box 17550
Denver, CO 80217
(303) 779-5455

**Connecticut**
Connecticut State Medical Society
160 St. Ronan St.
New Haven, CT 06511
(203) 865-0587

**Delaware**
Medical Society of Delaware
1925 Lovering Ave.
Wilmington, DE 19806
(302) 652-6512

**District of Columbia**
D.C. Medical Society
2215 M St., NW
Washington, DC 20037
(202) 466-1800

**Florida**
Florida Medical Association
760 Riverside Ave.
P.O. Box 2411
Jacksonville, FL 32204
(904) 356-1571

**Georgia**
Georgia Medical Association
938 Peachtree St., NE
Atlanta, GA 30309
(404) 876-7535

**Hawaii**
Hawaii Medical Association
1360 S. Bevetania
Honolulu, HI 96814
(808) 536-7702

**Idaho**
Idaho Medical Association
P.O. Box 2668
Boise, ID 83701
(208) 344-7888

**Illinois**
Illinois Medical Society
20 N. Michigan Ave.
Suite 700
Chicago, IL 60602
(312) 782-1654

**Indiana**
Indiana State Medical Association
322 Canal Walk
Indianapolis, IN 46202
(317) 261-2060

**Iowa**
Iowa Medical Society
1001 Grand Ave.
W. Des Moines, IA 50265
(515) 223-1401

**Kansas**
Kansas Medical Society
623 SW 10th Ave.
Topeka, KS 66612
(913) 235-2383

**Kentucky**
Kentucky Medical Association
301 N. Jurstbourne Parkway
Suite 200
Louisville, KY 40222
(502) 426-6200

**Louisiana**
Louisiana State Medical Society
3501 N. Causeway
Metairie, LA 70002
(504) 832-9815

**Maine**
Maine Medical Association
P.O. Box 190
Manchester, ME 04351
(207) 622-3374

**Maryland**
Maryland Medical Society
1211 Cathedral St.
Baltimore, MD 21201
(410) 539-0872

**Massachusetts**
Massachusetts Medical Society
1440 Main St.
Waltham, MA 02154
(617) 893-4610

**Michigan**
Michigan Medical Society
120 W. Saginaw St.
E. Lansing, MI 48823
(517) 337-1351

**Minnesota**
Minnesota Medical Association
Suite 300
3433 Broadway St. NW
Minneapolis, MN 55413
(612) 378-1875

**Mississippi**
Mississippi Medical Association
735 Riverside Dr.
Jackson, MS 39202
(601) 354-5433

**Missouri**
Missouri Medical Association
113 Madison St.
P.O. Box 1028
Jefferson, MO 65102
(314) 636-5151

**Montana**
Montana Medical Association
2021 11th Ave., Suite #1
Helena, MT 59601
(406) 443-4000

**Nebraska**
Nebraska Medical Association
233 S. 13th St., Suite #1512
Lincoln, NE 68508
(402) 474-4472

**Nevada**
Nevada Medical Association
3660 Baker West #3101
Reno, NV 89509
(702) 825-6788

**New Hampshire**
New Hampshire Medical Society
7 North State St.
Concord, NH 03301
(603) 224-1909

**New Jersey**
New Jersey Medical Society
2 Princess Rd.
Lawrenceville, NJ 08648
(609) 896-1766

**New Mexico**
New Mexico Medical Society
7770 Jefferson NE, Suite #400
Albuquerque, NM 87109
(505) 828-0237

**New York**
New York Medical Society
420 Lakeville Rd.
Lakesuccess, NY 11042
(516) 488-6100

**North Carolina**
North Carolina Medical Society
P.O. Box 27167
Raleigh, NC 27611
(919) 833-3836

**North Dakota**
North Dakota Medical Association
P.O. Box 1198
Bismarck, ND 58502
(701) 223-9475

**Ohio**
Ohio State Medical Association
1500 Lake Shore Dr.
Columbus, OH 43017
(614) 486-2401

**Oklahoma**
Oklahoma State Medical Association
601 NW Expressway
Oklahoma City, OK 73118
(405) 843-9571

**Oregon**
Oregon State Medical Association
5210 South Corbett
Portland, OR 97201
(503) 226-1555

**Pennsylvania**
Pennsylvania State Medical Society
777 E. Park Dr.
P.O. Box 8820
Harrisburg, PA 17105
(717) 558-7750

**Rhode Island**
Rhode Island State Medical Society
106 Francis St.
Providence, RI 02903
(401) 331-3207

**South Carolina**
South Carolina State Medical Association
P.O. Box 11188
Columbia, SC 29211
(803) 798-6207

**South Dakota**
South Dakota State Medical Association
1323 S. Minnesota Ave.
Sioux Falls, SD 57105
(605) 336-1965
Share Care is a special program in South Dakota for low income

Medicare recipients in which doctors accept Medicare payment in full (no deductibles or co-payments). 50-60% of the doctors in the state participate. You can apply for a card with the Association.

### Tennessee

Tennessee State Medical Association
P.O. Box 120909
Nashville, TN 37212
(615) 385-2100
They have the Tennessee Medical Access Program for people over 65 and a referral program through half of the county health agencies.

### Texas

Texas State Medical Association
401 W. 15th St.
Austin, TX 78701
(512) 370-1300
The local societies can refer you to places in your area for free or low-cost care.

### Utah

Utah State Medical Association
540 E. 500 S.
Salt Lake City, UT 84102
(801) 355-7477

### Vermont

Vermont State Medical Association
Box 1457
Montpelier, VT 05601
(802) 223-7898

### Virginia

Virginia State Medical Society
4205 Dover Rd.
Richmond, VA 23221
(804) 353-2721
Some local societies have information regarding pilot programs in their areas, as well as the Medallion Program for Medicaid-managed care.

### Washington

Washington State Medical Association
2033 6th Ave., Suite 900
Seattle, WA 98121
(206) 441-9762

### West Virginia

West Virginia State Medical Association
4307 MacCorkle Ave., SE
Charleston, WV 25304
(304) 925-0342

### Wisconsin

Wisconsin State Medical Association
P.O. Box 1109
Madison, WI 53701
(608) 257-6781

### Wyoming

Wyoming State Medical Association
P.O. Drawer 4009
Cheyenne, WY 82003
(307) 635-2424

# Handicapped and Disabled: The Best Places To Start For Help

If you are disabled or handicapped and need help becoming more independent, there are hundreds of sources of free help and money from federal, state, local, private, and non-profit organizations.

The help available ranges from free information services, self-help groups (for specific disabilities and disabilities in general), free legal aid, and independent living programs, to free money for education, job training, living expenses, transportation, equipment and mobility aids. You can even get money to have your home retrofitted to make it more accessible to your specific handicap. And if you're denied any of these programs or services, there are several free sources of legal help to make sure that you get what you're entitled to.

The three best places where you should begin your search for information about services and money programs for the disabled and handicapped are:

The Social Security Administration
Your State Office of Vocational Rehabilitation
Client Assistance Programs

In this Section, you'll find descriptions and listings of contacts for these three programs, along with several additional best places for self-help and aid for handicapped or disabled individuals.

## Free Money For The Disabled Who Have Worked In The Past

If you're disabled and expect to be so for at least one year, and have worked long enough and recently enough under Social Security, you may be eligible for Social Security Disability Insurance Benefits (DIB). If you are found entitled to DIB, you will receive a monthly check in an amount based on your prior earnings.

If you start back to work after receiving DIB, you have nine months (not necessarily consecutive), to earn as much as you can without affecting your benefits. (The nine months of work must fall within a five-year period before your trial work period can end.) After your trial work period ends, your work is evaluated to see if it is "substantial." This means that your earnings are more than $500.00. For 36 months after a successful trial work period, if you are still disabled, you will be eligible to receive a monthly benefit without a new application for any month your earnings drop below $500.00

Your Medicare coverage will continue for 39 months beyond the trial work period. If your Medicare coverage stops because of your work, you may purchase it for a monthly premium. For more information on "quarters of coverage" and the trial work period:

☎ Contact:
The Social Security Administration
(800) 772-1213

## Free and Low-Cost Medical Insurance For the Disabled Who Have Worked In the Past

If you qualify for the Disability Insurance Benefits (DIB) described above, and have been receiving these payments for at least two years, you will also qualify to receive Medicare Part A for free which provides insurance coverage for hospitalization. You can also receive Medicare Part B for a monthly premium of $46.10. This provides insurance coverage for your doctor visits and testing services. This is the same Medicare coverage those over 65 receive. Remember, there are deductibles and limits of coverage. For instance, doctor visits are covered after you meet the $100 deductible for the year, after which Medicare will pay 80% of the approved rate, and you are responsible for the other 20%. To apply for this medical insurance or to receive the Medicare Handbook which provides detailed information on coverage:

☎ Contact:
The Medicare Hotline
800-638-6833

## Cash For Dependents Of the Disabled

If you are eligible for Disability Insurance Benefits (DIB) described above, your dependents (wife, husband, children, or and in some cases, grandchildren) may also be eligible for payments on your record. To find out if your dependent is eligible:

☎ Contact:
The Medicare Hotline
(800) 772-1213

## Money For The Disabled Who Have Not Worked In The Past

If you are disabled but do not have enough work under Social Security for Disability Insurance Benefits (DIB), you may still be eligible to receive Supplemental Security Income (SSI) benefits if your income and resources are low enough. To see if you are eligible for SSI:

☎ Contact:
The Social Security Administration
(800) 772-1213

## What To Do When Benefits Are Denied

If you are denied any of the above-mentioned Social Security cash benefits--which often happens regardless of the disability or its severity--you can get free legal help to appeal the Social Security Administration's decision on your application. Contact your state or local Department of Welfare and request the name and address of the nearest Legal Services Corporation (LSC) program, and also contact your nearest State Client Assistance Program (CAP) office. Both programs offer low-income individuals free legal help and representation in appealing application decisions. The CAP program will either provide you with free legal help and representation for your appeal or they will help you find such aid. Unlike legal help offered under the Legal Services Corporation, CAP services are not determined by your income. On the chance that neither of these agencies seem to be able to help you, contact the Disability Rights Education and Defense Fund (DREDF) at (415) 644-2555 or (415) 841-8645.

## Free Money for Education and Job Training

If your disability stops you from being able to keep a full-time job or from being able to competitively look for a job, your state's Office of Vocational Rehabilitation (OVR) can help. OVR can give you up to $6,000 each year for job training or education. You can use this grant money, which you do not have to pay back, to cover any expenses related to your training or education, including tuition and fees, travel expenses, books, supplies, equipment (computers, motorized wheelchairs, etc.), a food allowance, tutoring fees, photocopies, and so on. For more information, contact your state's Office of Vocational Rehabilitation listed below.

## Help For the Handicapped to Find Or Create a Job

Your state Office of Vocational Rehabilitation (OVR) also acts as an employment agency for the disabled and can contact employers for you who have looked favorably on hiring the disabled. OVR will act as a liaison between you and a prospective employer and help them to create a job for you by providing needed disability-related job equipment, providing needed transportation or other mobility equipment, or by providing any other help you might need to be able to work at a job for which you're qualified. For example, OVR has provided books in braille and braille-to-speech conversion equipment, and computer-robotics equipment that have allowed disabled individuals to work. For more information, contact your state's Office of Vocational Rehabilitation listed at the end of this section.

## Help For the Handicapped Already On the Job

If you are working and become disabled or handicapped, your state Office of Vocational Rehabilitation (OVR) can provide you with the equipment, transportation, education, training and other help you might need to keep your job. For example, many times a disability can put someone in a wheelchair. OVR can provide you with a motorized wheelchair so you can continue in your job. Contact your state Office of Vocational Rehabilitation listed at the end of this section for more information.

## Medical Help For the Disabled/Handicapped

Your state Office of Vocational Rehabilitation can pay for (or help you pay for) any medical testing or treatment that can be expected to help you, as a handicapped or disabled individual, have a more healthy, prosperous, independent, and fulfilling life. Contact your state Office of Vocational Rehabilitation listed at the end of this section for more information.

## What To Do When OVR Benefits Are Denied

The first place to start when your state Office of Vocational Rehabilitation denies you handicap or disability benefits is your nearest state Client Assistance Program (CAP) office. CAP is a free information, referral, and legal service that helps disabled or handicapped individuals appeal a denial by OVR (or other agency). For a variety of reasons, it is not uncommon for a disabled individual to be turned down for services by OVR even when he/she is in fact eligible to receive them. It is sometimes helpful to get a photocopy of section 103 of Chapter 34 of the

*Code of Federal Regulations of the U.S. Department of Education* from your local or county library. These are the federal guidelines that each state OVR must follow when determining eligibility. This part of the code is only a few pages and can help you explain to the Client Assistance Program officer why you believe you are eligible even though you've been denied. CAP can take your appeal process from the first stages and all the way to the U.S. Supreme Court if necessary--and it won't cost you a penny.

It is also sometimes helpful to contact the state Office of Vocational Rehabilitation (OVR) itself and make the executive director aware of your circumstances. When it appears that progress via CAP is stalled or has been dragging on for months, it can also be very helpful to contact the regional commissioner of the Rehabilitation Services Administration (RSA), a branch of the Office of Special Education Programs of the U.S. Department of Education. RSA is responsible for overseeing and funding the state OVR agencies and is generally receptive to a short explanatory phone call and letter from those who believe they can concisely and clearly show that they have been wrongly denied OVR services. If they think you've got a case, they'll contact the OVR in question and make sure that they review your application more favorably.

To get in touch with an RSA official, contact the U.S. Department of Education, Office of Special Education and Rehabilitative Services, RSA, Washington, DC 20202: (202) 205-8870 or (202) 205-5482, and ask for the address and phone number of the regional commissioner for the ED-OSERS-RSA office serving your area.

## Three Important Tips When Appealing an OVR Denial Of Services

1. If your state Office of Vocational Rehabilitation (OVR) denies you services based on other similar cases in which they have denied other prospective clients, it is important and effective to argue that such reasons for denial are not allowable under federal regulations. The 34 Code of Federal Regulations Chapter III section 361.31(b)(1) states clearly that the barriers faced by a disabled individual are unique to each individual and to each individual set of circumstances.

2. If you have previously been accepted by your state Office of Vocational Rehabilitation (OVR) as a client and you have gained employment but your disability has not improved and you lose employment due to no fault of your own, then OVR can again provide you with their services to help you regain employment. For more specifics consult again the 34 Code of Federal Regulations, Chapter III and check under the *Post-Employment Services* sections and *Supported Employment* sections.

3. If you're currently receiving Social Security Disability (SSD), make sure that your state Office of Vocational Rehabilitation (OVR) and Client Assistance Program (CAP) are aware of this fact. Because of the more restrictive SSD definition of what it means to be disabled (compared to OVR), being on SSD almost always automatically qualifies an SSD recipient for OVR services. It is very hard for OVR to argue otherwise.

## Free Legal Help and Information Services For the Handicapped

If you think you've been wrongly denied benefits or discriminated against because of a disability or handicap, the Client Assistance Program (CAP) will help you fight for your rights when you're denied various types of disability benefits from any disability program. They will help you directly and/or put you in contact with the agencies that can help you. Your state CAP office is listed at the end of this section.

## More Free Legal Help for the Disabled

A national non-profit law and policy center, the Disability Rights Education and Defense Fund (DREDF) can provide you with direct legal representation and act as co-counsel in cases of disability-based discrimination. They also educate legislators and policy makers on issues affecting the rights of people with disabilities. Contact: Disability Rights Education and Defense Fund (DREDF), 2212 Sixth St., Berkeley, CA 94710; (510) 644-2555 (Voice/TDD).

## Information Clearinghouse For All Types Of Disabilities

The Clearinghouse On Disability Information will answer your questions on a wide range of disability topics and send you all kinds of information about services for disabled and handicapped individuals at the national, state, and local levels. They have several free publications, including *Office Of Special Education and Rehabilitative Services (OSERS) News In Print* newsletter, which describes OSERS programs, research, and topical information on a broad range of disability issues. The *Summary of Existing Legislation Affecting Persons With Disabilities* is available for all federal laws through 1991. The *Pocket Guide to Federal Help For Individuals with Disabilities* is a general handy beginning reference. Contact: Clearinghouse On Disability Information, Office Of Special Education and Rehabilitative Services, Communication and Information Services, U.S. Department Of Education, Room 3132 Switzer Bldg., Washington, DC 20202-2524; (202) 205-8723, or (202) 205-8241.

## Additional Resources

### Higher Education and Adult Training For People With Handicaps

National Clearinghouse on Postsecondary
Education for Individuals with Handicaps
One Dupont Circle, NW
Suite 800
Washington, DC 20036 (202) 939-9320 (Voice/TDD)
(800) 544-3284 (outside D.C.)

The Higher Education and Adult Training for People with Handicaps (HEATH) Resource Center is a clearinghouse and information exchange center for resources on postsecondary education programs and the disabled. Topics include educational support services, policies, procedures, adaptations, and opportunities on American campuses, vocational-technical schools, adult education programs, independent living centers, and other training organizations after high school. Another clearinghouse, National Information Center for Children and Youth with Disabilities, handles the concerns of younger disabled persons through secondary school.

## Rehabilitation Information Hotline

National Rehabilitation Information Center (NARIC)
8455 Colesville Road
Suite 935
Silver Spring, MD 20910

(800) 346-2742

The National Rehabilitation Information Center, a library and information center on disability and rehabilitation, collects and disseminates the results of federally funded research projects. NARIC also maintains a vertical file of pamphlets and fact sheets published by other organizations. NARIC has documents on all aspects of disability and rehabilitation including, physical disabilities, mental retardation, psychiatric disabilities, independent living, employment, law and public policy and assistive technology.

Their user services include the ABLEDATA database which describes thousands of assistive devices, from eating utensils to wheelchairs. A listing of fewer than 20 products is free; NARIC charges $5 for up to 100 products, and $5 for each additional hundred products.

## Free Information for Employers Who Hire the Handicapped

Job Accommodation Network (JAN)
Suite 1
918 Chestnut Ridge Road
Morgantown, WV 26506-6080

(800) 526-7234
(800) 526-2262 (Canada)

The Job Accommodation Network (JAN) brings together free information about practical ways employers can make accommodations for employees and job applicants with disabilities. The Network offers comprehensive information on methods and available equipment that have proven effective for a wide range of accommodations, including names, addresses, and phone numbers of appropriate resources.

## State Vocational Rehabilitation (OVR) Agencies

### Alabama
Lamona H. Lucas, Director
Division of Rehabilitation Services
P.O. Box 11586
2129 E. South Blvd.
Montgomery, AL 36116
(205) 281-8780

### Alaska
Keith Anderson, Director
Division of Vocational Rehabilitation
801 West 10th St.
Suite 200
Juneau, AK 99801-1894
(907) 465-2814

### American Samoa
Peter P. Galea'i, Director
Division of Vocational Rehabilitation
Dept. of Human Resources
American Samoa Government
Pago Pago, AS 96799
10288011684 - 633-2336

### Arizona
Roger Hodges, Administrator
Rehabilitation Services Admin.
Dept. of Economic Security
1789 W. Jefferson
2nd Floor, NW
Phoenix, AZ 85007
(602) 542-3332

### Arkansas
Bobby C. Simpson, Director
Division of Rehabilitation Services
P.O. Box 3781
Arkansas Dept. of Human Services
Little Rock, AR 72203
(501) 296-1600

James C. Hudson, Director
Division of Services for the Blind
Dept. of Human Services
P.O. Box 3237
411 Victory Street
Little Rock, AK 72203
(501) 324-9270

### California
Brenda Premo, Director
Dept. of Rehabilitation
830 K Street Mall
P. O. Box 94422
Sacramento, CA 95814
(916) 445-3971

### Colorado
Anthony Francavilla, Manager
Division of Vocational Rehabilitation
Dept. of Social Services
110 16th Street, 2nd Floor
Denver, CO 80202
(303) 620-4152

**Connecticut**
John F. Halliday, Director
Bureau of Rehab. Services
Dept. of Human Resources
10 Griffin Rd., North
Windsor, CT 06095
(203) 298-2003

George A. Precourt, Director
Board of Education and Services for the Blind
Dept. of Human Resources
170 Ridge Rd.
Wethersfield, CT 06109
(203) 566-5800

**Delaware**
Michelle Pointer, Director
Division of Vocational Rehabilitation
Dept. of Labor, Elwyn Building
321 East 11th St.
Wilmington, DE 19801
(302) 577-2850

Dianne L. Post, Director
Div. for the Visually Impaired
Biggs Building
Health & Social Services Campus
1901 N. Dupont Highway
New Castle, DE 19720
(302) 577-4731

**District of Columbia**
Ruth Royall Hill, Administrator
D.C. Rehabilitation Services Administration
Commission on Social Services
Dept. of Human Services
605 G Street, NW, Room 1111
Washington, DC 20001
(202) 727-3227

**Florida**
Tamira Bibb Allen, Director
Division of Vocational Rehabilitation
Dept. of Labor and Employment Security, Building A
2002 Old St. Augustine Rd.
Tallahassee, FL 32399-0696
(904) 488-6210

Whit Springfield, Director
Division of Blind Services
Dept. of Education
2540 Executive Center Circle, W
Douglas Building
Tallahassee, FL 32301
(904) 488-1330

**Georgia**
Yvonne Johnson, Director
Division of Rehabilitation Services,
Dept. of Human Resources
878 Peachtree Street, NE
Room 706
Atlanta, GA 30309
(404) 350-4700

**Guam**
Norbert Ungacto, Acting Director
Dept. of Vocational Rehabilitation
Government of Guam
122 Harmon Plaza, Room B201
Harmon Industrial Park, Guam 96911
10288-011-671-646-9468

## Hawaii

Neil Shim, Administrator
Division of Vocational
Rehabilitation
Dept. of Human Services
Bishop Trust Bldg.
1000 Bishop St., Room 605
Honolulu, HI 96813
(808) 586-5355

## Idaho

George J. Pelletier, Jr.,
Administrator
Division of Vocational Rehab.
Len B. Jordon Building
Room 150
650 West State
Boise, ID 83720
(208) 334-3390

Edward J. McHugh, Director
Idaho Commission for the Blind
341 W. Washington St.
Boise, ID 83702
(208) 334-3220

## Illinois

Andrey McCrimon, Director
Illinois Dept. of Rehab. Services
623 E Adams St.
P.O. Box 19429
Springfield, IL 62794-9429
(217) 782-2093

## Indiana

Cheryl Sullivan, Director
Division of Aging and
Rehabilitation Services
Indiana Family and Social
Services Admin.
P.O. Box 7083
402 W. Washington St.
Room W341
Indianapolis, IN 46207-7083
(317) 232-1147

## Iowa

Marge Knudsen, Administrator
Division of Vocational
Rehabilitation Services
Dept. of Education
510 E. 12th St.
Des Moines, IA 50319
(515) 281-6731

R. Creig Slayton, Director
Department for the Blind
524 4th St.
Des Moines, IA 50309-2364
(515) 281-1334

## Kansas

Glen Yancey, Commissioner
Dept. of Social & Rehabilitation
Services
300 Southwest Oakley Street
Biddle Bldg.
1st Floor
Topeka, KS 66606
(913) 296-3911

## Kentucky

Sam Serraglio, Commissioner
Dept. of Vocational
Rehabilitation
500 Mero St.
Frankfort, KY 40601
(502) 564-4566

Priscilla Rogers
Director

Kentucky Dept. for the Blind
427 Versailles Rd.
Frankfort, KY 40601
(502) 573-4754

### Louisiana

May Nelson, Director
Rehabilitation Services
Dept. of Social Services
8225 Florida Blvd.
P.O. Box 94371
Baton Rouge, LA 70806
(504) 925-4131

### Maine

Margaret Brewster
Acting Director
Bureau of Rehabilitation
Dept. of Human Services
35 Anthony Ave.
Augusta, ME 04333-0011
(207) 624-5300

### Maryland

James S. Jeffers
Division of Vocational
Rehabilitation
Administrative Offices
2301 Argonne Dr.
Baltimore, MD 21218
(410) 554-3000

### Massachusetts

Elmer C. Bartels, Commissioner
Massachusetts Rehabilitation
Commission
Fort Point Place
27-43 Wormwood St.
Boston, MA 02210-1606
(617) 727-2172

Charles Crawford, Commissioner
Massachusetts Commission for
the Blind
88 Kingston St.
Boston, MA 02111-2227
(617) 727-5550, ext. 4503

### Michigan

Peter Griswold, Director
Michigan Rehabilitation Services
Dept. of Education
P.O. Box 30010
Lansing, MI 48909
(517) 373-3391

Philip E. Peterson, Director
Commission for the Blind
Dept. of Labor
201 N. Washington Square
Lansing, MI 48909
(517) 373-2062

### Minnesota

R. Jane Brown, Commissioner
Div. of Rehabilitation Services
Dept. of Jobs and Training
390 N. Robert Street, 5th Floor
St. Paul, MN 55101
(612) 296-5616

Richard Davis
Acting Assistant Commissioner
State Services for the Blind
1745 University Avenue
St. Paul, MN 55104
(612) 642-0508

### Mississippi

Nell C. Carney, Executive
Director
Dept. of Rehabilitation Services

1281 Hwy. 51
Madison, MS 39110
(601) 853-5100

**Missouri**
Don L. Gann, Assistant Commissioner
Dept. of Elementary and Secondary Education
Division of Vocational Rehab.
2401 E. McCarty St.
Jefferson City, MO 65101
(314) 751-3251

Dwain Hovis, Interim Deputy Director
Rehabilitation Services for the Blind
Division of Family Services
619 E. Capitol
Jefferson City, MO 65101
(314) 751-4249

**Montana**
Joe A. Mathews, Administrator
Dept. of Social and Rehabilitation Services
Rehabilitation/Visual Services Division
P.O. Box 4210, 111 Sanders
Helena, MT 59604
(406) 444-2590

**Nebraska**
Frank Lloyd, Associate Commissioner & Director
Division of Vocational Rehabilitation Services
State Dept. of Education
301 Centennial Mall South
6th Floor
Lincoln, NE 68509
(402) 471-3654

James S. Nyman, Director
Services for Visually Impaired
Dept. of Public Institutions
4600 Valley Rd.
Lincoln, NE 68510-4844
(402) 471-2891

**Nevada**
Stephen A. Shaw, Administrator
Rehabilitation Division
Dept. of Human Resources, Room 502
505 E. King St.
Carson City, NV 89710
(702) 687-4440

**New Hampshire**
Paul Leather, Director
Division of Vocational Rehabilitation
State Dept. of Education
78 Regional Dr.
Building 2
Concord, NH 03301-9686
(603) 271-3471

**New Jersey**
Thomas Jennings, Director
Division of Vocational Rehabilitation Services
Dept. of Labor & Industry
John Fitch Plaza
135 E. State St., CN-398
Trenton, NJ 08625
(609) 292-5987

Jamie Casabianca-Hillton
Executive Director

Commission for the Blind and
Visually Impaired
Dept. of Human Services
153 Halsey Street, 6th Floor
P.O. Box 47017
Newark, NJ 07101
(201) 648-2324

**New Mexico**

Terry Brigance, Director
Division of Vocational
Rehabilitation
State Dept. of Education
435 St. Michael Dr., Bldg. D
Santa Fe, NM 87503
(505) 827-3511

Arthur Schreiber, Director
Commission for the Blind
PERA Building
Room 553
Santa Fe, NM 87503
(505) 827-4479

**New York**

Lawrence Gloeckler, Deputy
Commissioner
Vocational Educational Services
for Individuals with Disabilities
New York State Education Dept.
One Commerce Plaza, 16th Floor
Albany, NY 12234
(518) 474-2714

Eugene Luini, Assistant
Commissioner
Dept. of Social Services
Commission for the Blind &
Visually Handicapped
1 Commercial Plaza, Room 724
99 Washington Ave.
Albany, NY 12210
(518) 473-1801

**North Carolina**

Phil Beck, Director
Division of Vocational
Rehabilitation Services
Dept. of Human Resources
State Office
P.O. Box 26053
Raleigh, NC 27611
(919) 733-3364

John B. DeLuca, Director
Division of Services for the
Blind
Dept. of Human Resources
309 Ashe Ave.
Raleigh, NC 27606
(919) 733-9822

**North Dakota**

Gene Hysjulien, Director
Office of Vocational
Rehabilitation
Dept. of Human Services
Administrative Office
400 E. Broadway Ave.
Suite 303
Bismarck, ND 58501-4038
(800) 755-2745

**Ohio**

Robert L. Rabe, Administrator
Ohio Rehabilitation Services
Commission
400 E. Campus View Blvd.
Columbus, OH 43235-4604
(614) 438-1210
(Voice/TDD)

**Oklahoma**
Jerry Dunlap, Administrator
Rehabilitation Services Division
Dept. of Human Services
P.O. Box 36659
Oklahoma City, OK 73136
(405) 522-6006

**Oregon**
Joil Southwell, Administrator
Vocational Rehabilitation Division
Dept. Of Human Resources
500 Summer St.
Salem, OR 97310
(503) 945-5880

Charles Young, Administrator
Commission for the Blind
535 SE 12th Ave.
Portland, OR 97214
(503) 378-8479

**Pennsylvania**
Gil Selders, Executive Director
Office of Vocational Rehabilitation
Dept. of Labor & Industry Bldg.
7th & Forster Sts.
Harrisburg, PA 17120
(717) 787-5244

Norman E. Witman, Director
Bureau of Blindness & Visual Services
Dept. of Public Welfare
1401 North 7th St.
P.O. Box 2675
Harrisburg, PA 17105
(717) 787-6176

**Puerto Rico**
Eliam Olliveras, Assistant Secretary
Vocational Rehabilitation
Dept. of Social Services
P.O. Box 191118
San Juan, PR 00919-1118
(809) 725-1792

**Rhode Island**
Raymond Carroll, Asst. Administrator
Office of Vocational Rehabilitation Services
Dept. of Human Services
40 Fountain St.
Providence, RI 02903
(401) 421-7005

**South Carolina**
P. Charles LaRosa, Jr., Commissioner
Vocational Rehabilitation Dept.
P.O. Box 15
1410 Boston Ave.
West Columbia, SC 29171-0015
(803) 822-4300

Donald Gist, Commissioner
Commission for the Blind
1430 Confederate Ave.
Columbia, SC 29201
(803) 734-7520

**South Dakota**
David Miller, Director
Division of Rehabilitation Services
East Highway 34
c/o 500 East Capitol

Pierre, SD 57501-5070
(605) 773-3195

Grady Kickul, Director
Division of Service to the Blind
and Visually Impaired
East Highway 34
c/o 500 East Capitol
Pierre, SD 57501-5070
(605) 773-4644

**Tennessee**
Jack Van Hooser, Acting
Commissioner
Division of Rehabilitation
Services
Dept. of Human Services
Citizen Plaza Building
400 Deadrick St., 15th Floor
Nashville, TN 37248
(615) 741-2521

**Texas**
Vernon M. Arrell, Commissioner
Texas Rehabilitation Commission
4900 N. Lamar, Room 7100
Austin, TX 78751-2316
(512) 483-4001

Pat D. Westbrook, Executive
Director
Texas Commission for the Blind
Administration Bldg.
4800 North Lamar
P.O. Box 12866
Austin, TX 78711
(512) 459-2600

**Utah**
R. Blaine Peterson, Executive
Director
Utah State Office of
Rehabilitation
250 E. 500 South
Salt Lake City, UT 84111
(801) 538-7530

**Vermont**
Diane Dalmasse, Director
Vocational Rehabilitation
Division
Agency of Human Services
Osgood Building
Waterbury Complex
103 S. Main St.
Waterbury, VT 05676
(802) 241-2186

Steven R. Stone, Acting Director
Division for the Blind &
Visually Impaired
Agency of Human Services
Osgood Building
Waterbury Complex
103 S. Main St.
Waterbury, VT 05676
(802) 241-2210

**Virgin Islands**
Caterine Mall, Administrator
Division of Disabilities
& Rehabilitation Services
Dept. of Human Services
1403 Hospital Rd.
St. Thomas, VI 00802
(809) 774-0930

**Virginia**
Howard Gordon, Commissioner
Dept. of Rehabilitative Services
Commonwealth of Virginia
8004 Franklin Farms Dr.

P.O. Box K300
Richmond, VA 23288
(804) 662-7000

John Vaughn, Commissioner
Dept. for the Visually Handicapped
Commonwealth of Virginia
397 Azalea Ave.
Richmond, VA 23227-3697
(804) 371-3145

**Washington**
Jeanne Munro, Director
Division of Vocational Rehabilitation
Dept. of Social & Health Services
P.O. Box 45340
Olympia, WA 98504-5340
(206) 438-8000

Shirley Smith, Director
Dept. of Services for the Blind
400 S, Evergreen Park Dr.
Olympia, WA 98504-0933
(206) 586-1224

**West Virginia**
William Dearien, Director
Division of Vocational Rehabilitation
State Board of Rehabilitation
State Capitol Complex
P.O. Box 50890
Charleston, WV 25305
(304) 766-4601

**Wisconsin**
Judy Norman-Nunnery, Administrator
Div. of Vocational Rehabilitation
Dept. of Health and Social Services
Room 850
1 West Wilson, 8th Floor
P.O. Box 7852
Madison, WI 53702
(608) 266-1562

**Wyoming**
Bob Clabby, Administrator
Division of Vocational Rehabilitation
Dept. of Employment
Room 1417
1100 Herschler Bldg.
Cheyenne, WY 82002
(307) 777-7359

## State Client Assistance Program (CAP)

The first place to start when your state Office of Vocational Rehabilitation denies you handicap or disability benefits is your nearest state Client Assistance Program (CAP) office. CAP is a free information, referral, and legal service that helps disabled or handicapped individuals appeal a denial by OVR (or other agency). CAP can take your appeal process from the first stages and all the way to the U.S. Supreme Court if necessary--and it won't cost you a penny.

**Alabama**
Jerry Norsworthy
Dept. of Rehabilitation Services
Division of Rehabilitation
and Crippled Services
2129 E. South Blvd
P.O. Box 11586
Montgomery, AL 36116
(205) 281-8780

**Alaska**
Pam Stratton, CAP Director
ASSIST
2900 Boniface Pkwy., #100
Anchorage, AK 99504-3195
(907) 333-2211

**American Samoa**
Minareta Thompson, Director
Client Assistance and P&A
Program
P.O. Box 3937
Pago Pago, AS 96799
10288-011-684-633-2441

**Arizona**
Leslie Cohen, CAP Director
Arizona Center for Disability
Law
3208 E. Ft. Lowell Rd.
Suite 106
Tucson, AZ 85716
(602) 327-9547

**Arkansas**
Dale Turrentine, CAP Director
Advocacy Services, Inc.
Evergreen Place, Suite 201
1100 North University
Little Rock, AR 72207
(501) 296-1775

**California**
Anna Claybourne, Director
Client Assistance Program
830 K Street Mall, Room 220
Sacramento, CA 95814
(916) 322-5066

**Colorado**
Kimberly Ericson, CAP
Coordinator
The Legal Center
455 Sherman St., Suite 130

Denver, CO 80203
(303) 722-0300

**Connecticut**
Susan Werboff, CAP Director
Office of P&A for Handicapped
& DD Persons
60 Weston Street
Hartford, CT 06120-1551
(203) 297-4300

**Delaware**
Carol Glasspool, CAP Director
254 E. Camden-Wyoming Ave.
Camden, DE 19934
(302) 698-9336

**District of Columbia**
Toni Fisher, CAP Director
I.P.A.C.H.I.
4455 Connecticut Ave., NW
Suite B100
Washington, DC 20008
(202) 966-8081

**Florida**
Steve Howells, CAP Program
Director
Advocacy Center for Persons
with Disabilities
Webster Bldg.
2671 Executive Center Circle
West, #100
Tallahassee, FL 32301-5024
(904) 488-9070

**Georgia**
Phil D. Payne, CAP Director
Division of Rehabilitation
Services
2 Peachtree St., NE, Room 305
Atlanta, GA 30309
(800) 822-9727

**Guam**
Fidela Limtiacho, President of
the Board
Parent Agencies Network
130 Rehabilitation Center St.
Koro, Guam 96911
10288-011-671-475-3101

**Hawaii**
Executive Director
Protection and Advocacy Agency
1580 Makaloa Street, Suite 1060
Honolulu, HI 96814
(808) 949-2922

**Idaho**
Shawn DeLoyola, Director
Co-Ad, Inc.
4477 Emerald Dr. Suite B-100
Boise, ID 83706
(208) 336-5353

**Illinois**
Cynthia Grothaus, Manager
Illinois Client Assistance Project
100 N. First Street, 1st Floor
Springfield, IL 62702
(217) 782-5374

**Indiana**
Amy Ames, Executive Director
Indiana Advocacy Services
850 North Meridian, Suite 2-C
Indianapolis, IN 46204
(317) 232-1150

**Iowa**
Don Westergard, CAP Director
Division of Persons with Disabilities
Lucas State Office Bldg.
Des Moines, IA 50319
(515) 281-3957

**Kansas**
Mary Reyer, Director
Client Assistance Program
Biddle Bldg., 1st Floor
300 SW Oakley
Topeka, KS 66606
(913) 296-1491

**Kentucky**
Drane High, Director
Client Assistance Program
Capitol Plaza Tower, 9th Floor
Frankfort, KY 40601
(502) 564-8035
(800) 633-6283

**Louisiana**
Susan Howard, CAP Director
Advocacy Center for the Elderly and Disabled
210 O'Keefe
Suite 700
New Orleans, LA 70112
(504) 522-2337

**Maine**
Paul Vestal, Director
Maine Advocacy Services
P.O. Box 2007
Augusta, ME 04338-2007
(207) 626-2774
(800) 452-1948

**Maryland**
Peggy Dew, CAP Program Director
State Dept. of Education
Division of Vocational Rehabilitation
2301 Argon Dr.
Baltimore, MD 21218
(410) 554-3221

**Massachusetts**
Barbara Lybarger, Director
Client Assistance Program
Office of Handicapped Affairs
One Ashburton Place, Room 1305
Boston, MA 02108
(617) 727-7440

**Michigan**
Duncan O. Wyeth, CAP Director
Department of Rehabilitation Services
P.O. Box 30008
Lansing, MI 48909
(517) 373-8193

Robert Utrup, CAP Advocate
Commission for the Blind
201 N. Washington Sq.
2nd Floor, Victor Bldg.
P.O. Box 30015
Lansing, MI 48909
(517) 373-6425

**Minnesota**
Roseann Eshback, CAP Project Coordinator
Minnesota Legal Aid
430 First Ave., North, Suite 300

Minneapolis, MN 55401
(612) 332-1441

**Mississippi**
Pat La Rose, Director
Easter Seals Society
P.O. Box 4958
3226 N. State St.
Jackson, MS 39296-4958
(601) 982-7051

**Missouri**
Michael Finkelstein, Interim Director
Missouri P&A Services
925 S. Country Club Dr., Unit B-1
Jefferson City, MO 65109
(314) 893-3333

**Montana**
Lynn Wislow, CAP Director
Montana Advocacy Program
P.O. Box 1680
Helena, MT 59624
(406) 444-3889
(800) 245-4743

**Nebraska**
Victoria L. Rasmussen, CAP Director
Division of Rehabilitation Services
Department of Education
301 Centennial Mall South
Lincoln, NE 68509
(402) 471-3656

**Nevada**
William E. Bauer, Director
Client Assistance Program
Suite 108
1755 E. Plumb Lane
Reno, NV 89408
(702) 688-1440

**New Hampshire**
Christy Goodrich, CAP Ombudsman
Governor's Commission for the Disabled
57 Regional Dr.
Concord, NH 03301-9686
(603) 271-2773

**New Jersey**
Ellen Lence, CAP Coordinator
Department of Public Advocate
Office for Advocacy of DD
216 S. Broad St., 3rd Floor
Trenton, NJ 08608
(609) 292-9742
(800) 992-7233

**New Mexico**
Joyce Pomo, CAP Coordinator
Protection & Advocacy System, Inc.
1720 Louisiana Blvd., NE, Suite 204
Albuquerque, NM 87110
(505) 256-3100

**New York**
Michael Peluso, CAP Director
State Commission on Quality of Care for the Mentally Disabled
99 Washington Ave, Suite 1002
Albany, NY 12210
(518) 473-7378

**North Carolina**
Kathy Brack, CAP Director
Division of Vocational
Rehabilitation Services
P.O. Box 26053
Raleigh, NC 27611
(919) 733-3364

**North Dakota**
Dennis Lyon, CAP Director
Office of Vocational
Rehabilitation
Dept. of Human Services
400 East Broadway
Suite 303
Bismarck, ND 58501
(701) 328-3970

**Ohio**
Joyce Clemons, CAP
Administrator
Governor's Office of Advocacy
for People with Disabilities
30 East Broad Street
Room 1201
Columbus, OH 43266-0400
(614) 466-9956

**Oklahoma**
Steve Stokes, Director
Oklahoma Office of
Handicapped Concerns
4300 N. Lincoln Blvd., Suite 200
Oklahoma City, OK 73105
(405) 521-3756

**Oregon**
Kim Marks, CAP Director
Oregon Disabilities Commission
1257 Perry St., SE
Salem, OR 97310
(503) 721-0135
(800) 746-7398

**Pennsylvania**
Alice Paylor, Regional Manager
Client Assistance Program
Medical Center East
211 N. Whitfield, Suite 215
Pittsburgh, PA 15206
(412) 363-7223
(800) 525-7223

Stephen Pennington, Statewide
Director
Client Assistance Prog. (SEPLS)
110 Center, Suite 800
1617 JFK Blvd
Philadelphia, PA 19103
(215) 557-7112
(800)742-8877

**Puerto Rico**
Paul Jimenez, CAP Program
Coordinator
Ombudsman for the Disabled
P.O. Box 5163
Hato Rey, PR 00919-5163
(809) 758-1049

**Rhode Island**
Ted Mello, CAP Director
Rhode Island P&A System, Inc.
151 Broadway, 3rd Floor
Providence, RI 02903
(401) 831-3150

**South Carolina**
Larry Barker, CAP Director
Office of the Governor

308 Brown Bldg.
1205 Pendleton
Columbia, SC 29201
(803) 782-0639
(800) 922-5225

**South Dakota**
Nancy Schade, CAP Director
South Dakota Advocacy Services
221 S. Central Ave.
Pierre, SD 57501
(605) 224-8294
(800) 658-4782

**Tennessee**
Dan Suggs, Director
Tennessee P&A, Inc.
P.O. Box 121257
Nashville, TN 37212
(615) 298-1080

**Texas**
Judy Sokolow, CAP Coordinator
Advocacy, Inc.
7800 Shoal Creek Blvd.
Suite 171-E
Austin, TX 78757
(512) 454-4816

**Utah**
Nancy Friel, CAP Director
Legal Center for People With Disabilities
455 East 400 South, Suite 410
Salt Lake City, UT 84101
(801) 363-1347
(800) 662-9080

**Vermont**
Judy Dixon, Director
Client Assistance Program
Vermont Legal Aid
P.O. Box 1367
Burlington, VT 05402
(802) 863-2871
(800) 747-5022

**Virginia**
Russell Cutchins, CAP Manager
Department for the Rights of the Disabled
101 N. 14th Street, 17th Floor
Richmond, VA 23219
(804) 225-2042
(800) 552-3962

**Virgin Islands**
Camille Ayala, Executive Director
Virgin Islands Advocacy Agency
7A Whim St., Suite 2
St. Croix, VI 00840
(809) 776-4303

**Washington**
Jerry Johnsen, Director
Client Assistance Program
P.O. Box 22510
Seattle, WA 98122
(206) 721-4049

**West Virginia**
Susan Edwards, CAP Director
West Virginia Advocates
Litton Bldg., 4th Floor
1287 Quarrier St.
Charleston, WV 25301
(304) 346-0847
(800) 950-5250

**Wisconsin**

Linda Vegoe, Acting CAP Director
Governor's Commission for People With Disabilities
1 W Wilson St., Suite 558
Madison, WI 53707
(608) 266-5378

**Wyoming**

Kriss Smith, CAP Director
Wyoming P&A System, Inc.
2424 Pioneer Ave., Suite 101
Cheyenne, WY 82001
(307) 638-7668
(307) 632-3496
(800) 821-3091

# Free and Low-cost Dental Care For Rich and Poor

Don't let your teeth fall out just because you can't afford to go to a dentist. There are hundreds of programs across the country that offer free and low-cost dental care for all kinds of people, ***often regardless of your income level***. If you know where and when to look, you may be able to get:

- free dentures for your grandmother,
- free fillings when you're between jobs,
- braces for kids at 80% discounts, or
- free dental implants by the best doctors in the world.

Most health insurance plans don't include dental coverage, which means people often go without regular dental care simply because they think they can't afford it. But you may not be aware of the hundreds of programs that are designed for people like you--programs that actually require that you *don't* have dental insurance so that you can qualify to receive free or large discounts on your dental care.

Here are some general examples of the kinds of programs funded all across the country:

## Dental Care for the Elderly

You'll find that most states have special programs just for the elderly, especially those who have trouble finding money to pay for dental care on a limited income. Often dentists donate their time and services to make sure the elderly are taken care of. See the state-by-state listing below.

## Dental Schools for Everyone

The best-kept secrets about low-cost dental care are the 53 dental schools across the country. They offer quality dental care at a fraction of the cost of private dentists. Many will even set up a repayment plan for you if you can't afford to pay the bill. Also, researchers at many dental schools receive big money from the federal government to do cutting edge dental research, and these researchers often need patients to work on for free. Be sure to ask about any clinical research underway at the dental school nearest you. See state-by-state listing below.

## Free and Low Cost Dental Clinics

Many state and local health departments support dental clinics which offer their services for free or on a sliding fee scale basis. Services are usually limited to those with limited income or those with special needs. See state-by-state listing below.

## Free Dental Care for Children

Almost every state runs some kind of dental care program to make sure that kids keep their teeth in good shape. Many of these programs offer their services for free or at huge discounts based upon your ability to pay. See state-by-state listing below.

## Dental Care for Disabled and Handicapped

There are special programs just for those with mental or physical disabilities, including those with mental retardation, cerebral palsy, multiple sclerosis, and much more. Many states also have special programs that offer free care for children born with cleft palates. See state-by-state listing below.

## Dentures for Young and Old

Don't sit around with false teeth that keep falling out when you eat or hurt so badly that you can't keep them in your mouth. Many states have discount denture programs where you can receive big savings on false teeth, no matter what your age. See state-by-state listing below.

## Free Tooth Implants and Impacted Molar Removal

These are just two of the many subjects that top dental researchers are studying at the National Institute of Dental Research which is part of the National Institutes of Health in Bethesda, Maryland. Also underway are studies on facial pain, taste disorders, herpes simplex, and dry mouth conditions. Patients who participate in these clinical trials receive their dental care free of charge. For information about the clinical studies program at the National Institutes of Health, you or your doctor can contact: Clinical Center, National Institutes of Health, Bethesda, MD 20892, 301-496-2563.

## Dentists Who Get Government Grants to do Work for Free

Washington is not the only place where doctors receive government grants to conduct dental research and treat patients for free. Each year hundreds of dental schools and other dental research facilities around the country receive money to work on everything from gum disease to denture satisfaction. You can contact the following office to receive information about on-going or up-coming dental research in your area.

National Institute of Dental Research
Research Data and Management
Information Section
5333 Westbard Ave., Room 539
Bethesda, MD 20814
301-594-7645

Another method of finding these doctors is by contacting the "Dental Schools" and "State Institutions Receiving Government Grants for Dental Research" in the state-by-state listing below. Dental schools normally receive a good portion of available research and the other listing represents those who received grant money last year.

## Dentists on Wheels

If you have trouble getting around because of a handicap or other infirmity, some states, like Illinois, Arizona, and Missouri, have mobile dental vans that will actually come to your home or nursing home and provide you with dental care right there on the spot.

## Dental Societies - Dentists Who Volunteer

Each state's Dental Society keeps track of free and low-cost dental programs in their state, so it's a good idea to call them if you have any questions or if you're interested in learning about any new dental programs that start up. Some Dental Societies also act as a clearinghouse for identifying dentists who volunteer their services to those facing emergencies or those who have other special problems. See the state-by-state listing below.

## State-by-State Listing

## Alabama

**Dental Programs**
Department of Public Health
Dental Health Division
434 Monroe St.
Montgomery, AL 36130 (205) 242-5760

Call your nearest Community Health Center or Clinic for information on reduced fees for dental care. Usually clinics offer a sliding fee scale--qualifications vary. For example, some clinics will treat only children and senior citizens.

**Dental School**
School of Dentistry . . . . . . . . . . . . . Annual patient visits: 49,617.
University of Alabama
1919 Seventh Ave., South (205) 934-2700
Birmingham, AL 35394 children: (205) 934-4546

**Dental Society**
Alabama Dental Association
836 Washington Ave.
Montgomery, AL 36104-3893 (205) 265-1684

| **Government Grants for Dental Research** | Grants |
|---|---|
| Oakwood College | $4,644 |
| University of Alabama at Birmingham<br>Birmingham, AL | $4,502,593 |

## Alaska

**Dental Programs**
Social Services
Department of Public Health

P.O. Box 110610
Juneau, AK 99811-0610 (907) 561-4211

Limited dental care is available. Call your Community Health Center to get information about whether they offer dental.

Anchorage Neighborhood Health Center
1217 East 10th Ave.
Anchorage, AK 99501 (907) 257-4600

Call or write Anchorage Neighborhood Health Center to get information on reduced-fee dental services for adults and children. A sliding fee scale based on income is available.

Senior Citizen Discounts
Anchorage Dental Society
3400 Spenard Rd., Suite 10
Anchorage, AK 99503 (907) 279-9144

There are no special programs through the Dental Society; however, they do keep a list of referrals of dentists who will give discounts to senior citizens.

**Dental Society**
Alaska Dental Society
3400 Spenard Rd., Suite 10
Anchorage, AK 99503-3783 (907) 277-4675

## Arizona

**Dental Programs**
Department of Health Services
Office of Dental Health
1740 West Adams St.
Phoenix, AZ 85007 (602) 542-1866

Low cost dental services are available through various Dental Clinics. They also offer a Homebound program for people who can no longer leave their homes (they will go to nursing homes). Individuals must contact the Office of Dental Health to get eligibility requirements.

*Mobile Dental Treatment Trailers* equipped as dental operatories, are stationed at elementary school campuses to provide dental preventive and restorative treatment to eligible children in the community.

*Fluoride and Sealant Programs* are also available through the public schools. Some Indian Health Centers offer dental for tribal members.

McDowell Clinic
1314 E. McDowell St.
Phoenix, AZ 85006 (602) 252-1909

The McDowell Clinic provides basic dental work for individuals with HIV. The Area on Aging has contracted with the Office of Dental Health to provide dental services using portable equipment set up at local Senior Centers. Eligibility to access these services is determined by AAA.

**Dental Society**
Arizona State Dental Association
4131 N. 36th St.
Phoenix, AZ 85018-4761 (602) 957-4777

## Arkansas

**Dental Programs**
Department of Health
Dental Division
4815 West Markham
Little Rock, AR 72201 (501) 661-2279

Limited dental care is available. Three clinics offer dental care at a reduced fee. Low-income is a major factor in determining eligibility. They will also see anyone who is in severe pain due to an emergency. All hospitals keep a listing of dentists who volunteer to treat emergencies. No special programs are available for handicapped or elderly.

**Dental Society**
Arkansas State Dental Association
920 W. 2nd St., #103
Little Rock, AR 72201-2125 (501) 372-3368

**Government Grants for Dental Research** Grants
University of Arkansas at Fayetteville . . . . . . . . . . . . . $102,389
Fayetteville, AR

## California

**Dental Programs**
Health Services Department
Oral Health
714 P St.
Sacramento, CA 95814 (916) 445-0174

Very limited dental care is available through some local Health Centers or Clinics on a sliding fee scale. You'll have to call each individually to see if dental is available.

Senior-Dent
California Dental Association
1201 K Street Mall
P.O. Box 13749 (916) 443-0505
Sacramento, CA 95853 (800) 736-7071

The *Senior-Dent Program* offers dental care at reduced fees to all qualified senior citizens. To qualify you must meet three eligibility requirements: 1) be 60 or older; 2) have an annual income of $16,000 or less; 3) not be receiving dental benefits from Denti-Cal or a dental insurance plan. Participating dentists offer at least a 15% discount. Call for additional information and a participating dentist.

**Dental Schools**
School of Dentistry . . . . . . . . . . . . . Annual patient visits: 52,017.
University of California-San Francisco

707 Parnassus Ave.
San Francisco, CA 94143 (415) 476-1891

School of Dentistry . . . . . . . . . . . . . Annual patient visits: 71,627.
University of California, Los Angeles
School of Dentistry
10833 LeConte Ave.
Los Angeles, CA 90024-1668 (310) 206-3904

School of Dentistry . . . . . . . . . . . . . Annual patient visits: 31,000.
University of Southern California
325 W. 34th St.
Los Angeles, CA 90089 (213) 740-2800

School of Dentistry . . . . . . . . . . . . Annual patient visits: 105,500.
Loma Linda University
11092 Anderson St.
Loma Linda, CA 92350 (909) 824-4675

**Dental Society**
California Dental Association
P.O. Box 13749
Sacramento, CA 95853-4749 (916) 443-0505

| **Government Grants for Dental Research** | Grants |
|---|---|
| University of California Davis<br>Davis, CA | $206,426 |
| University of California Irvine<br>Irvine, CA | $156,173 |
| University of California Los Angeles<br>Los Angeles, CA | $2,114,827 |
| University of California San Diego<br>San Diego, CA | $296,906 |
| University of California San Francisco<br>San Francisco, CA | $4,932,104 |
| Children's Hospital of Los Angeles<br>Los Angeles, CA | $321,069 |

| | |
|---|---|
| Molecular Research Institute | $39,936 |
| Xoma Corporation | $248,538 |
| Society for the Advancement of Chicanos/Native Americans | $20,000 |
| Scripps Research Institute | $248,333 |
| University of Southern California | $4,680,275 |
| SRI International | $131,726 |

## Colorado

**Dental Programs**
Department of Health
Family and Community Health Services
Dentistry
4300 Cherry Creek Dr., South, A4
Denver, CO 80222 (303) 692-2360

Call your local Health Department or Clinic to get information about reduced fee dental care. When dental care is offered, it is usually on a sliding fee scale based on income. Some will treat both children and adults.

Handicapped Children and Cleft Palate Program
4300 Cherry Creek Dr. South
Denver, CO 80222 (303) 692-2370

This program is for children under the age of 21. Call to get qualifications and additional information. Services are free of charge or on a sliding fee scale.

Dental Care for the Handicapped
Donated Dental Services
1800 Glenarm Pl., Suite 500
Denver, CO 80202 (303) 298-9650

Certain handicapped individuals who meet the following guidelines may be eligible to receive free or low-cost dental care. Patients must meet the following guidelines: 1) mentally or physically disabled including mental retardation, cerebral palsy, MS, or other disabilities; 2) Colorado resident; 3) each patient is screened to find those in most need; limited income due to handicap is a major factor. Call for additional information.

Old Age Pension Dental Program
Family and Community Health Services
Dentistry, Ptarmigan Building
4300 Cherry Creek Dr. North
Denver, CO 80222 (303) 692-2360

The *Old Age Pension Dental Program* is a cooperative effort to provide dental services to a segment of elderly that have an urgent need. Most services offered are denture-related. Individuals must be low income and at least 60 years old. Call to get additional information.

**Dental School**
School of Dentistry . . . . . . . . . . . . . Annual patient visits: 36,770.
University of Colorado Medical Center
4200 East Ninth Ave.
Denver, CO 80262 (303) 270-8751

**Dental Society**
Colorado Dental Association
3690 S. Yosemite Ave., Suite 100
Denver, CO 80237-1808 (303) 740-6900

**Government Grants for Dental Research** Grants
University of Colorado Health Sciences Center . . . . . . . . $386,078

## Connecticut

**Dental Programs**
Department of Health
Dental Health Division
150 Washington Street
Hartford, CT 06106 (203) 566-4800

Call your nearest Local Health Department or Clinic to find out information about reduced fees for dental care. Most clinics offer a sliding fee schedule and will accept Medicaid and insurance, though low-income is usually a requirement. Handicap access is also available. Preventive programs are run through the various public school systems and nursing homes. Area dentists volunteer their services to provide low-income elderly with reduced-fee dental care.

**Dental School**
School of Dental Medicine . . . . . . . . Annual patient visits: 19,496.
University of Connecticut
263 Farmington Ave. adults: (203) 679-3400
Farmington, CT 06032 children: (203) 679-3231

**Dental Society**
Connecticut Dental Association
62 Russ St.
Hartford, CT 06106-1589 (203) 278-5550

**Government Grants for Dental Research** Grants
University of Connecticut Health Center . . . . . . . . . . $2,199,626
Yale University . . . . . . . . . . . . . . . . . . . . . . . . . . . $347,094

## Delaware

**Dental Programs**
Division of Public Health
William Center Dental Clinic
805 River Rd.
Dover, DE 19901 (302) 739-4755

Children in pain, as well as children on Medicaid, are treated. There is very limited reduced fee dental care available in Delaware; however, there are two clinics that treat children and adults on a sliding fee scale. Call (302) 428-2269 to get additional information and qualifications.

Nemours Health Clinic
1801 Rockland Rd.
Wilmington, DE 19803 (800) 292-9538
(302) 651-4400

The Nemours Health Clinic offers a Dental Program for senior citizens over 65. There are income requirements, so be sure to call for additional information.

**Dental Society**
Delaware Dental Society
1925 Lovering Ave.
Wilmington, DE 19806-2147 (302) 654-4335

**Government Grants for Dental Research** Grants
University of Delaware . . . . . . . . . . . . . . . . . . . . . . . . $114,322

## District of Columbia

**Dental Programs**
Department of Public Health
Dental Health Division
1660 L Street, NW
Washington, DC 20036 (202) 673-6765

Low income is a major factor in determining eligibility for free and low-cost dental care through the DC government. For information on this very limited dental care, you'll need to call your local clinic. You must be under 21 for most dental clinic programs, and a sliding fee scale is used, based on your ability to pay.

**Dental School**
College of Dentistry . . . . . . . . . . . Annual patient visits: 128,886.
Howard University
600 W St., NW
Washington, DC 20059 (202) 806-0100

**Dental Society**
District of Columbia Dental Society
502 C St., NE
Washington, DC 20002-5810 (202) 547-7613

The Society will give referrals to clinics that offer low-cost dental care. There are no programs for the elderly.

| **Government Grants for Dental Research** | **Grants** |
|---|---|
| American Association for Dental Research | $40,000 |
| Georgetown University | $333,083 |

## Florida

**Dental Programs**
Department of Health and Rehabilitative Services
Public Health Dental Program
1317 Winewood Blvd.
Tallahassee, FL 32399-0700 (904) 487-1845

Call your local County Health Department or Clinic for information on low cost dental care. Clinics usually offer a sliding fee scale. Qualifications vary and emphasis is on children. Guidelines are 200% of poverty standards but offer sliding fee scale based on ability to pay.

**Dental School**
College of Dentistry . . . . . . . . . . . . Annual patient visits: 47,441.
University of Florida
Gainesville, FL 32610 (904) 392-4261
geriatric clinic: (904) 392-9820

**Dental Society**
Florida Dental Association
1111 E. Tennessee St., Suite 102
Tallahassee, FL 32308-6914 (800) 877-9922
(904) 681-3629

| **Government Grants for Dental Research** | **Grants** |
|---|---|
| Florida State University | $312,249 |
| University of Florida | $5,023,030 |
| University of South Florida | $156,335 |
| Mount Sinai Medical Center<br>Miami Beach, FL | $182,058 |

## Georgia

**Dental Programs**
Department of Human Resources
Oral Health Section
Two Peachtree St., 6th floor
Atlanta, GA 30303 (404) 657-2574

Call your local Health Department or Clinic to get information on low-cost dental care. Most will treat children and adults, but low-income is a major factor in determining your eligibility. Fluoride and Sealant Programs are available through various public school systems.

**Dental School**
School of Dentistry . . . . . . . . . . . . . Annual patient visits: 16,676.
Medical College of Georgia
1459 Laney Walker Blvd.
Augusta, GA 30912 (706) 721-2696

**Dental Society**
Georgia Dental Association
2801 Buford Hwy, Suite T60
Atlanta, GA 30329 (404) 636-7553

| **Government Grants for Dental Research** | **Grants** |
|---|---|
| University of Georgia | $129,312 |
| Georgia Institute of Technology | $237,653 |
| Medical College of Georgia | $1,310,555 |
| Morehouse School of Medicine | $95,875 |
| Emory University | $1,191,993 |

## Hawaii

**Dental Programs**
Department of Health
Dental Health Division
1700 Lanakila Ave., Room 203
Honolulu, HI 96817 (808) 832-5710

Dental care is available for very low income individuals who are in the GAP Group, which includes children and adults. A sliding fee scale is used to determine what you pay based on your income. Dental care is also available for the mentally or physically handicapped, as well as homeless individuals. To be treated, you must meet certain criteria, which you can get by calling your local clinic.

**Dental Society**
Hawaii Dental Association
1000 Bishop St., Suite 805
Honolulu, HI 96813-4281 (808) 536-2135

## Idaho

**Dental Programs**
Department of Health and Welfare
Dental Program
P.O. Box 83720
Boise, ID 83720-0036 (208) 334-5966

Idaho has a limited dental care program for low-income individuals, but it is very limited for adults. Some restorative dental work is performed. Emergency service for women or children under the age of 21 is available. Call for eligibility requirements. Also, contact your nearest Community Health Center or Clinic to see if they offer dental assistance. Their fee scales are usually a sliding fee schedule, based on your ability to pay. *Preventive Programs* are offered through the public school system and some nursing homes, which are designed to help educate these groups on the importance of preventing dental problems before they occur.

Senior Care Program
Boise City/Ada County
3010 W. State St., Suite 120
Boise, ID 83703-5949 (208) 345-7783

The *Dental Access Program* helps low-income people receive assistance with the cost of dentures, denture repair, and extractions. Those eligible include: 1) Age 60 or older; 2) Residents of southwest Idaho; 3) Have limited or fixed income and no available resources to pay for dental work; 4) Must have a dental need that is denture related, 5) No Medicaid.

**Dental Society**
Idaho Dental Association
1220 W. Hays St.
Boise, ID 83702-5315 (208) 343-7543

## Illinois

**Dental Programs**
Department of Public Health
Dental Health Division
535 West Jefferson St.
Springfield, IL 62761-0001 (217) 785-4899

Call your local clinics or health centers to get information about reduced-fee dental services. Income is a major factor used to determine your eligibility, and sliding fee schedules are used based your ability to pay. Preventative programs are available for children through the various school systems.

Total Dent Program
Illinois Dental Society
P.O. Box 376
Springfield, IL 62705 (800) 252-2930

The *Total Dent Program* is designed to help low- or fixed-income individuals receive needed dental care at a discount rate. To qualify, you must meet ALL of the following requirements: 1) You cannot be eligible for the Public Aide Dental Program or other dental insurance coverage; 2) You must meet Title 20 income requirements; 3) You must be willing to sign a form certifying the above. Dentists who participate in this program offer a fee reduction of at least 20% to participating Illinois residents. Call for additional information.

Denture Referral Service
Illinois Dental Society
P.O. Box 376
Springfield, IL 62705 (217) 523-8495

The Illinois Retired Teachers Foundation sponsors the *Denture Referral Service* program, which provides dentures to eligible participants. Although you do NOT have to be a retired teacher to participate, you do need to fulfill the following requirements: 1) Resident of Illinois; 2) 65 years or older; 3) Have no public assistance or private dental insurance; 4) You must qualify for the Illinois *Circuit Breaker Program* which requires earnings of less than $14,000 per year.

Portable Dental Equipment
Illinois Dental Society
P.O. Box 376
Springfield, IL 62705 (217) 525-1406

In order to provide needed dental care for the homebound, elderly and physically and mentally handicapped, the Illinois State Dental Society maintains ten portable dental equipment units located throughout the state. Any licensed dentist in the state of Illinois may use the equipment to provide on-site dental care to these special individuals.

**Dental Schools**

Dental School . . . . . . . . . . . . . . . . Annual patient visits: 96,044
Northwestern University

240 E. Huron, 1st Floor
Chicago, IL 60611 (312) 908-5950
This school has a geriatric clinic.

School of Dental Medicine . . . . . . . . Annual patient visits: 33,258
Southern Illinois University
2800 College Ave.
Building 263
Alton, IL 62002 (618) 474-7000

College of Dentistry . . . . . . . . . . . . Annual patient visits: 70,510
University of Illinois
801 S. Paulina
Chicago, IL 60612 (312) 996-7558
This school also has a program for geriatrics. A doctor with an assistant will visit nursing homes and retirement homes.

**Dental Society**
Illinois Dental Society
P.O. Box 376
Springfield, IL 62705-0376 (217) 525-1406

| **Government Grants for Dental Research** | **Grants** |
|---|---|
| American Dental Association Health Foundation | $1,582,463 |
| University of Illinois at Chicago<br>Chicago, IL | $478,079 |
| University of Illinois Urbana-Champaign | $289,735 |
| College of Medicine at Rockford | $192,754 |
| Southern Illinois University at Edwardsville<br>Edwardsville, IL | $96,135 |
| University of Health Science/Chicago Medical School | $141,680 |
| University of Chicago<br>Chicago, IL | $116,230 |
| Northwestern University | $955,631 |
| Rosary College | $66,838 |

## Indiana

**Dental Programs**
Department of Public Health
Dental Health Division
P.O. Box 1964
Indianapolis, IN 46206 (317) 383-6417

The Dental Program offers reduced-fee dental care. Anyone with low income is eligible. Comprehensive care is available for children, and some limited care for adults. Call your local heath center for more information.

Senior Smile Program
Dental Care for Senior Citizens
Indiana Dental Association
P.O. Box 2467
Indianapolis, IN 46204 (317) 634-2610

Dental care at reduced fees is available at participating dentists to those who meet the following guidelines: 1) 65 or older; 2) have no private dental insurance nor federal, state or other dental health insurance; 3) income no more than $10,000/single or $14,000 for married couples. Call the Indiana Counsel on Aging at (317) 254-5465 for more information.

Donated Dental Services
Dental Care for Handicapped
P.O. Box 872
Indianapolis, IN 46206 (317) 631-6022

Participating dentists provide free and low-cost dental care to handicapped individuals who meet the following guidelines: 1) mentally or physically disabled including mental retardation, cerebral palsy, MS, or other disabilities; 2) live in Indiana; 3) each patient screened to find those in most need. Limited income due to handicap is a major factor in determining eligibility.

**Dental School**
School of Dentistry . . . . . . . . . . . . . Annual patient visits: 58,495.

Indiana University
1121 West Michigan St.
Indianapolis, IN 46202 (317) 274-7957
clinic (children): (317) 274-8111
(adults): (317) 274-3547

**Dental Society**
Indiana Dental Association
P.O. Box 2467
Indianapolis, IN 46206-2467 (317) 634-2610

| **Government Grants for Dental Research** | **Grants** |
| --- | --- |
| Indiana University-Purdue University at Indianapolis . . Indianapolis, IN | $1,310,525 |

## Iowa

**Dental Programs**
Department of Public Health
Dental Division
Lucas State Office Building
Des Moines, IA 50319-0075 (515) 281-5787

Call local Clinics or Health Centers to get information about reduced-fee dental services. A sliding fee schedule is most often used, and most services are for children. Very limited adult care is available with low-income levels used to determine eligibility.

Iowa Dental Elderly Access Program (IDEA)
Iowa Dental Association
505 Fifth Ave., Suite 333
Des Moines, IA 50309-2379 (515) 282-7250

This program makes dental services available to Iowa Senior Citizens with limited financial means. Those eligible: 1) 65 or older; 2) Residents of Iowa; 3) Income is 225% or less of the Federal income poverty level; 4) Have no medical or dental insurance coverage for the dental procedures being requested.

Discounts off the dentists regular fee will be made available and are determined on an individual basis in consultation with a participating dentist. Call to get more information and an application.

**Dental School**
College of Dentistry . . . . . . . . . . . . Annual patient visits: 56,817.
University of Iowa
Dental Building
Iowa City, IA 52242-1001 (319) 335-7499
Special care clinic for Geriatrics and Handicapped: (319) 335-7373

**Dental Society**
Iowa Dental Association
505 Fifth Ave.
Suite 333
Des Moines, IA 50309-2379 (515) 282-7250

**Government Grants for Dental Research** **Grants**
University of Iowa . . . . . . . . . . . . . . . . . . . . . . . . . . $3,178,529
Iowa State University of Science and Technology . . . . . $153,010

## Kansas

**Dental Programs**
Department of Health and Environment
Dental Program
Landon State Office Building
900 SW Jackson, Room 665
Topeka, KS 66612-1290 (913) 296-1500

A Health Clinic in Wichita offers reduced-fee dental services for individuals with low income. A sliding fee scale is used. There is also a Fluoride Rinse Program available in the public school systems where needed. Dental care for children on Medicaid is available.

Senior Care Program
Kansas Dental Association
5200 SW Huntoon St.
Topeka, KS 66604-2398 (800) 432-3583
(913) 272-7360

Dental care at reduced fees is available by participating dentists to those who meet the following guidelines: 1) 60 years or older; 2) have no private, federal or state dental insurance; 3) income no more than $10,000/single or $15,000 for married couples. Fees vary but are reduced. Call for additional information.

**Dental Society**
Kansas Dental Association
5200 SW Huntoon St.
Topeka, KS 66604-2398 (913) 272-7360

**Government Grants for Dental Research** **Grants**
University of Kansas Medical Center . . . . . . . . . . . . . . $260,451

## Kentucky

**Dental Programs**
Department of Health
Dental Health Division
275 East Main St.
Frankfort, KY 40621-0001 (502) 564-3246

Call your nearest Health Clinic for information on who offers free and low-cost dental care. Income is a major factor used in determining eligibility. There are three such programs now running in Kentucky. All ages are treated using a sliding fee scale to determine ability to pay.

Jefferson County Dental
Park Duval Health Facility
1817 South 34th St.
Louisville, KY 40211 (502) 774-4401

Those eligible to participate in the dental care program at this facility must meet the following guidelines: 1) Must be a resident of Jefferson County; 2) Must meet low-income guidelines; 3) Must pay on a sliding fee scale based on income level.

Kentucky Physicians Program
Kentucky Health Care Access Foundation
125 East Maxwell Street
Lexington, KY 40508 (800) 633-8100

Under the Kentucky Physicians Program, all dental work is done by volunteer dentists. Those eligible is receive treatment include: 1) Individuals with no insurance, no Medicaid and be within the Federal Poverty Guidelines; 2) Must be registered as a program participant. The first visit is free. Pharmacies donate medication based on need. Call to get additional information.

Denture Access Program
Kentucky Dental Association
1940 Princeton Dr.
Louisville, KY 40205-1873 (502) 459-5373

The Denture Access Program offers full dentures at a reduced rate. There are no age requirements to participate. Call for additional information and a referral to a participating dentist.

**Dental Schools**

College of Dentistry . . . . . . . . . . . . Annual patient visits: 38,723.
University of Kentucky
801 Rose St.
Lexington, KY 40536

For appointments to the college clinic: (606) 323-6525

The university has some programs for the elderly, and a few satellite programs where they go to nursing homes.

Kentucky Clinic Dentistry
A219 Kentucky Clinic
740 South Limestone adults: (606) 233-5562
Lexington, KY 40536-0284 children: (606) 233-6261

The residency program includes pediatric and general practice residency. They will also see medical card patients. The program is not income-based.

University of Louisville . . . . . . . . . . Annual patient visits: 65,914.
School of Dentistry adults: (502) 852-5096
Louisville, KY 40292 children: (502) 852-5642

**Dental Society**
Kentucky Dental Association
1940 Princeton Dr.
Louisville, KY 40205-1873 (502) 459-5373

| **Government Grants for Dental Research** | **Grants** |
|---|---|
| University of Kentucky . . . . . . . . . . . . . . . . . . . . . . . . | $279,052 |
| University of Louisville . . . . . . . . . . . . . . . . . . . . . . . .<br>Louisville, KY | $346,981 |

## Louisiana

**Dental Programs**
Department of Public Health
Dental Health Division
1300 Perdido Street AE13
New Orleans, LA 70112 (504) 896-1337

The Dental Program offers reduced-rate dental care through your nearest clinic. Louisiana State University offers dentures for those in need, and also restorative work for those under 18 years of age. Anyone with low income under the age of 21 is eligible for these programs. This office also provides referrals for patients with AIDS. For the 24-hour Emergency Dental Service, call (504) 897-8250 for more information.

Donated Dental Services
Dental Care for Handicapped
NFDH-Louisiana

LSDU Dept. Pediatric Dentistry
1100 Florida Ave. Box 139
New Orleans, LA 70119 (504) 948-6141

Certain handicapped individuals who meet the following guidelines can receive reduced-rate and free dental care through this programs: 1) mentally or physically disabled including mental retardation, cerebral palsy, MS, or other disabilities; 2) live in Louisiana; 3) each patient must be screened to find those in most need--limited income due to handicap is a major factor in determining eligibility.

Special Children Dental Clinic
200 Henry Clay Ave.
New Orleans, LA 70118 (504) 896-1337

This program is for children that are in a handicapped children's program - on Medicaid. Treatment is free.

**Dental School**
School of Dentistry . . . . . . . . . . . . . Annual patient visits: 47,247.
Louisiana State University
1100 Florida Ave.
Building 101
New Orleans, LA 70119 (504) 947-9961

**Dental Society**
Louisiana Dental Association
320 Third St.
Suite 201
Baton Rouge, LA 70801 (504) 336-1692

| **Government Grants for Dental Research** | **Grants** |
|---|---|
| Louisiana State University Medical Center . . . . . . . . . . New Orleans, LA | $780,684 |
| Louisiana State University A&M College . . . . . . . . . . . Baton Rouge, LA | $115,951 |
| Optimizing Corrosion Testing of Dental Alloys . . . . . . Tulane University of Louisiana | $127,461 |

# Maine

**Dental Programs**
Department of Human Services
Division of Dental Health
Bureau of Health
State House Station # 11
Augusta, ME 04333 (207) 287-3121

Call your nearest Community Health Center or Clinic for information on reduced fees for dental care. Usually fees are based on a sliding scale. Insurance is accepted. Both children and adults are eligible. *American Indian/Alaska Native Tribal Programs* offer direct and/or referral medical/dental services for registered members of federally recognized American Indian/Alaska Native Tribes. These are tribally-directed programs and may differ significantly in eligibility requirements and services.

Senior Dent Program
Maine Dental Association
P.O. Box 215
Manchester, ME 04351 (207) 622-7900

The Senior Dent program offers comprehensive dental care to low-income elderly at reduced fees. Those eligible must: 1) be residents of Maine; 2) be 62 or older; 3) Have no dental benefits under a private insurance plan or the Medicaid program; 4) Have an annual income that qualifies them for *Maine's Low Cost Drug Program*. Those eligible will receive at least a 15% discount from the usual and customary fees.

**Dental Society**
Maine Dental Association
P.O. Box 215
Manchester, ME 04351-0215 (207) 622-7900

## Maryland

**Dental Programs**
Maryland State Health Department
Dental Health Division - Baltimore
201 West Preston St.
Baltimore, MD 21201-2399 (800) 492-5231

Under the Maryland Access to Care program, low-income individuals under 21 or over 65 years of age. The program offers reduced fee dental care. Fee schedule for care is based on ability to pay.

Under 21 Dental Care
Exler and Jacobs D.D.S. P.A.
P.O. Box 12121
Baltimore, MD 21281 (410) 563-1671

Baltimore has clinics available for those qualified under the age of 21. Call for more information.

Senior Dent Program
Dental Care for Senior Citizens
Maryland State Dental Association
6450 Dobbin Rd.
Columbia, MD 21045-5824 (410) 964-2880

Senior citizens over 65 years of age living in MD and who meet certain income eligibility requirements may qualify for low-cost dental care. Call for qualifications and more information.

Dental Care for Handicapped
Donated Dental Services
6450 Dobbin Rd.
Columbia, MD 21045-5824 (410) 964-1944

Certain handicapped individuals who meet the following guidelines may be eligible to receive free or low-cost dental care: 1) mentally or physically disabled including mental retardation, cerebral palsy, MS, or other disabilities; 2) Maryland resident; 3) each patient is screened to find those in most need: limited income due to handicap is a major factor. Call Lois Bidel for more information.

**Dental School**
Baltimore College of Dental Surgery . Annual patient visits: 57,865.
University of Maryland
666 W. Baltimore St.
Baltimore, MD 21201 (410) 706-5603

**Dental Society**
Maryland Dental Association
6450 Dobbin Rd.
Columbia, MD 21045-5824 (410) 964-2880

| Government Grants for Dental Research | Grants |
|---|---|
| U.S. National Institute of Dental Research | $138,800 |
| University of Maryland Baltimore Co. Campus Baltimore, MD | $237,488 |
| University of Maryland Baltimore Prof. School Baltimore, MD | $1,319,996 |
| Henry M. Jackson Foundation for the Advancement Mil/Med | $35,500 |
| Quantex Corporation | $355,486 |
| Federation of American Soc. for Experimental Biology | $3,000 |
| American Society for Cell Biology | $3,000 |
| Johns Hopkins University | $687,693 |
| U.S. PHS Public Advisory Groups | $200,000 |

## Massachusetts

**Dental Programs**
Department of Health and Hospitals
Community Dental Programs
1010 Massachusetts Ave.
Boston, MA 02118 (617) 534-4717

Eighteen Health Center Programs throughout Boston offer low-cost dental care usually on a sliding fee scale based on your income. Requirements vary, so be sure to call to get additional information. Some hospitals offer limited dental.

Developmentally Disabled Program
150 Tremont Street
Boston, MA 02111 (617) 727-0732

This program offers dental care for individuals who are mentally retarded, have cerebral palsy, and those who are physically disabled. Call for additional information.

Dentistry for All
Massachusetts Dental Society
83 Speen St.
Natick, MA 07160-4144 (508) 651-7511

The *Dentistry for All Program* is a reduced-fee dental program for low-income individuals who have no dental coverage of any kind. Call to get additional information.

**Dental Schools**

Harvard School of Dental Medicine . . Annual patient visits: 26,270.
188 Longwood Ave.
Boston, MA 02115 (617) 432-1423

School of Graduate Dentistry . . . . . . Annual patient visits: 34,324.
Boston University
100 E. Newton St.
Boston, MA 02118 (617) 638-4671

School of Dental Medicine . . . . . . . . Annual patient visits: 87,522.
Tufts University
One Kneeland St.
Boston, MA 02111 (617) 956-6547

**Dental Society**

Massachusetts Dental Society
83 Speen St.
Natick, MA 01760-4144 (508) 651-7511

**Government Grants for Dental Research** **Grants**

New England Medical Center Hospitals, Inc. . . . . . . . . $421,987

Hampshire College . . . . . . . . . . . . . . . . . . . . . . . . . . . $98,921
Beth Israel Hospital . . . . . . . . . . . . . . . . . . . . . . . . . $113,085
Boston, MA
University of Massachusetts Medical School . . . . . . . . . . $866,893
Boston University . . . . . . . . . . . . . . . . . . . . . . . . . . . $1,192,463
Boston, MA
Children's Hospital . . . . . . . . . . . . . . . . . . . . . . . . . . $234,721
Boston, MA
Abiomed, Inc. . . . . . . . . . . . . . . . . . . . . . . . . . . . . . $260,373
Spire Corporation . . . . . . . . . . . . . . . . . . . . . . . . . . . $308,131
Cambridge Scientific, Inc. . . . . . . . . . . . . . . . . . . . . . $232,579
Forsyth Dental Center . . . . . . . . . . . . . . . . . . . . . . . . $6,008,592
Endicott College . . . . . . . . . . . . . . . . . . . . . . . . . . . . $102,457
Health Programs International, Inc. . . . . . . . . . . . . . . . . $50,000
Harvard University . . . . . . . . . . . . . . . . . . . . . . . . . . $2,522,817
Harvard, MA
Massachusetts General Hospital . . . . . . . . . . . . . . . . . . $124,137
CBR Laboratories, Inc. . . . . . . . . . . . . . . . . . . . . . . . $396,191
Tufts University Boston . . . . . . . . . . . . . . . . . . . . . . . $477,341
Boston, MA

## Michigan

**Dental Programs**
Department of Public Health
Dental Health Division
3423 Martin Luther King Jr., Blvd.
P.O. Box 30195
Lansing, MI 48909 (517) 335-8898

There are no direct dental services through the State Health Department. You must call your local or county health department for participating clinics and qualifications.

Senior Dent Program
Michigan Dental Association
230 North Washington Square, Suite 208

Lansing, MI 48933 (800) 589-2632

Dental care at reduced fees are available to senior citizens who meet the following guidelines: 1) 65 or older; 2) have no private dental insurance nor federal, state or other dental health insurance; 3) meet certain low-income requirements. Fees vary, and procedures covered include all types of dental care except full dentures. Over 800 dentists in Michigan participate.

Discount Dentures
Michigan Dental Association
230 North Washington Square, Suite 208
Lansing, MI 48933 (800) 589-2632

Under the *Professionally Acceptable Economy Denture Service (PAEDS)*, qualified patients can receive reduced-fees on full dentures (upper, lower or both) provided by licensed dentists. It also includes examination and x-rays. Those: 1) no age or income eligibility requirements. 2) must call the above number for additional information. Fees vary but are always at a reduced rate. Payment is handled through patient and dentist.

**Dental Schools**

School of Dentistry . . . . . . . . . . . . . Annual patient visits: 47,152.
University of Detroit-Mercy
2985 E. Jefferson Ave.
Detroit, MI 48207 (313) 446-1800

School of Dentistry . . . . . . . . . . . . . Annual patient visits: 88,035.
University of Michigan
1011 North University
Ann Arbor, MI 48109-1078 (313) 763-6933

**Dental Society**

Michigan Dental Association
230 Washington Square North, Suite 208
Lansing, MI 48933-1392 (517) 372-9070

| **Government Grants for Dental Research** | **Grants** |
|---|---|
| University of Michigan at Ann Arbor . . . . . . . . . . . .<br>Ann Arbor, MI | $5,108,084 |
| Wayne State University . . . . . . . . . . . . . . . . . . . . . . . | $367,880 |

## Minnesota

**Dental Programs**
State Health Department
Dental Division
717 Delaware Street SE
Minneapolis, MN 55440 (612) 623-5441

Call your Local Health Clinic to find out who offers dental care on a reduced-fee scale. Also contact "First Call for Help," (612) 224-1133, for additional information on clinics. Low-income is a major factor in determining eligibility.

Senior Partners Care Dental Program
Minnesota Senior Federation
Iris Park Place
1885 University Ave. W., Suite 190 (800) 365-8765
St. Paul, MN 55104 (612) 642-1398

The *Senior Partners Care Dental Program* is designed to bridge the Medicare gap, with participating dentists agreeing to provide a 20% discount for all professional dental services. Those eligible must: 1) join the Minnesota Senior Foundation; 2) be 55 or older and retired; 3) meet the annual income criteria of less than 200% of poverty ($1100/single or $1500/ couple per month in 1992); 4) have less than $21,000 in liquid assets (cash savings, stocks, CDs, etc.); 5) NOT be a part of any dental plan.

**Dental School**
School of Dentistry . . . . . . . . . . . . . Annual patient visits: 34,078
University of Minnesota
515 SE Delaware St.
Minneapolis, MN 55455 (612) 625-2495

**Dental Society**
Minnesota Dental Association
2236 Marshall Ave.
St. Paul, MN 55104-5792 (612) 646-7454

| **Government Grants for Dental Research** | **Grants** |
|---|---|
| University of Minnesota Twin Cities | $3,548,413 |
| LAI Laboratories, Inc. | $241,190 |

## Mississippi

**Dental Programs**
Department of Health
Dental Health Division
P.O. Box 1700/2423
North State St.
Jackson, MS 39215-1700 (601) 960-7500

Very limited dental care is available through the County Health Departments. The *Childrens Medical Program* offers dental to children with disabilities, including cleft palate, on a reduced sliding fee scale. A *Mouthrinse Program* is available through the public school system. The *Dental Corrections Program* purchases dental services for indigent children under the age of 18 years who have severe dental problems and are not eligible for financial assistance from other sources. Call Ernest Griffin or Dr. Joseph Young at (601) 960-7479 for additional information.

Low-Cost Denture Referral Program
Mississippi Dental Association
2630 Ridgewood Rd.
Jackson, MS 39216-4920 (601) 982-0442

Under this denture program, patients and dentists negotiate the reduced cost for services based on the patients' ability to pay. Call for additional information.

**Dental School**
School of Dentistry . . . . . . . . . . . . . Annual patient visits: 15,097.
University of Mississippi
2500 North State St.
Jackson, MS 39216 (601) 984-6155

**Dental Society**
Mississippi Dental Association
2630 Ridgewood Rd.
Jackson, MS 39216-4920 (601) 982-0442

| **Government Grants for Dental Research** | **Grants** |
|---|---|
| University of Mississippi . . . . . . . . . . . . . . . . . . . . . . . | $71,765 |
| University of Mississippi Medical Center . . . . . . . . . . . . | $70,833 |

## Missouri

**Dental Programs**
Department of Public Health
Dental Health Division
P.O. Box 570
Jefferson City, MO 65102 (314) 751-6247

Call your nearest health center or clinic for information on reduced fees for dental care. Usually clinics offer a sliding fee scale, and qualifications vary, though low income is a major factor considered. Fluoride Rinse Programs are available through the public school system.

Missouri Elks Program for the Handicapped
Truman Medical Center East
7900 Lee's Summit Rd.
Kansas City, MO 64139 (816) 373-1486

This program offers dental care for physically challenged adults and children through three mobile units, which provide in-home care for those unable to get out on their own. Call for information on eligibility guidelines.

Dental Care for Senior Citizens
Senior Care Program
Missouri Dental Association
230 W. McCarty
P.O. Box 1707 (800) 688-1907
Jefferson City, MO 65102-1707 in KC: (816) 333-5454
in St. Louis: (314) 965-5960

This program provides low-cost dental care to seniors who meet the following eligibility requirements: 1) 60 years or older; 2) income no more than $15,000 (single) or $20,000 (for married couples); 3) you cannot be currently receiving dental care through any public aid program or insurance plan. Participating dentists have agreed to provide a minimum of a 25% discount on services; however, the dentist may charge the usual fee for the initial office visit and examination.

**Dental School**
School of Dentistry . . . . . . . . . . . . . Annual patient visits: 7,500.
University of Missouri
650 E. 25th St.
Kansas City, MO 64108-2795 (816) 235-2100

**Dental Society**
Missouri Dental Association
P.O. Box 1707
Jefferson City, MO 65102-1707 (314) 634-3436

**Government Grants for Dental Research** **Grants**
University of Missouri Columbia . . . . . . . . . . . . . . . . $453,079
Columbia, MO
University of Missouri Kansas City . . . . . . . . . . . . . . $1,449,322
Kansas City, MO
Jewish Hospital of St. Louis . . . . . . . . . . . . . . . . . . . $231,507
St. Louis, MO
St. Louis University . . . . . . . . . . . . . . . . . . . . . . . . . $217,071
St. Louis, MO
Washington University . . . . . . . . . . . . . . . . . . . . . . . $838,516

## Montana

**Dental Programs**
Health Services Division
Dental Department
Health and Environment Sciences
P.O. Box 200901
Cogswell Building
Helena, MT 59620-0901 (406) 444-0276

Through the Maternal and Child Health department, counties can choose how they wish to use funds for dental care, so call your county health department to find out about treatments. Also Fluoride and Mouthrinse Programs are available for those who are in need.

**Dental Society**
Montana Dental Association
P.O. Box 1154
Helena, MT 59624-1154 (406) 443-2061

## Nebraska

**Dental Programs**
Health Department
Dental Health Division
301 Centennial Mall South
P.O. Box 95007
Lincoln, NE 68509-5007 (402) 471-2822

Call your local Clinic to find out if they offer dental care. Low-income is a major factor in determining eligibility, and fees are usually based on a sliding scale. Children are a first priority.

Senior Dent Program
Nebraska Dental Association
3120 O Street
Lincoln, NE 68510-1599 (402) 476-1704.

The *Senior Dent Program* offers dental care at a reduced fee for senior citizens. There are eligibility requirements that include being at least 65 years of age. Cal to find out additional information.

**Dental Schools**

School of Dentistry . . . . . . . . . . . . . Annual patient visits: 61,218.
Creighton University
2802 Webster Ave.
Omaha, NE 68178 (402) 280-2865

College of Dentistry . . . . . . . . . . . . Annual patient visits: 17,599.
University of Nebraska Medical Center
40th and Holdrege Sts.
Lincoln, NE 68583 adults: (402) 472-1333
children: (402) 472-1305

**Dental Society**

Nebraska Dental Association
3120 O St.
Lincoln, NE 68510-1599 (402) 476-1704

| **Government Grants for Dental Research** | **Grants** |
|---|---|
| University of Nebraska Lincoln . . . . . . . . . . . . . . . . . .<br>Lincoln, NE | $115,576 |
| Creighton University . . . . . . . . . . . . . . . . . . . . . . . . . | $198,704 |

## Nevada

**Dental Programs**

Nevada Health Department
Family Services
505 East King St.
Carson City, NV 89710 (702) 687-4740

Call your County Health Department to see if they offer dental. Only very limited, low-cost dental care is available to adults other than possibly extractions due to pain. Most often, programs are only for children. *First Call for Help* will refer you for assistance based on what is available. In Reno, call (702) 329-4630. In Las Vegas, call (702) 369-4397. Clark County Dental Society keeps a list of dentists who offer discounts to senior citizens. Call (702) 255-7873 to get a referral.

Children's Special Health Care Program
505 East King St., Room 205
Carson City, NV 89710 (702) 687-4885

Children to the age of 12 are treated, but you must call for additional information and qualifications.

Geriatric Health Clinic
1001 East 9th St.
Reno, NV 89512 (702) 328-2482

This clinic does referrals only.

**Dental Society**
Nevada Dental Association
6889 W. Charleston #B
Las Vegas, NV 89117 (702) 255-4211

## New Hampshire

**Dental Programs**
Department of Health and Welfare
Dental Division
6 Hazen Dr.
Concord, NH 03301 (603) 271-4685

New Hampshire has a very limited dental care program for those of low-income. Children are a first priority. Call the toll-free Helpline at (800) 852-3345, ext. 4238 to find out about other possible dental assistance. Some state technical colleges offer dental Hygiene Programs.

Denture Program
New Hampshire Dental Society
P.O. Box 2229
Concord, NH 03302-2229 (603) 225-5961

The *Denture Program* offers dentures to anyone who needs them at a reduced rate. There are financial guidelines that need to be met, but the program is for all ages. Call the above number for additional information.

**Dental Society**
New Hampshire Dental Society
P.O. Box 2229
Concord, NH 03302-2229 (603) 225-5961

## New Jersey

**Dental Programs**
Department of Health
Dental Health Division, CN 364
Trenton, NJ 08625-0364 (609) 292-1723

Some area hospitals offer dental care on a sliding fee scale based on income, but most services offered are for children. Only limited care is available for adults. Also a limited number of clinics in some towns offer dental care, also using a sliding fee scale.

Senior Dent
New Jersey Dental Association
One Dental Plaza
P.O. Box 6020
North Brunswick, NJ 08902-6020 (908) 821-9400

The *Senior Dent* program offers increase access to Dental Care for senior citizens by offering at least a 15% discount on services. Those eligible: 1) you must have a PAA (Pharmacy) card; 2) be age 65 or older; 3) have annual income of less than $15,700 (single) or $19,250 (married couple; 4) have no dental insurance or Medicaid benefits. Call the State Division on Aging for additional information at (800) 792-8820.

Donated Dental Services
One Dental Plaza
North Brunswick, NJ 08902-4313 (908) 821-2977

Donated Dental Services offers comprehensive dental care for handicapped individuals. Those eligible: 1) the mentally or physically disabled including mental retardation, cerebral palsy, MS or other disabilities; 2) New Jersey residents; 3) each patient is screened to find those in most need. Limited income due to disability is a major factor in determining eligibility.

**Dental School**
New Jersey Dental School . . . . . . . . Annual patient visits: 58,615.
University of Medicine and Dentistry
110 Bergen St.
Newark, NJ 07103 (201) 982-4300

**Dental Society**
New Jersey Dental Association
One Dental Plaza
P.O. Box 6020
North Brunswick, NJ 08902-6020 (908) 821-9400

| Government Grants for Dental Research | Grants |
|---|---|
| University of Medicine and Dentistry of NJ | $932,720 |
| University of Med/Dent NJ<br>R.W. Johnson Medical School | $90,991 |
| Rutgers The State University New Brunswick<br>New Brunswick, NJ | $46,424 |

## New Mexico

**Dental Programs**
Department of Health
Dental Division
1190 Saint Francis Dr.
Santa Fe, NM 87502-6110 (505) 827-2389

Call your nearest Community Health Center or Clinic for information on reduced fees for dental care. Most clinics will charge according to ability to pay, and children are usually a priority. Carrie Tingley Hospital treats mentally disadvantaged and disabled; call (505) 843-7493 for additional information. There are also some Indian Health Centers that offer dental care to tribal members.

Community Dental Services, Inc.
2116 Hinkle SE
Albuquerque, NM 87102 (505) 765-5683
Community Dental Services offers reduced-fee dental services based on income.

**Dental Society**
New Mexico Dental Association
3736 Eubank Blvd., NE, #1A
Albuquerque, NM 87111-3556 (505) 294-1368

| **Government Grants for Dental Research** | **Grants** |
|---|---|
| Lovelace Medical Foundation . . . . . . . . . . . . . . . . . . . . | $395,309 |
| University of New Mexico Albuquerque . . . . . . . . . . .<br>Albuquerque, NM | $161,584 |

## New York

**Dental Programs**
New York State Department of Health
Dental Division
Corning Tower
194 Washington Ave.
Albany, NY 12237-0619 (518) 474-1961
The *Dental Rehabilitation Program* is designed to correct severe physically handicapping dental defects for children up to the age of 21. The *Preventive Dentistry Program* provides dental care for high risk and underserved children. Call to get additional

information and qualifications for either of these programs. *Community-Based Fluoride and Sealant Programs* are also available.

New York City Department of Health
Dental Health
93 Worth Street, Room 1001
New York, NY 10013 (212) 566-8166

Clinics throughout the city boroughs offer free dental care to children. Call the above number to get additional information about services offered. A recording will give you phone numbers of clinics so that you can choose the one most convenient. Also, some private and city hospitals offer reduced-fee dental services on a sliding fee scale for adults based on income. Call your nearest hospital to get additional information and see if they offer dental care.

Senior Citizens Dental Access Program
Dental Society of New York State
7 Elk St.
Albany, NY 12207-1023 (518) 465-0044

The *Dental Access Program* offers reduced-fee dental services for senior citizens. Those eligible: 1) 65 or older; 2) have no public assistance or private insurance; 3) live in New York.

**Dental Schools**

School of Dental and Oral Surgery . . Annual patient visits: 53,255.
Columbia University
630 W. 168th St.
New York, NY 10032 (212) 305-5665

College of Dentistry . . . . . . . . . . . Annual patient visits: 269,095.
New York University
345 E. 24th St.
New York, NY 10010 (212) 998-9800
Geriatric Clinic: (212) 998-9767

School of Dental Medicine . . . . . . . . Annual patient visits: 15,321.
State University of New York at Stony Brook
Rockland Hall
Health Science Center (516) 632-8989
Stony Brook, NY 11794 children: (516) 632-8967
adults: (516) 632-8974
geriatric clinic: (516) 632-9245

School of Dental Medicine . . . . . . . . Annual patient visits: 78,000.
State University of New York at Buffalo
325 Squire, 3435 Main St. (716) 829-2821
Buffalo, NY 14214-3008 children: (716) 829-2723
adults: (716) 829-2720

**Dental Society**
Dental Society of New York
7 Elk St.
Albany, NY 12207-1023 (518) 465-0044

| **Government Grants for Dental Research** | **Grants** |
|---|---|
| Beth Israel Medical Center<br>New York, NY | $667,312 |
| Cornell University Ithaca<br>Ithaca, NY | $213,700 |
| Cornell University Medical Center | $173,364 |
| Mount Sinai School of Medicine | $211,600 |
| Columbia University New York<br>New York, NY | $1,640,918 |
| Eastman Dental Center | $1,614,286 |
| Hospital for Special Surgery | $291,266 |
| Montefiore Medical Center<br>Bronx, NY | $300,452 |
| New York Academy of Sciences | $10,000 |
| State University of New York at Albany<br>Albany, NY | $142,942 |
| State University New York Stony Brook<br>Stony Brook, NY | $946,316 |

State University of New York at Buffalo . . . . . . . . . . $5,741,273
Buffalo, NY
Health Science Center at Syracuse . . . . . . . . . . . . . . . . . $94,120
Syracuse, NY
New York University . . . . . . . . . . . . . . . . . . . . . . . $1,189,424
Rensselaer Polytechnic Institute . . . . . . . . . . . . . . . . . . $42,963
University of Rochester . . . . . . . . . . . . . . . . . . . . . . $3,480,294
Rochester, NY
Naylor Dana Institute for Disease Prevention . . . . . . . . $148,457

## North Carolina

**Dental Programs**
Health and Natural Resources Environment
Dental Department
1815-8 Capital Blvd.
Raleigh, NC 27604 (919) 733-3853

Call your nearest County Health Clinic to see if they offer dental care at a reduced cost. When offered, it is usually on a sliding fee scale and most often for children. Prevention and education are the main focus with *Fluoride and Sealant Programs* throughout the various public school systems.

Senior Smile Program
North Carolina Dental Association
P.O. Box 12047
Raleigh, NC 27605-2047 (919) 832-1222

The *Senior Smile Program* offers reduced-fee dental care for senior citizens. This program works under the American Dental Association (ADA). The ADA toll-free number for this program is (800) 621-8099. Call for more information.

**Dental School**
School of Dentistry . . . . . . . . . . . . . Annual patient visits: 30,395.
University of North Carolina
104 Brauer Hall
Chapel Hill, NC 27599 (919) 966-1161

**Dental Society**
North Carolina Dental Society
P.O. Box 12047
Raleigh, NC 27605-2047 (919) 832-1222

| Government Grants for Dental Research | Grants |
|---|---|
| University of North Carolina Charlotte<br>Charlotte, NC | $96,650 |
| University of North Carolina Chapel Hill<br>Chapel Hill, NC | $5,219,258 |
| Winston-Salem State University<br>Winston-Salem, NC | $6,179 |
| Duke University | $424,146 |

## North Dakota

**Dental Programs**
Health Department
Maternal and Child Health Department
600 E. Blvd. Ave.
Bismarck, ND 58505-0200 (701) 224-2372

Crippled Children Services offers dental and health care for those in need. Some Indian Health Centers offer dental for tribal members. The Fargo Homeless Project offers emergency dental work for the homeless. No programs other than Medicaid offer dental care, and no clinics offer dental.

Senior Dent
North Dakota Dental Association
Box 1332
Bismarck, ND 58502 (701) 223-8870

The *Senior Dent* program makes a full range of Dental Services available to financially eligible North Dakotans age 55 or older at a reduced fee. Those eligible must: 1) be 55 or older; 2) Not be covered by medical assistance or enrolled in a dental insurance plan; 3) have income that is 125% or less of federal poverty guidelines. Fees vary, but dentists have agreed to offer at least a 33% discount off their regular fees. Contact your local Senior Citizen Center for more information.

**Dental Society**
North Dakota Dental Association
P.O. Box 1332
Bismarck, ND 58502-1332 (701) 223-8870

## Ohio

**Dental Programs**
State Health Department
Dental Health Division
246 North High
Columbus, OH 43215 (614) 466-4180

Ohio offers a *Sealant and Fluoride Mouthrinse Program* through the public school system.

Access to Dental Care Programs
Ohio Dental Association
1370 Dublin Rd.
Columbus, OH 43215-1098 (800) MY-SMILE

The Ohio Dental Association coordinates numerous Access to Dental Care Programs. Free or low-cost dental care is available through the *Access to Dental Care for Children with Special Health Care Needs (CSHCN)* program. This program assists local agencies to increase access to needed oral health services for this special needs group. Funds are also used to provide comprehensive services for high risk children and/or women of childbearing age, otherwise known as *Child and Family Health Projects (CFSHP)*. Primary Care is also available through some County Health Departments and Clinics. Call for additional information and qualifications.

Dental Services for the Handicapped
Donated Dental Services
421 E. 4th St.
Cincinnati, OH 45202 (513) 621-2517

Free and low-cost dental care is available to the handicapped and elderly is they meet the following guidelines: 1) Mentally or physically disabled including mental retardation, cerebral palsy, MS or other disabilities; 2) individuals may also be elderly living on a fixed income; 3) each patient is screened to find those in most need. Limited income due to handicap is a major factor in determining eligibility.

Greater Cincinnati Oral Health Council
635 W. Seventh St.
Cincinnati, OH 45203 (513) 621-0248

A charter agency of the United Way, the Public Dental Service Society's dental care programs help special groups such as children from low-income families, the homeless, the aging and those with disabling conditions. 1) *Dental Sealant Program*: sealants are applied to low-income and handicapped children of Cincinnati. 2) *Head Start*: provides dental education, consultation and preventive treatment for children of disadvantage families. 3) *Homeless Program*: provides dental care for homeless adults and children. 4) *Dental Registry for the Elderly and Handicapped*: a computerized referral service matches patients with special needs with a dentist who can accommodate these needs.

**Dental Schools**

College of Dentistry . . . . . . . . . . . . Annual patient visits: 51,476.
Ohio State University
305 W. 12th Ave.
Columbus, OH 43210 (614) 292-2751

School of Dentistry . . . . . . . . . . . . . Annual patient visits: 86,630.
Case Western Reserve University
2123 Abington Rd.
Cleveland, OH 44106 (216) 368-3200

**Dental Society**
Ohio Dental Association
1370 Dublin Rd.
Columbus, OH 43215-1098 (614) 486-2700

| Government Grants for Dental Research | Grants |
|---|---|
| Case Western Reserve University | $597,100 |
| Medical College of Ohio at Toledo<br>Toledo, OH | $642,940 |
| University of Cincinnati<br>Cincinnati, OH | $344,197 |
| Ohio State University | $801,513 |

## Oklahoma

**Dental Programs**
State Department of Health
Dental Health Services
1000 Northeast Tenth St.
Oklahoma City, OK 73117-1299 (405) 271-5502

Call your local Health Center or hospital to see if dental is offered. When offered, it is usually on a sliding fee scale, and in some instances only for children.

Children's Hospital
P.O. Box 26307
Oklahoma City, OK 73126 (405) 271-4750

Handicapped children or those with medical problems can get dental care. Call for additional information.

Care-Dent Program
Oklahoma Dental Society
629 West I-44 Service Rd.
Oklahoma City, OK 73118 (800) 876-8890

*Care-Dent* offers savings to those who need denture service. Dentists also provide a thorough examination. Call for a participating dentist and more information.

Senior Dent Program
Oklahoma Dental Society
629 West I-44 Service Rd. (800) 876-8890
Oklahoma City, OK 73118 (405) 848-8873

The *Senior Dent Program* offers complete, professional dental care at a reduced fee to those seniors who meet the following guidelines: 1) 65 or older; 2) have no dental insurance; 3) income no more than $8,000/single or $12,000 for a married couple. Dentists offer a 20% discount to qualifying senior citizens. Call for more information.

Disabled Program
4024 North Lincoln Blvd., Suite 101 (800) 522-9510
Oklahoma City, OK 73105-5220 (405) 424-8092

The *D-Dent Program* offers free dental care for the physically disabled. You must apply, and applicants are carefully screened.

**Dental School**
College of Dentistry . . . . . . . . . . . . Annual patient visits: 45,615.
University of Oklahoma
Health Sciences Center
P.O. Box 26901
Oklahoma City, OK 73190-3044 (405) 271-6056

**Dental Society**
Oklahoma Dental Association
629 W. Interstate 44 Service Rd.
Oklahoma City, OK 73118-6032 (405) 848-8873

**Government Grants for Dental Research** **Grants**
University of Oklahoma Health Sciences Center . . . . . . $338,458

## Oregon

**Dental Programs**
Department of Health
Dental Health Division

800 NE Oregon St.
Portland, OR 97232 (503) 731-4098

Community Access Programs offer reduced-fee dental care to low-income individuals using a sliding fee schedule. Call your nearest Health Clinic for more information. The program requires enrollment at most clinics before treatment can begin. Under the *King Fluoride Program*, children are provided school-based fluoride mouthrinses and tablets.

Low-Cost Denture Program
107 Oakway Center, Suite C
Eugene, OR 97401 (503) 686-1175

Under this program, residents of Lake County, 55 years or older, and who meet the following guidelines may be eligible to receive low-cost denture care, including full upper and lower dentures, partials, reclines and repairs: 1) receive no public assistance; 2) income no more than $7,500 (single) or $10,500 (married couples). Call for additional qualifications and information.

Dental Care for Senior Citizens
Senior Smile Dental Service
Multnomah Dental Society
1618 W First, Suite 317
Portland, OR 97201 (503) 223-4738

Under this program, low income seniors over 60 years old, who live in Multnomah County may be eligible to receive both general and specialized dental care at a 50% reduced fee. Call for more information and to register.

Dental Care for Handicapped
Donated Dental Services
CDRC
P.O. Box 574, Room 2205
Portland, OR 97207 (503) 241-7075

Certain Oregon residents who are mentally or physically handicapped (cerebral palsy given first priority), or elderly may qualify for low-cost dental care under this program. Eligibility screening is required.

**Dental School**
School of Dentistry . . . . . . . . . . . . . Annual patient visits: 44,900.
Sam Jackson Park
Oregon Health Sciences University
611 SW Campus Dr.
Portland, OR 97201 (503) 494-8867

**Dental Society**
Oregon Dental Association
17898 SW McEwan Rd.
Portland, OR 97224-7798 (503) 620-3230

| **Government Grants for Dental Research** | **Grants** |
|---|---|
| University of Oregon . . . . . . . . . . . . . . . . . . . . . . . . | $207,311 |
| Oregon Health Sciences University . . . . . . . . . . . . . . . | $636,122 |

## Pennsylvania

**Dental Programs**
Department of Public Health
Dental Health Division
500 South Broad Street
Philadelphia, PA 19146 (215) 875-5666

The Dental Program offers reduced-rate dental care through your nearest clinic. Insurance is accepted and fee set according to financial situation. Anyone with low income is eligible, but children are first priority.

Dental Care for Senior Citizens
Access to Care Program
3501 North Front St.
Harrisburg, PA 17110 (717) 234-5941

Under this program, individuals 65 or over can receive at least a minimum of 15% discount on dental care through 1,700 participating dentists across PA. To be eligible, you must: 1) have no private dental insurance nor federal, state or other dental health assistance; 2) have income no more than $13,000 (single) or $16,200 (married couples). Call the PA Counsel on Aging at (800) 692-7256 for more program information.

Dental Care for Handicapped (Philadelphia only)
Donated Dental Services
Fidelity Bank Bldg.
123 S. Broad St., 22nd Floor
Philadelphia, PA 19109-1022 (215) 546-0300

Certain low-income mentally or physically handicapped residents of Philadelphia may qualify to receive free or low-cost dental care. Each patient is screened to find those most in need: limited income due to handicap is a major factor.

**Dental Schools**

School of Dentistry . . . . . . . . . . . . . Annual patient visits: 77,665.
Temple University
3223 N. Broad St.
Philadelphia, PA 19140 (215) 707-2900

School of Dental Medicine . . . . . . . . Annual patient visits: 85,000.
University of Pennsylvania
4001 W. Spruce St.
Philadelphia, PA 19104 (215) 898-8961

School of Dental Medicine . . . . . . . . Annual patient visits: 59,570.
University of Pittsburgh
3501 Terrace St.
Salk Hall
Pittsburgh, PA 15261 (412) 648-8760

**Dental Society**

Pennsylvania Dental Association
P.O. Box 3341
Harrisburg, PA 17105-3341 (717) 234-5941

| **Government Grants for Dental Research** | **Grants** |
|---|---|
| Pennsylvania State University-University Park . . . . . . . <br>University Park, PA | $379,184 |
| University of Pittsburgh at Pittsburgh . . . . . . . . . . . . <br>Pittsburgh, PA | $1,509,555 |
| Drexel University . . . . . . . . . . . . . . . . . . . . . . . . . . . | $122,068 |
| Thomas Jefferson University . . . . . . . . . . . . . . . . . . . | $616,651 |
| University of Pennsylvania . . . . . . . . . . . . . . . . . . . | $4,312,531 |
| Philadelphia College of Osteopathic Medicine . . . . . . . . <br>Philadelphia, PA | $104,491 |
| Temple University . . . . . . . . . . . . . . . . . . . . . . . . . . | $498,997 |
| Medical College of Pennsylvania . . . . . . . . . . . . . . . . . | $94,254 |

## Rhode Island

**Dental Programs**

Department of Public Health
Oral Health Division
3 Capital Hill
Providence, RI 02908-5097 (401) 277-2588

The dental program offers reduced-fee basic dental care (not crowns or bridges, for example). Call your nearest clinic for more information. Most insurance are accepted and the pay schedule is according to situation. Anyone with low-income can qualify.

Travelers Aide Society for the Homeless
177 Union St.
Providence, RI 02903 (401) 521-2255

The Travelers Aid Society offers dental care for the homeless. Call Linda Dziobeck for more information.

Dental Care for Handicapped
Independence Square
500 Prospect St.
Pawtucket, RI 02860 (401) 728-9448

Through the *Donated Dental Services Program*, free and low-cost dental care is available to the handicapped that meet the following guidelines: 1) mentally or physically disabled including mental retardation, cerebral palsy, MS, or other disabilities; 2) live in Rhode Island; 3) each patient must be screened to find those in most need. Limited income due to handicap is a major factor in determining eligibility.

South County
Health Center of South County
One River St.
Wakefield, RI 02879 (401) 783-0853

Basic dental treatments for all ages are available. Call Herb Manfield for more information.

Child Dental Care
Saint Josephs Hospital
21 Peace St.
Providence, RI 02907 (401) 456-4324

Basic dental treatments are available for children who are patients of the hospital, with a sliding fee schedule used to determine costs. Start-up date: February, 1995.

**Dental Society**
Rhode Island Dental Association
200 Centerville Rd.
Warwick, RI 02886-4339 (401) 732-6833

| **Government Grants for Dental Research** | **Grants** |
| --- | --- |
| Gordon Research Conferences | $9,000 |

## South Carolina

**Dental Programs**
Department of Health and Environmental Control
2600 Bull St.
Columbia, SC 29201 (803) 734-4972

A program through the public school system offers dental care for children. Applications are picked up at participating schools, but not during the summer. Call your local Health Center or Clinic to find out if they offer dental care, dental usually it is for children.

Primary Care Center
P.O. Box 6923
Columbia, SC 29260 (803) 738-9881

Some Primary Care Clinics or Centers offer dental on a sliding fee scale based on income. Call to get additional information.

Senior Care Dental Program
South Carolina Dental Association
120 Stonemark Ln.
Columbia, SC 29210-3841 (803) 750-2277

The *Senior Care Program* offers dental care to senior citizens at a reduced fee. The minimum discount is 20%, and there are specific eligibility guidelines, which you can get from your local Council on Aging or Commission on Aging (Buford: 803-524-1787) or the Dental Society at (803) 750-2277.

**Dental School**

College of Dental Medicine . . . . . . . Annual patient visits: 25,315.
Medical University of South Carolina
171 Ashley Ave.
Charleston, SC 29425 (803) 792-2611

**Dental Society**

South Carolina Dental Association
120 Stonemark Ln.
Columbia, SC 29210-3841 (803) 750-2277

| **Government Grants for Dental Research** | **Grants** |
|---|---|
| University of South Carolina at Columbia . . . . . . . . . . Columbia, SC | $113,498 |
| Medical University of South Carolina . . . . . . . . . . . . . | $180,824 |

## South Dakota

**Dental Programs**
Department of Health
Dental Division
Anderson Building
445 E. Capitol Ave.
Pierre, SD 57501 (605) 773-3361

Although comprehensive dental care is not offered through local Health Centers, the *Emergency Care Referral Program* can put you in touch with dental care in emergency situations.

Indian Health Program
Indian Health Services
Federal Building
115 4th Ave. SE
Aberdeen, SD 57401 (605) 226-7501

Dental care is available at no charge for Indians enrolled in a tribe. Call the office above for additional information and find out locations for treatment.

**Dental Society**
South Dakota Dental Association
P.O. Box 1194
Pierre, SD 57501-1194 (605) 224-9133

## Tennessee

**Dental Programs**
Department of Health
Oral Health Services
Tennessee Tower, 11th Floor
3128 Ave. North
Nashville, TN 37247-5410 (615) 741-7213

Contact your Local Health Center or Clinic to find out if they offer reduced-fee dental services. Low income is a major factor in determining eligibility, and a sliding fee scale is most often used. Qualifications vary, and care is primarily for children. Emergency care is offered to adults to alleviate pain. Although there are no special programs for the elderly or disabled, they will be treated based on the above income criteria.

**Dental Schools**

School of Dentistry . . . . . . . . . . . . . Annual patient visits: 7,972.
Meharry Medical College
1005 D.B. Todd Blvd.
Nashville, TN 37208 (615) 327-6669

College of Dentistry . . . . . . . . . . . . Annual patient visits: 52,551.
University of Tennessee
875 Union Ave.
Memphis, TN 38163 (901) 448-6257

**Dental Society**

Tennessee Dental Association
P.O. Box 120188
Nashville, TN 37212-0188 (615) 383-8962

| **Government Grants for Dental Research** | **Grants** |
|---|---|
| University of Tennessee at Memphis . . . . . . . . . . . . . . Memphis, TN | $488,255 |
| Meharry Medical College . . . . . . . . . . . . . . . . . . . . . . | $319,364 |

## Texas

**Dental Programs**

Department of Health
Dental Health Services
1100 West 49th St.
Austin, TX 78756 (512) 458-7323

The dental program administered by the Bureau of Dental Health Services provides emergency dental treatment for eligible children through the age of 18. A family's income for financial eligibility must correspond to 133% of the federal poverty level, and services must not be available from some other sources. Services are provided through several delivery methods, including mobile and portable dental units, fixed clinics, and fee-for-service arrangements with providers.

Senior Dent
Texas Dental Association
1946 South Interregional
Austin, TX 78704

*Senior Dent* offers reduced-cost dental care to those who are: 1) 65 or older; 2) not be receiving federal, state, or other dental health insurance; 3) have a total household income of less than $12,000 or acceptance by the participating dentist because of special circumstances. Call for more information.

In Texas, several regional offices of the Texas Public Health Office have additional information on reduced-fee dental care in their regions. Call or write the appropriate region to get additional information.

Region 1
Texas Public Health
1109 Kemper St.
Lubbock, TX 79403 (806) 744-3577

Region 3
Texas Public Health
2561 Matlock Road
Arlington, TX 76015-1621 (817) 792-7224

Region 4 & 5 North
Texas Public Health
1517 West Front St.
Tyler, TX 75702 (903) 595-3585

Region 6
Texas Public Health
10500 Forum Place Drive, Suite 123
Houston, TX 77036-8599 (713) 995-1112

Region 7
Texas Public Health
2408 South 37th St.
Temple, TX 76504 (817) 778-6744

Region 8
Texas Public Health
1021 Garnerfield Rd.
Uvalde, TX 78801 (210) 278-7173

Region 11
Texas Public Health
601 West Sesame Drive
Harlingen, TX 78550 (210) 423-0130

**Dental Schools**

Baylor College of Dentistry . . . . . . . Annual patient visits: 75,411.
3302 Gaston Ave.
Dallas, TX 75246 (214) 828-8100

Health Science Center . . . . . . . . . . Annual patient visits: 113,153.
Dental Branch
University of Texas
6516 John Freeman Ave.
Houston, TX 77030 (713) 792-4056

Health Science Center . . . . . . . . . . Annual patient visits: 124,783.
Dental School
University of Texas
7703 Floyd Curl Dr.
San Antonio, TX 78284 (210) 567-3222

**Dental Society**
Texas Dental Association
P.O. Box 3358
Austin, TX 78764-3358 (512) 443-3675

| **Government Grants for Dental Research** | **Grants** |
|---|---|
| Baylor College of Medicine | $93,118 |
| Texas College of Osteopathic Medicine | $106,601 |
| University of Texas Medical Center Br Galveston<br>Galveston, TX | $309,649 |
| University of Texas MD Anderson Cancer Center | $149,455 |
| University of Texas Health Science Center Houston<br>Houston, TX | $1,777,299 |
| University of Texas Health Science Center<br>San Antonio, TX | $4,409,412 |
| Baylor College of Dentistry | $563,581 |

## Utah

**Dental Programs**
Department of Health
Dental Health Division
288 North 1460 West
Salt Lake City, UT 84116 (801) 538-6179

A few Community Health Centers offer dental care for people with low income, usually using a sliding-fee scale. The Homeless Shelter in Utah has a dental clinic that offers free dental care for the homeless. The Indian Health Care Clinic offers dental for Native Americans. Under the *Dental House Calls Program*, reduced-fee dental care is available from volunteer dentists for the handicapped or elderly who are unable to leave their homes. The Medicaid dental program is very extensive for children and adults.

**Dental Society**
Utah Dental Association
1151 E. 3900 South, #B160
Salt Lake City, UT 84124-1216 (801) 261-5315

| **Government Grants for Dental Research** | **Grants** |
|---|---|
| University of Utah . . . . . . . . . . . . . . . . . . . . . . . . . . . | $424,976 |

## Vermont

**Dental Programs**
Department of Health
Dental Division
108 Cherry St.
P.O. Box 70
Burlington, VT 05402 (802) 863-7200

Limited dental care is available. The *Dr. Dinosaur Program* is available for children up to 18 years of age who have a family income of 225% of poverty level. Call for additional information.

Island Pond Health Center
P.O. Box 425
Island Pond, VT 05846 (802) 723-4300

This nonprofit Health Center in northeastern Vermont offers eligible residents of specific towns dental care for a reduced fee based on a sliding scale based on their income from the previous year. Fees range from 100% coverage for preventive dental services and 50% coverage for all other services that they provide. No specialty services, such as orthodontics, are available. Call to get additional information and to find out if Health Care Inc. has reduced fee dental care available in your town.

**Dental Society**
Vermont Dental Society
132 Church St.
Burlington, VT 05401-8401 (802) 864-0115

| **Government Grants for Dental Research** | **Grants** |
|---|---|
| University of Vermont and State Agricultural College . . | $417,410 |

## Virginia

**Dental Programs**
Health Department
Dental Division
1500 E. Main, Room 239
Richmond, VA 23219 (804) 786-3556

Community Health Centers offer dental care at a reduced-fee based on income. Although children are a first priority, adults are treated on an emergency basis. There are approximately 90 such Centers across VA that offer dental care.

**Dental School**
School of Dentistry . . . . . . . . . . . . . Annual patient visits: 61,722
Virginia Commonwealth University
Box 980566
Richmond, VA 23298 (804) 828-9095

**Dental Society**
Virginia Dental Association
P.O. Box 6906
Richmond, VA 23230-0906 (804) 358-4927

| Government Grants for Dental Research | Grants |
|---|---|
| Virginia Commonwealth University | $2,609,933 |
| University of Virginia Charlottesville<br>Charlottesville, VA | $378,373 |
| Hampton University | $3,294 |
| Virginia Polytechnic Institute and State University | $238,172 |

## Washington

**Dental Programs**
State Health Department
Dental Division
P.O. Box 47867
Olympia, WA 98504-7867 (206) 664-3427

Call your nearest Health Department or Clinic to find out if they offer free or discount dental care. When dental care is offered, it is usually for children and senior citizens, with only limited care for adults. A sliding fee scale is used, and low income is a factor in determining what you're charged. Ask to speak with Connie Mix or Bob Blacksmith to get additional information on these programs.

Seattle-King County Dental Society
2201 Sixth Ave., Suite 1306
Seattle, WA 98121-1832 (206) 443-7607

The Seattle-King County Dental Society has a listing of clinics and programs that offer free or minimal cost dental care. Contact them for a free copy.

Elderly and Disabled
Washington State Dental Association
2033 Sixth Avenue #333
Seattle, WA 98121 (206) 448-1914

Under the *Access Program for the Elderly and Disabled*, dental care at a reduced cost is available from participating dentists who meet the following guidelines: 1) 65 or older; 2) have no dental insurance; 3) income no more than $15,670/single or $19,765 for a family; 4) for the disabled, the same criteria for eligibility applies, but there is no age restriction. Eligibility must be re-certified every 12 months. Fees are reduced by at least 25% for patients meeting the criteria. Call or write for an application.

**Dental School**

School of Dentistry . . . . . . . . . . . . . Annual patient visits: 45,500.
University of Washington
Health Science Building
Northeast Pacific St.
Seattle, WA 98195 (206) 543-5830

**Dental Society**

Washington Dental Association

2033 6th Ave., Suite 333
Seattle, WA 98121-2514 (206) 448-1914

| **Government Grants for Dental Research** | **Grants** |
|---|---|
| Gemtech, Inc. | $264,000 |
| Washington State University | $76,250 |
| University of Washington | $6,038,456 |

## West Virginia

**Dental Programs**
Department of Health and Human Resources
Dental Information
State Capital Complex, Bldg. 6
Charleston, WV 25305 (304) 926-1700

Very limited dental care is available through the Health Department other than Medicaid: however, below you'll find other contacts that do offer reduced-fee services.

Low-Income Adults

Linkline
One United Way Square

Charleston, WV 25301 (800) 540-8659
(304) 340-3510

*Linkline* offers reduced-fee dental services for adults 19 to 59, but you must first apply to the program and be accepted. Low income is a major factor in determining your eligibility.

Tiskewah Dental Clinic
600 Florida St.
Charleston, WV 25302 (304) 348-6613

This dental clinic treats children year-round, and senior citizens during the summer free of charge. Call to find out if you might qualify.

**Dental School**
School of Dentistry . . . . . . . . . . . . . Annual patient visits: 27,522.
West Virginia University
The Medical Center
Morgantown, WV 26505 (304) 598-4810

**Dental Society**
West Virginia Dental Association
1002 Kanawha Valley Building
300 Capitol St.
Charleston, WV 25301-1794 (304) 344-5246

**Government Grants for Dental Research** **Grants**
West Virginia University . . . . . . . . . . . . . . . . . . . . . . . $196,600

## Wisconsin

**Dental Programs**
Division of Health
1 West Wilson
Madison, WI 53701 (608) 266-5152

Very limited reduced-fee dental care is available in Wisconsin. Call your local Health Center or Clinic to find out if dental is available.

Wisconsin Dental Society
111 East Wisconsin Ave., Suite 1300
Milwaukee, WI 53202 (414) 276-4520

The Wisconsin Dental Society has been working with County Dental Society's to come up with programs to assist the underserved with reduced fee dental services. Keep in contact with them to find out of any new programs that you might qualify for.

**Dental School**
School of Dentistry . . . . . . . . . . . . . Annual patient visits: 48,235.
Marquette University

604 N. 16th St.
Milwaukee, WI 53233 (414) 288-6500

**Dental Society**
Wisconsin Dental Association
111 E. Wisconsin Ave., Suite 1300
Milwaukee, WI 53202-4811 (414) 276-4520

| **Government Grants for Dental Research** | **Grants** |
|---|---|
| University of Wisconsin Madison, Madison, WI | $483,738 |
| Marquette University | $109,378 |

## Wyoming

**Dental Programs**
State Health Department
Dental Division
Hathaway Building, 4th Floor
Cheyenne, WY 82002 (307) 777-7945

The *Marginal Program* for low-income children provides dental care up to 19 years of age. You must apply and be accepted to be eligible. The *Cleft Palate Clinic* offers free diagnostic treatment and referrals. The *Sealant Program* provides sealant treatment for children of low-income families. The *Elderly Program* offers reduced fees for those low-income adults 65 or older. There is no reduced-fee dental care for those individuals 20 to 64 except through *Title 19 Emergency Care* program.

**Dental Society**
Wyoming Dental Association
330 S. Center St., Suite 322
Casper, WY 82601-2875 (307) 234-0777

# Free Prescription Drugs

## Free Medications From Drug Companies

Leave it to the government to know where you can get free Halcion, AZT, Valium or Motrin but not make any effort to tell you about it. The U.S. Senate's Special Committee on Aging recently published a report on how certain eligible groups, including the elderly and the poor, can actually get their much needed prescription drugs free of charge directly from the companies that manufacture them. Here's what the committee discovered:

Taking prescription medications is often a matter of life and death for millions of Americans, yet many just can't afford the drugs they need simply because they're too expensive. Many are forced to choose between paying for food or their medications, especially the elderly. The relative lack of prescription drug insurance has been compounded by prescription cost increases that can actually surpass the rate of inflation by four times.

Though not widely known, drug companies have programs that offer many prescription drugs free of charge to poor and other vulnerable groups that cannot afford them. However, these free drug programs are being used by only a small number of people that could truly benefit from them. And to add to this, the programs often require long waiting times for qualified patients to receive their free medications from drug manufacturers.

The Pharmaceutical Manufacturer's Association (PMA) has established a *Directory of Prescription Drug Indigent Programs*, which lists up-to-date information on individual manufacturers' patient programs. Although the directory does not always identify the drugs manufactured, it still should be your first call.

☎ Contact:
Pharmaceutical Manufacturer's Association
(800) PMA-INFO

The following pages contain an alphabetical list of all drugs currently covered under Prescription Drug Indigent Programs, as well as the manufacturer that supplies them. We have also included some helpful tips and questions you should ask when contacting the programs:

1) If a drug is not listed in the directory, it still may be provided by the company. You should call the manufacturer directly to check.

2) Ask about the eligibility requirements. Some companies require that you have a limited income or no insurance coverage, while others require only that you get a doctor's referral.

3) Ask about the enrollment process. Many drug companies require a phone call or letter from your doctor.

4) If your doctor refuses to call or does not believe the program will work, contact the drug companies yourself and find out about the application process. You will still need a doctor to fill the application, but you can at least get the forms, and then encourage your doctor to complete them. If your doctor still refuses, maybe you can find another doctor who will.

5) Find out how you will receive the prescription drugs, and how you can get refills. Most companies send the medications directly to your doctor. There have been some problems with delays in receiving the drugs, so check to see

what the company's shipping schedule is, and what you or your doctor should do if there is a problem.

## A to Z Drug Listing

In this Section you'll find a comprehensive A to Z listing of all the drugs that are available to certain qualified groups free of charge directly from the manufacturers.

Each company determines the eligibility criteria for its program. Often, determination is based on the patient's income level and lack of insurance.

**Unless specified below, manufacturers require a phone call or written statement from your doctor's office requesting the medication.**

First, find the drug you need and the corresponding manufacturer. Next, look up the address and telephone number of the appropriate drug manufacturer from the *Directory of Pharmaceutical Manufacturers*, which follows the A to Z drug listing.

Your doctor will need to contact the drug company to find out about how to receive the drug free of charge. Remember, although they want your doctor to call, if your doctor refuses, make the call yourself. After they enroll you in the program, the drug manufacturer will send the medication directly to your doctor who will pass it along to you.

Important Note: More drugs are constantly being added to this list. If you do not find your drug listed here, contact the manufacturer of the drug to see if your drug is included in this program.

## Alphabetical Listing of Drugs

| *Drug* | *Manufacturer* |
|---|---|
| **A —** | |
| Accrupril | Parke-Davis |
| Aci-Jel | Ortho |
| Actigall | Ciba-Geigy |
| Actimmune | Genentech |
| Activase | Genentech |
| Adriamycin PFS | Adria |
| Adrucil | Adria |
| Aldactazide | Searle |
| Aldactone | Searle |
| Aldomet | Merck |
| ALT/S | Hoechst-Roussel |
| Altace | Hoechst-Roussel |
| Alupent | Boehringer |
| Amoxil | SmithKline Beecham |
| Anafranil | Ciba-Geigy |
| Anaprox | Syntex |
| Ansaid | Upjohn |
| Antivert | Pfizer |
| Anturane | Ciba-Geigy |
| Anusol HC | Parke-Davis |
| Apresazide | Ciba-Geigy |
| Apresoline | Ciba-Geigy |
| Aralen | Sanofi Winthrop |
| Aredia | Ciba-Geigy |
| Artane | Lederle |
| Asacol | Procter & Gamble |
| Atrovent | Boehringer |
| Axid | Eli Lilly |

*If your drug is not listed here, it is still worthwhile to contact the manufacturer.*

| | |
|---|---|
| Augmentin | SmithKline Beecham |
| Axid | Eli Lilly |
| AZT (Retrovir) | Burroughs-Wellcome |
| Azulfidine | Pharmacia |
| Azulfidine En-Tab | Pharmacia |

## B —

| | |
|---|---|
| Bactrim | Hoffman-LaRoche |
| Bactrim DS | Hoffman-LaRoche |
| Bactroban | SmithKline Beecham |
| Beconase | Glaxo |
| Beconase AQ | Glaxo |
| Berelan | Lederle |
| Betagen | Allergan |
| Betaseron | Berlex |
| Betaspace | Berlex |
| BICNU | Bristol-Myers |
| Blenoxance | Bristol-Myers |
| Bleph-10 | Allergan |
| Blephamide | Allergan |
| Botox | Allergan |
| Breonesin | Sanofi Winthrop |
| Brethaire | Ciba-Geigy |
| Brethine | Ciba-Geigy |
| Bronkometer | Sanofi Winthrop |
| Bucladin-S | ICI |
| BuSpar | Bristol-Myers |

## C —

| | |
|---|---|
| Calan | Searle |
| Calan SR | Searle |
| Capoten | Bristol-Myers |
| Capozide | Bristol-Myers |
| Carafate | Marion Merrell Dow |
| Cardene | Syntex |
| Cardizem | Marion Merrell Dow |

*If your drug is not listed here, it is still worthwhile to contact the manufacturer.*

| | |
|---|---|
| Cardizem CD | Marion Merrell Dow |
| Cardizem SR | Marion Merrell Dow |
| Cardura | Pfizer |
| Cataflam | Ciba-Geigy |
| Catapres | Boehringer |
| Ceclor | Eli Lilly |
| CEENU | Bristol-Myers |
| Ceftin | Glaxo |
| Cefzil | Bristol-Myers |
| Ceredase | Genzyme |
| Cipro | Miles |
| Claforan | Hoechst-Roussel |
| Cleocin | Upjohn |
| Clinoril | Merck |
| Clozaril | Sandoz |
| Cogentin | Merck |
| Cognex | Parke-Davis |
| Compazine | SmithKline Beecham |
| Cordarone | Wyeth-Ayerst |
| Corgard | Bristol-Myers |
| Corzide | Bristol-Myers |
| Coumadin | DuPont Merck |
| Cyclospasmol | Wyeth-Ayerst |
| Cytadren | Ciba-Geigy |
| Cytotec | Searle |
| Cytovene | Syntex |
| Cytoxan | Bristol-Myers |

## D —

| | |
|---|---|
| Dalmane | Hoffman-LaRoche |
| Danocrine | Sanofi Winthrop |
| Dantrium | Norwich-Eaton |
| Desferal | Ciba-Geigy |
| Desyrel | Bristol-Myers |
| Diabeta | Hoechst-Roussel |

*If your drug is not listed here, it is still worthwhile to contact the manufacturer.*

| | |
|---|---|
| Diabinese | Pfizer |
| Diamox | Lederle |
| Didronel | Procter & Gamble |
| Dienestrol | Ortho |
| Diflucan | Pfizer |
| Dilantin | Parke-Davis |
| Dipentum | Pharmacia |
| Diprolene | Schering |
| Diprosone | Schering |
| Dolobid | Merck |
| Drisdol | Sanofi Winthrop |
| Duragesic | Janssen |
| Duricef | Bristol-Myers |
| Dyazide | SmithKline Beecham |
| Dymelor | Eli Lilly |
| DynaCirc | Sandoz |

## E —

| | |
|---|---|
| E-Mycin | Upjohn |
| Efudex (Fluorouracil Injection) | Hoffman-LaRoche |
| Eldepryl | Sandoz |
| Emcyt | Pharmacia |
| Eminase | SmithKline Beecham |
| Entex | Procter & Gamble |
| Epifrin | Allergan |
| Epogen | Amgen |
| Ergamisol | Janssen |
| Erycette | Ortho |
| Esidrix | Ciba-Geigy |
| Esimil | Ciba-Geigy |
| Estrace | Bristol-Myers |
| Estraderm | Ciba-Geigy |
| Eulexin | Schering |
| Extel | Procter & Gamble |



*If your drug is not listed here, it is still worthwhile to contact the manufacturer.*

## F —

| | |
|---|---|
| Famvir | SmithKline Beecham |
| Feldene | Pfizer |
| Flexeril | Merck |
| Floxin | Ortho |
| Fludara | Berlex |
| FML | Allergan |
| Folex | Adria |
| Folex PFS | Adria |
| Foscavir | Astra USA |
| Fulvicin | Schering |

## G —

| | |
|---|---|
| Gantrisin | Hoffman-LaRoche |
| Gantanol | Hoffman-LaRoche |
| Gastrocrom | Fisons |
| Glucotrol | Pfizer |
| Grifulvin Suppositories | Ortho |

## H —

| | |
|---|---|
| Habitrol | Ciba-Geigy |
| Halcion | Upjohn |
| Haldol | McNeil |
| Hismanal | Janssen |
| Hivid | Hoffman-LaRoche |
| HMS | Allergan |
| Humulin | Eli Lilly |
| Hydraea | Immunex |
| Hytakerol | Sanofi Winthrop |

## I —

| | |
|---|---|
| Idamycin | Adria |
| Ifex | Bristol-Myers |

*If your drug is not listed here, it is still worthwhile to contact the manufacturer.*

| | |
|---|---|
| Iletin | Eli Lilly |
| Imodium | Janssen |
| IMOGAM Rabies | Connaught |
| IMOVAX Rabies | Connaught |
| Imuran | Burroughs-Wellcome |
| Indocin | Merck |
| Insulin Products | Eli Lilly |
| Interferon-A Recombinant | Hoffman-LaRoche |
| Intron-A | Schering |
| Ismelin | Ciba-Geigy |
| Isoptin | Knoll |
| Isordil | Wyeth-Ayerst |
| Isuprel | Sanofi Winthrop |

## K —

| | |
|---|---|
| K-Lyte | Bristol-Myers |
| Keflex | Eli Lilly |
| Kerlone | Searle |
| Kinesed | ICI |
| Klonopin | Hoffman-LaRoche |
| Klotrix | Bristol-Myers |
| Kytril | SmithKline Beecham |

## L —

| | |
|---|---|
| Lamprene | Ciba-Geigy |
| Lanoxin | Burroughs-Wellcome |
| Lasix | Hoechst-Roussel |
| Lescol | Sandoz |
| Leucovorin Calcium | Lederle |
| Leukine | Immunex |
| Leustatin | Ortho-Biotech |
| Librium | Hoffman-LaRoche |
| Lidex | Syntex |
| Limbritol | Hoffman-LaRoche |
| Lincocin | Upjohn |
| Lindane Lotion/Shampoo | Reed and Carnrick |



*If your drug is not listed here, it is still worthwhile to contact the manufacturer.*

| | |
|---|---|
| Lioresal | Ciba-Geigy |
| Lithobid | Ciba-Geigy |
| Lodosyn | DuPont Merck |
| Loniten | Upjohn |
| Lo/Ovral | Wyeth-Ayerst |
| Lopid | Parke-Davis |
| Lopressor | Ciba-Geigy |
| Lopressor/HCT | Ciba-Geigy |
| Loprox | Hoechst-Roussel |
| Lorelco | Marion Merrell Dow |
| Lotensin | Ciba-Geigy |
| Lotensin HCT | Ciba-Geigy |
| Lotrimin | Schering |
| Lotrisone | Schering |
| Loxapine | Lederle |
| Ludiomil | Ciba-Geigy |
| Lyophilized Cytoxan | Bristol-Myers |
| Lysodren | Bristol-Myers |

## M —

| | |
|---|---|
| Macrobid | Procter & Gamble |
| Macrodantin | Procter & Gamble |
| Marax | Pfizer |
| Marinol Capsules | Roxane |
| Maxaquin | Searle |
| Maxzide | Lederle |
| Meclan | Ortho |
| Medrol | Upjohn |
| Megace | Bristol-Myers |
| Mepron | Burroughs-Wellcome |
| Mesnex | Bristol-Myers |
| Metrodin | Ares-Serono |
| Mevacor | Merck |
| Micronase | Upjohn |
| Minipress | Pfizer |

*If your drug is not listed here, it is still worthwhile to contact the manufacturer.*

| | |
|---|---|
| Minizide | Pfizer |
| Minocin | Lederle |
| Monistat | Ortho |
| Monistat Derm | Ortho |
| Monopril | Bristol-Myers |
| Motrin | Upjohn |
| Mutamycin | Bristol-Myers |
| Myambutol | Lederle |
| Mycobutin | Pharmacia |
| Mycostatin | Bristol-Myers |
| Mytelase | Sanofi Winthrop |

## N —

| | |
|---|---|
| Naphcon-A | Allergan |
| Naprosyn | Syntex |
| Nasalide | Syntex |
| Natalins | Bristol-Myers |
| Natalins RX | Bristol-Myers |
| Navane | Pfizer |
| NebuPent | Fujisawa USA |
| NegGram | Sanofi Winthrop |
| Neosar | Adria |
| Neupogen | Amgen |
| Neurontin | Parke-Davis |
| Nicorette | Marion Merrell Dow |
| Nimotop | Miles |
| Nitrodisc | Searle |
| Nitrostat | Parke-Davis |
| Nizoral Tablets | Janssen |
| Nolvadex | Zeneca |
| Nordette | Wyeth-Ayerst |
| Normodyne | Schering |
| Norpace | Searle |
| Norpace CR | Searle |
| Noroxin | Merck |
| Norplant System | Wyeth-Ayerst |



*If your drug is not listed here, it is still worthwhile to contact the manufacturer.*

| | |
|---|---|
| Norspace | Searle |
| Nutropin | Genentech |

## O —

| | |
|---|---|
| Oculinium | Allergan |
| Ocusert | ALZA |
| Optimine | Schering |
| Oramorph SR Tablets | Roxane |
| Orinase | Upjohn |
| Ortho-Dienestrol | Ortho |
| Orudis | Wyeth-Ayerst |
| Ovcon | Bristol-Myers |

## P —

| | |
|---|---|
| Pancrease | McNeil |
| Parafon Forte DSC | McNeil |
| Paraplatin | Bristol-Myers |
| Parlodel | Sandoz |
| Pavabid | Marion Merrell Dow |
| PBZ | Ciba-Geigy |
| Pepcid | Merck |
| Periactin | Merck |
| Persa-Gel | Ortho |
| Persa-Gel W | Ortho |
| Persantine | Boehringer |
| Phenergan | Wyeth-Ayerst |
| PhisoHex | Sanofi Winthrop |
| Pilagan | Allergan |
| Plaquenil | Sanofi Winthrop |
| Platinol | Bristol-Myers |
| Plendil | Merck |
| Ponstel | Parke-Davis |
| Pravochol | Bristol-Myers |
| Premarin | Wyeth-Ayerst |
| Prilosec | Merck |

*If your drug is not listed here, it is still worthwhile to contact the manufacturer.*

| | |
|---|---|
| Primaquine | Sanofi Winthrop |
| Prinivil | Merck |
| Procan | Parke-Davis |
| Procan SR | Parke-Davis |
| Procardia | Pfizer |
| Procardia YL | Pfizer |
| Procrit | Ortho-Biotech |
| Progestasert | ALZA |
| Prograf capsules | Fujisawa USA |
| Prokine | Hoechst-Roussel |
| Pronestyl SR | Bristol-Myers |
| Propine | Allergan |
| Propulsid | Janssen |
| Proscar | Merck |
| Prostat | Ortho |
| Protropin | Genentech |
| Proventil | Schering |
| Provera | Upjohn |
| Prozac | Eli Lilly |
| Pyridium | Parke-Davis |

## Q —

| | |
|---|---|
| Questran | Bristol-Myers |
| Quinamm | Marion Merrell Dow |
| Quinaglute Dura-Tabs | Berlex |

## R —

| | |
|---|---|
| Regitine | Ciba-Geigy |
| Relafen | SmithKline Beecham |
| Rheumatrex | Lederle |
| Ridaura | SmithKline Beecham |
| Rifadin | Marion Merrell Dow |
| Rifamate | Marion Merrell Dow |
| Rifater | Marion Merrell Dow |
| Rimactane | Ciba-Geigy |
| Risperdal | Janssen |



*If your drug is not listed here, it is still worthwhile to contact the manufacturer.*

| | |
|---|---|
| Rocaltrol | Hoffman-LaRoche |
| Rocephin Injectable | Hoffman-LaRoche |
| Roxanol | Roxane |
| Rubex | Immunex |
| Rythmol | Knoll |

## S —

| | |
|---|---|
| Sandimmune | Sandoz |
| Sandoglobulin | Sandoz |
| Sandostatin | Sandoz |
| Santyl | Knoll |
| Sectral | Wyeth-Ayerst |
| Seldane | Marion Merrell Dow |
| Seldane D | Marion Merrell Dow |
| Septra | Burroughs-Wellcome |
| Septra DS | Burroughs-Wellcome |
| Ser-Ap-Es | Ciba-Geigy |
| Sinemet | DuPont Merck |
| Sinemet Cr | DuPont Merck |
| Sinequan | Pfizer |
| Slow-K | Ciba-Geigy |
| Sorbitrate | Zeneca |
| Spectazole | Ortho |
| Sporanox Capsules | Janssen |
| Sublingual | Parke-Davis |
| Sultrin | Ortho |
| Survanta | Abbott |
| Symmetrel | DuPont Merck |
| Synalar | Syntex |
| Synemol | Syntex |
| Synthroid | Boots |
| Sy Trexan | DuPont Merck |

## T —

| | |
|---|---|
| Tagamet | SmithKline Beecham |

| | |
|---|---|
| Tarabine | Adria |
| Tegretol | Ciba-Geigy |
| TEN-K | Ciba-Geigy |
| Tenormin | Zeneca |
| Tenoretic | Zeneca |
| Terazol | Ortho |
| Testoderm | ALZA |
| TheraCys | Connaught |
| Ticlid | Syntex |
| Timolol | Merck |
| Timoptic | Merck |
| Tenuate | Marion Merrell Dow |
| Tofranil | Ciba-Geigy |
| Tofranil-PM | Ciba-Geigy |
| Tolectin | McNeil |
| Tolinase | Upjohn |
| Topicort | Hoechst-Roussel |
| Toradol | Syntex |
| Trancopal | Sanofi Winthrop |
| Trandate | Glaxo |
| Transderm-Scop | Ciba-Geigy |
| Transdermal-Nitro | Ciba-Geigy |
| Trental | Hoechst-Roussel |
| Trexan | DuPont Merck |
| Tridesilon Cream | Miles |
| Trinalin | Schering |
| Triostat | SmithKline Beecham |
| Triphasil | Wyeth-Ayerst |

## V —

| | |
|---|---|
| Vagistat | Bristol-Myers |
| Valium | Hoffman-LaRoche |
| Vancenase | Schering |
| Vascor | McNeil |
| Vasodilan | Bristol-Myers |
| Vasoretic | Merck |



*If your drug is not listed here, it is still worthwhile to contact the manufacturer.*

| | |
|---|---|
| Vasotec | Merck |
| Ventoli | Glaxo |
| VePesid | Bristol-Myers |
| Verelan | Lederle |
| Vermox | Janssen |
| Vibramycin | Pfizer |
| Videx | Bristol-Myers |
| Vincasar | Adria |
| Vincasar PFS | Adria |
| Vistaril | Pfizer |
| Voltaren | Ciba-Geigy |

**W —**

| | |
|---|---|
| Wellcovorin | Burroughs-Wellcome |
| Winstrol | Sanofi Winthrop |
| Wytensin | Wyeth-Ayerst |

**X —**

| | |
|---|---|
| Xanax | Upjohn |

**Z —**

| | |
|---|---|
| Zantac | Glaxo |
| Zarontin | Parke-Davis |
| Zestoretic | Zeneca |
| Zestril | Zeneca |
| Zithromax | Pfizer |
| Zoladex | Zeneca |
| Zoloft | Pfizer |
| Zostrix | Knoll |
| Zovirax | Burroughs-Wellcome |
| Zyloprim | Burroughs-Wellcome |

# Directory of Pharmaceutical Manufacturer Indigent Patient Programs

## ABBOTT LABORATORIES/ROSS LABORATORIES

Survanta Lifeline
Medical Technology Hotlines
555 13th Street NW
Suite 7E
Washington, DC 20004-1109

(800) 922-3255
Fax: (202) 637-6690

## ADRIA LABORATORIES, INC.

Adria Laboratories
Patient Assistance Program
P.O. Box 9525
McLean, VA 22102

(800) 366-5570

**Products Covered by the Program**
Adriamycin PFS, Adrucil, Folex, Idamycin, Neosar, Tarabine, and Vincasar

**Other Product Information**
Two months' supply. Physician must certify patient is unable to afford the cost of the drug, and is unable to obtain assistance elsewhere.

## ALLERGAN PRESCRIPTION PHARMACEUTICALS

Allergan Patient Assistance Program
c/o Judy McGee
Physician Services Representative (T1-1D)
Allergan, Inc.

P.O. Box 19534 (800) 347-4500
Irvine, CA 92713-9534 Ext. 7791

**Products Covered by the Program**
Betagen (levobunolol HCl).25%; Betagen (levobunolol HCl) .5%, b.i.d., q.d.: Propine (dipivefrin HCl); Pilagan (pilocarpine nitrate) 1%; Pilagan (pilocarpine nitrate) 2%; Pilagan (pilocarpine nitrate) 4%; Epifrin .25%; Epifrin .5%; Epifrin 1%; Epifrin 2%

**Other Product Information**
Only Allergan chronic medications, glaucoma and dry-eye products will be available. Physicians may make new requests for new and existing patients as needed.

**Botox Division**

Botox Patient Assistance Program
Allergan, Inc.
2525 Dupont Dr.
Irvine, CA 92713 (800) 347-4500

**Products Covered by the Program**
Botox (botulinum toxin type A)

**Other Program Information**
Eligibility form to be completed by physician and patient. Patient eligibility form is submitted for each visit; the physician is then credited for the product needed. Physician must waive office fee to the patient. Eligibility forms are available from Botox Reimbursement Manager in Irvine, CA.

## ALZA PHARMACEUTICALS

Indigent Patient Assistance Program
Attn: Sales Service Department M6
ALZA Pharmaceuticals
P.O. Box 10950
Palo Alto, CA 94303-0802 (415) 962-4243

**Products Covered by the Program**
Testoderm, Ocusert, Progestasert

**Other Program Information**
The physician must request an Indigent Patient Application Kit from ALZA Pharmaceuticals. Due to state laws prohibiting sampling of controlled substances, the Indigent Program for Testoderm CIII is not available in New York, Ohio, Kentucky, Kansas and Georgia.

## AMGEN, INC.

**Name of Program**
Safety Net Program for Epogen
Medical Technology Hotlines (800) 272-9376
in Washington, DC (202) 637-6698

**Product Covered by the Program**
Epogen (For patients on dialysis only)

**Name of Program**
Safety Net Program for Neupogen
Medical Technology Hotlines (800) 272-9376
in Washington, DC (202) 637-6698

**Product Covered by the Program**
Neupogen

**Other Product Information**
Providers apply on behalf of the patient. Any administering physician, hospital, home health company or retail pharmacy may sponsor a patient by applying to the program on his or her behalf. The program is based on a 12-month patient year rather than a calendar year.

## ARES-SERONO, INC.

Gina Cella, Manager
Corporate Communications
Ares-Serono, Inc.
100 Longwater Circle (617) 982-9000
Norwell, MA 02061 Fax: (617) 982-1269

## ASTRA USA, INC.

FAIR Program (Foscavir Assistance and
Information Reimbursement)
1101 King St., Suite 600
Alexandria, VA 22314 (800) 488-3247

**Products Covered by the Program**
Foscavir (foscarnet sodium) Injection

**Other Product Information**
Patient is not covered for outpatient prescription drugs under private insurance or a public program. Patient's income must fall below level selected by the company. Patient may or may not be poor, but retail drug purchase would cause hardship. Patient is covered for outpatient prescription drugs, but may be eligible for assistance with deductibles or maximum benefit limits.

TOPROL-XL
ASTRA USA
Attention: Erin Flynn
50 Otis St.
Westboro, MA 01581 (800) 225-6333

## BERLEX LABORATORIES

**Name of Program**
Berlex Laboratories Cardiovascular Assistance Program
Berlex Laboratories (800) 423-7539

**Products Covered by the Program**
Betaspace (sotalol HCl) and Quinaglute Dura-Tabs (quinidine gluconate tablets)

**Name of Program**
Betaseron Support Program (800) 788-1467

**Products Covered by the Program**
Betaseron (Interferon beta-1b) for SC injection

**Name of Program**
Fludara PACT Program
(Patient Assistance for Cancer Treatment) (800) 473-5832

**Products Covered by the Program**
Fludara (fludarabine phosphate) for injection

**Eligibility**
Patients are eligible regardless of insurance status.

## BOEHRINGER INGLEHEIM PHARMACEUTICALS, INC.

Partners in Health Information Line
P.O. Box 368
Ridgefield, CT 06877-0368 (800) 556-8317

**Products Covered by the Program**
All products covered except controlled substances.

**Eligibility**
Patients must meet the following criteria: No prescription insurance coverage, patient ineligible for Medicaid/state assistance programs, annual income guidelines must be met.

**Other Program Information**
Prescription required for every request.

## BOOTS PHARMACEUTICALS, INC.

Boots Cares Program
Boots Pharmaceuticals, Inc.
30 Tri-State International Center
Suite 200
Lincolnshire, IL 60069-4415
Attn: Sandy Bauco

**Products Covered by the Program**
Synthroid Tablets (levothyroxine sodium, USP) only

**Eligibility**
Physician must submit appropriate documentation proving patient indigence to company. Decisions are made on a case-by-case basis.

## BRISTOL-MYERS SQUIBB COMPANY

Bristol-Myers Squibb
Patient Assistance Program
P.O. Box 9445
McLean, VA 22102-9998 (800) 736-0003
Fax: (703) 760-0049

**Names of Programs**
Indigent Patient Program
Cardiovascular Access Program
Cancer Patient Access Program
Videx Temporary Assistance Program ...... (800) 788-0123

**Products Covered by the Program**
Many Bristol-Myers Squibb Pharmaceutical Products.

**Eligibility**
Application forms are supplied by the company to physicians.

## BURROUGHS-WELLCOME CO.

Burroughs-Wellcome Co.
Patient Assistance Program
P.O. Box 52035
Phoenix, AZ 85072-9349 (800) 722-9294

**Products Covered by the Program**
All marketed Burroughs-Wellcome Co. prescription products.

**Eligibility**
Patient eligibility is tied to multiples of the federal poverty guidelines. Program drug benefits are provided primarily through pharmacies. Direct product shipment to the health care provider is available for injectable products.

## CIBA-GEIGY CORPORATION, PHARMACEUTICALS DIVISION

Patient Assistance Program
Ciba-Geigy Corporation
556 Morris Avenue, D-2058
Summit, NJ 07901 (800) 257-3273

**Products Covered by the Program**
Actigall; Anafranil; Anturane; Apresazide; Apresoline; Aredia; Brethaire; Brethine; Cataflam; Cytadren; Desferal; Esidrix; Esimil; Estraderm; Habitrol; Ismelin; Lamprene; Lioresal; Lopressor; Lopressor/HCT; Lotensin; Lotensin HCT; Ludiomil; PBZ; Regitine; Rimactane; Ser-Ap-Es; Slow-K; Tegretol; TEN-K; Tofranil; Tofranil-PM; Transderm-Scop; Transdermal-Nitro; Voltaren

**Other Product Information**
Application must be completed by the physician and patient. Anyone can request information and refer any patient.

## CONNAUGHT LABORATORIES, INC.

**Name of Program:**
Rabies Post-Exposure Indigent Patient Program
Rabies Product Manager
Connaught Laboratories, Inc.
Route 611, P.O. Box 187
Swiftwater, PA 18370-0187

**Products Covered by the Program**
IMOVAX Rabies, rabies vaccine; IMOGAM Rabies, rabies immune globulin (human)

**Name of Program:**
TheraCys Indigent Patient Program
TheraCys Product Manager
Connaught Laboratories, Inc.
Route 611, P.O. Box 187
Swiftwater, PA 18370-0187 (717) 839-4617

**Products Covered by the Program**
TheraCys BCG live intravesical

**Other Product Information**
Six doses are provided for one induction course of therapy. Connaught does not provide, under the program, for a full course of therapy - induction and maintenance - which may be as high as 11 doses.

## DU PONT MERCK PHARMACEUTICAL CO.

Darlene Samis
Du Pont Pharma
P.O. Box 80026
Wilmington, DE 19880-0026 (800) 474-2762

**Name of Program:**
DuPont Merck Pharmaceutical
Company Patient Assistance Program

Physicians requests should be directed to their local DuPont Merck Pharmaceutical Company sales representative.

**Products Covered by the Program**
All non-controlled prescription products.

## FISONS PHARMACEUTICALS

**Name of Program**
Fisons Respiratory Care Program
Fisons Pharmaceuticals
P.O. Box 1766
Rochester, NY 14603-1766

**Products Covered by the Program**
Assess Peak Flow Meter; Intal Inhaler (cromolyn sodium inhalation aerosol); Intal Nebulizer Solution (cromolyn sodium inhalation, USP); Tilade Inhaler (nedocromil sodium inhalation aerosol)

**Name of Program**
Gastrocrom Patient Assistance Program
Fisons Pharmaceuticals
P.O. Box 1766
Rochester, NY 14603-1766

**Products Covered by the Program**
Gastrocrom (cromolyn sodium, USP) Capsules

## FUJISAWA USA, INC.

**Name of Program**
NeubuPent Indigent Patient Program
Laura Cruz, NebuPent Product Manager
Fujisawa USA, Inc.
3 Parkway North Center
Deerfield, IL 60015-2548 (708) 317-8636

**Products Covered by the Program**
NebuPent (pentamidine isethionate)

**Eligibility**
This program is designed to provide NebuPent (pentamidine isethionate) to AIDS patients who would not otherwise be able to afford this treatment.

**Name of Program**
Prograf Patient Assistance Program
c/o Medical Technology Hotlines
P.O. Box 7710 (800) 4-PROGRAF
Washington, DC 20044-7710 (800 477-6472)
in the Washington DC area (202) 293-5563

**Products Covered by the Program**
Prograf capsules (tacrolimus, FK506)

## GENENTECH, INC.

Uninsured Patient Assistance Program
Genentech, Inc.
Mail Stop #13, P.O. Box 2586
S. San Francisco, CA 94083-2586 (800) 879-4747

**Products Covered by the Program**
Actimmune (interferon gamma-1b); Activase (alteplase recombinant); Protropin (somatrem for injection); Nutropin (somatropin for injection)

## GENZYME CORPORATION

William Aliski
Director of Reimbursement
Genzyme Corporation
1 Kendall Square (617) 252-7871
Cambridge, MA 02139 Fax: (617) 252-7600

## GLAXO INC.

Glaxo Inc. Indigent Patient Program
Laura N. Wright
Supervisor, Trade Communications
Glaxo, Inc.
P.O. Box 13438 (800) 452-9677
Research Triangle Park, NC 27709 Fax: (919) 248-7971

**Products Covered by the Program**
All current Glaxo products.

## HOECHST-ROUSSEL PHARMACEUTICALS INC.

HRPI Patient Access Program
Hoeschst-Roussel Pharmaceuticals, Inc.
Route 202-206
P.O. Box 2500
Somerville, NJ 08876-1258 (800) 422-4779
Attn: Field Force Development HRPI-BB

**Products Covered by the Program**
Altace; ALT/S; Claforan; Diabeta; Lasix; Loprox; Topicort; Trental

## HOFFMAN-LA ROCHE, INC.

Inge Shanahan
Medical Communications Associate
Roche Laboratories
340 Kingsland Street (800) 285-4489
Nutley, NJ 07110 Fax: (201) 235-2765

**Products Covered by the Program**
Valium, Librium, Limbritol, Dalmane, Hivid, Bactrim, Bactrim DS, Klonopin, Efudex (Fluorouracil Injectable), Gantrisin, Gantanol, Interferon 2A Recombinant, Rocephin Injectable, and Rocaltrol.

**Eligibility**
Eligibility limited to private practice outpatients who are considered by the physician to be medically indigent and who are not eligible to receive Roche drugs through any other third-party reimbursement program.

**Other Product Information**
The physician's signature and DEA number are required for all applications, whether or not the request is for a controlled prescription drug. Drugs are shipped to registered DEA addresses only.

## ICI PHARMACEUTICALS

Yvonne A. Graham, Manager
Professional Services
ICI Pharmaceuticals Group
P.O. Box 15197
Wilmington, DE 19850-5197 (302) 886-2231

## IMMUNEX CORPORATION

Patient Assistance Program
Michael L. Kleinberg, M.S., FASHP
Vice President of Professional Services
Immunex Corporation
51 University St. (206) 587-0430
Seattle, WA 98101 (800) 466-8639

**Products Covered by the Program**
All currently marketed Immunex Corporation prescription products.

**Eligibility**
Physician determines patient eligibility based on company guidelines. Patient may or may not be poor, but retail purchase would cause hardship and all other reimbursement options have been exhausted.

**Other Program Information**
A patient assistance program enrollment form is obtained by the physician from the company medical services representative.
Up to two refills are available.

## JANSSEN PHARMACEUTICA

Janssen Patient Assistance Program
1800 Robert Fulton Drive
Reston, VA 22091-4346 (800) 544-2987

**Products Covered by the Program**
Duragesic; Ergamisol (levamisole HCl); Hismanal; Imodium; Nizoral Tablets; Propulsid; Sporanox Capsules; Vermox

**Eligibility**
Less than $25,000 total annual household income. Patient can have Medicare or private insurance but cannot have prescription coverage.

Professional Services Department
Janssen Pharmaceutica Inc.
1125 Trenton-Harbourton Road
Office A3200
P.O. Box 200
Titusville, NJ 08560-0200 (800) 253-3682

Ellen McDonald
Assistant Product Manager
Janssen Pharmaceutica Inc.
40 Kingsbridge Rd. (908) 524-9409
Piscataway, NJ 08854 Fax: (908) 524-9118

## KNOLL PHARMACEUTICAL COMPANY

Knoll Indigent Patient Program
Knoll Pharmaceutical Company

30 N. Jefferson Road
Whippany, NJ 07981 (800) 524-2474

**Products Covered by the Program**
Isoptin (verapamil); Rythmol (propafenone); Santyl (collagenase)

## LEDERLE LABORATORIES

Lederle PARTNERS IN PATIENT CARE Assistance Program

Physicians requests should be directed to (800) LED-CARE or the company medical representative from Lederle or STORZ Ophthalmics who services the physician.

**Products Covered by the Program**
All oral pharmaceutical products except controlled drugs.

**Other Product Information**
This program is designed to assist private practice physicians and community pharmacists who are concerned with the care of patients who are financially burdened. The patient receives the complimentary medication through a community pharmacy, which is reimbursed through an existing third-party pay program.

## ELI LILLY AND COMPANY

Lilly Cares
Program Administrator
P.O. Box 9105
McLean, VA 22102-0105 (800) 545-6962

**Products Covered by the Program**
Most all Lilly prescription products and insulins (except controlled substances).

## MARION MERRELL DOW INC.

Indigent Patient Program
Marion Merrell Dow Inc.
P.O. Box 8600 (816) 966-4000
Kansas City, MO 64114 (800) 362-7466

**Products Covered by the Program**
All prescription products, except Rifadin, Rifamate, Rifater, Tenuate.

## McNEIL PHARMACEUTICAL

McNeil Patient Assistance Program
Thomas Schwend, R.Ph.
Manager
Medical Information and Patient Assistance Program Liaison
McNeil Pharmaceutical
P.O. Box 300, Route 202 South
Raritan, NJ 08869-0602 (800) 682-6532

**Products Covered by the Program**
Prescription products prescribed according to approved labeled indications and dosage regimens.

## MERCK HUMAN HEALTH DIVISION

Merck Patient Assistance Program
Merck & Co., Inc.
P.O. Box 4 (WP35-258) (800) NSC MERCK
West Point, PA 19486-0004 (800-672-6372)
215-652-5000
(collect calls accepted)

**Products Covered by the Program**
Many Merck products.

**Other Product Information**
Up to a three-month supply of the prescribed medications will be sent directly to the physician for distribution to the patient. Any subsequent request for the same patient require the same procedure.

## MILES INC. PHARMACEUTICAL DIVISION

Miles Inc. Indigent Patient Program
Miles Inc. Pharmaceutical Division
400 Morgan Lane
West Haven, CT 06516 (800) 998-9180

**Products Covered by the Program**
All Miles Inc. prescription medications used as recommended in prescribing information.

## NORWICH-EATON PHARMACEUTICALS (PROCTOR AND GAMBLE)

R. M. Brandt, Manager (607) 335-2079
Coverage and Reimbursement Fax: (607) 335-2020
(800) 448-4878

## ORTHO BIOTECH INC.

Financial Assistance Program (FAP) For PROCRIT (Epoetin alfa) and LEUSTATIN (cladribine) Injection/Ortho Biotech

The Ortho Biotech FAP Program
1800 Robert Fulton Drive (800) 553-3851
Suite 300 (800) 447-3437
Reston, VA 22091-4345 (800) 441-1366

**Products Covered by the Program**
Procrit (Epoetin alfa), for non-dialysis use; Leustatin (cladribine) Injection.

**Other Program Information**
Patient eligibility application forms are available from Ortho Biotech Product Specialists or by accessing the 800 number (800-553-3851). This call can help determine if a patient is eligible to enroll in the program.

## ORTHO PHARMACEUTICAL CORPORATION

Ortho Pharmaceutical Patient Assistance Program
Thomas Schwend, R.Ph.
Manager
Medical Information and Patient Assistance Program Liaison
P.O. Box 300, Route 202 South
Raritan, NJ 08869-0602 (800) 682-6532

**Products Covered by the Program**
Prescription products prescribed according to approved labeled indications and dosage regimens.

**Other Program Information**
Physicians should request free medication by written request. Requests must be accompanied by a signed and dated prescription and letter stating financial status and need. All medication will be sent to the physician for dispensing to the patient.

## PARKE-DAVIS

Parke-Davis Patient Assistance Program
P.O. Box 9945
McLean, VA 22102 (800) 755-0120

**Products Covered by the Program**
With a few exceptions, all Parke-Davis medications are available through this program. (Includes, but not limited to: Accrupril; Cognex; Dilantin; Lopid; Neutrontin; Nitrostat Sublingual; Procan SR: and Zarontin).

**Other Program Information**
Patient or patient's representative can call the toll-free number. Enrollment screening will be handled entirely over the phone. If eligible, the patient will receive a prescription card which, along with a written prescription from his/her physician, can be taken to any pharmacy participating in the PCS RECAP program. The pharmacist will dispense up to a 90-day supply of Parke-Davis medication free of charge. Patient must reapply at six months.

## PFIZER INC

Pfizer Indigent Patient Program
P.O. Box 25457
Alexandria, VA 22314-5457 (800) 646-4455

**Products Covered by the Program**
All Pfizer outpatient products, except Diflucan and Zithromax are covered by this program. (Diflucan is covered under the Diflucan Patient Assistance Program).

**Roerig Division**

**Name of Program**
Diflucan Patient Assistance Program

Physician Requests Should be Directed to:
Diflucan Patient Assistance Program (800) 869-9979

**Products Covered by the Program**
Diflucan (fluconazole)

**Eligibility**
Patient must not have insurance or other third-party coverage, including Medicaid, and must not be eligible for a state's AIDS drug assistance program. Patient must have an income of less than $25,000 a year without dependents, or less than $40,000 a year with dependents.

**Name of Program**
Sharing the Care
Pfizer Inc.
13th Floor
235 E. 42nd St.
New York, NY 10017 (800) 984-1500

**Products Covered by the Program**
Pfizer single-source products.

The program, a joint effort of Pfizer, the National Governors' Association and the National Association of Community Health Centers, works solely through community, migrant and homeless health centers certified by the federal government as meeting criteria of Section 329, 339, or 340 of the Public Health Service Act. Center must have an in-house pharmacy to participate. To be eligible, patient must be a patient of a participating health center and must be uninsured, not eligible for government entitlement programs that cover pharmaceuticals, and at or below federal poverty line.

**Other Product Information**
Product is dispensed at health center pharmacy.

**Name of Program**
Arkansas Health Care Access Program

Physician Requests Should be Directed to:
Ms. Pat Keller
Program Director
Arkansas Health Care Access Foundation
P.O. Box 56248
Little Rock, Arkansas 72215 (800) 950-8233
(501) 221-3033

**Products Covered by the Program**
All Pfizer products are covered.

**Eligibility**
Must be an Arkansas resident to qualify. Eligible individuals are certified by the Arkansas Local County Department of Human Services as being Arkansas residents below the federal poverty guidelines, who do not have health insurance benefits and do not qualify for any government entitlement programs. No co-payment or cost-sharing is required from the patient. Physician must waive his or her fee for the initial visit. This program does not apply to individuals during hospital inpatient stays.

**Other Program Information**
Physicians should contact the Arkansas Health Care Access Foundation for further information.

**Name of Program**
Kentucky Health Care Access Program

Physician Requests Should be Directed to:
Keith Knapp
Executive Vice President
Kentucky Health Care Access Foundation
12700 Shelbyville Road (800) 633-8100
Louisville, KY 40243 (502) 244-4214

**Products Covered by the Program**
All Pfizer products are covered.

**Eligibility**
Must be a Kentucky resident to qualify. Eligible individuals are certified by the Kentucky Cabinet for Human Resources as Kentuckians below the federal poverty guidelines, who do not have health insurance benefits and do not qualify for any government entitlement programs. No co-payment or cost-sharing is required from the patient. Physician must waive his or her fee for the initial visit. This program does not apply to individuals during hospital inpatient stays.

**Other Program Information**
Physicians should contact the Kentucky Health Care Access Foundation for further information.

**Name of Program**
Commun-I-Care

Physicians Requests Should be Directed to:
Ms. Parker Sparrow, Director
Commun-I-Care
P.O. Box 12054 (803) 779-4875
Columbia, SC 29211 (800) 763-0059

**Products Covered By the Program**
All Pfizer products are covered.

**Eligibility**
Eligible individuals must be South Carolina residents. Individuals are certified by Commun-I-Care as below the federal poverty line and not covered by any government entitlement programs. No copayment or cost-sharing is required from the patient. Physician must waive his or her fee.

**Other Program Information**
Physicians should contact Commun-I-Care for further information.

## PHARMACIA INC.

**Name of Program**
Pharmacia Patient Assistance Program by Mycobutin
P.O. Box 9525
McLean, VA 22102 (800) 795-9759

**Products Covered By the Program**
Mycobutin (rifabutin capsules)

**Other Program Information**
Requests for assistance are initiated by a patient or a patient's physician calling the toll-free number.

**Name of Program**
Pharmacia Patient Assistance Program
P.O. Box 9525
McLean, VA 22102 (800) 366-5570

**Products Covered by the Program**
Adriamycin PFS (doxorubicin hydrochloride injection, USP); Adrucil (fluorouracil injection, USP); Azulfadine (sulfasalazine tablets, USP); Azulfidine En-Tab (sulfasalazine USP enteric-coated tablets); Dipentum (olsalazine capsules); Emcyt (estramustine phosphate sodium tablets); Folex PFS (methotrexate sodium injection, USP); Idamycin (idarubicin hydrochloride for injection); Neosar (cyclophosphamide for injection, USP); Vincasar PFS (vincristine sulfate injection, USP)

**Other Product Information**
Requests for assistance are initiated by a patient or a patient's physician calling the toll-free number. Applications are mailed directly to the patient's physician. The patient must complete the financial section of the application. Product is shipped to physician only.

## PROCTOR & GAMBLE PHARMACEUTICALS, INC.

Proctor & Gamble Pharmaceuticals, Inc.
17 Eaton Avenue
Norwich, NY 13815
Attn: Customer Service Department (800) 448-4878

**Products Covered by the Program**
Asacol, Dantrium Capsules, Didronel, Entex, Macrodantin, Macrobid

**Other Product Information**
The quantity of product supplied depends on diagnosis and need, but generally one month's supply is provided for a chronic medication. Refills require a new prescription and application from the physician. The prescription medication is sent directly to the physician, who provides it to the patient.

## REED AND CARNRICK/BLOCK DRUG COMPANY

Conrad Erdt
Customer Service Associate
Reed and Carnrick Pharmaceutical Company
One New England Ave. (908) 981-0070
Piscataway, NJ 08854 Fax: (908) 981-1391

## RHONE-POULENC RORER INC.

Rhone-Poulenc Rorer Indigent Access Program
Barbara Cappuccio
Medical Affairs
Rhone-Poulenc Rorer Inc.
500 Arcola Road
Collegeville, PA 19426 (610) 454-8298

**Products Covered by the Program**
All products are eligible, with some limitations on supply.

**Eligibility**
Program is administered on a case-by-case basis and generally honors all applications for assistance. The physician is requested to send in a valid prescription along with some information confirming the patient's indigent status and ineligibility for any other form of outpatient pharmaceutical insurance coverage.

## ROCHE LABORATORIES

A Division of Hoffman-La Roche Inc.

Roche Medical Needs Programs
Daria Osborne
Supervisor, Product Communications
Roche Laboratories
340 Kingsland St.
Nutley, NJ 07110 (800) 285-4484

**Products Covered by Program**
Total product line.

**Eligibility**
Physicians make the determination. Those eligible are private practice outpatients who are considered to be medically indigent and who are not eligible to receive Roche drugs through another third-party drug reimbursement program.

**Other Program Information**
Roche Medical Needs Program forms are required and can be obtained from the Professional Services Department. Physician's signature and DEA number are required on application. Repeat requests require additional applications.

## ROXANE LABORATORIES, INC

Patient Assistance Program
1101 King St., Suite 600
Alexandria, VA 22314 (800) 274-8651

**Products Covered by the Program**
Marinol (dronabinol) Capsules 2.5 mg in the Prescription Pre-Pac bottle of 60's only; Oramorph SR (morphine sulfate sustained release) Tablets 30 mg, 60 mg, and 100 mg; Roxanol (morphine sulfate concentrated oral solution) 20 mg/mL and 120 mL bottles;

Roxanol 100 (morphine sulfate concentrated oral solution) 100 mg/5mL and 240 mL bottles.

**Eligibility**
Product will be provided free of charge to patients through their physician or pharmacist, provided the patient is uninsured and the patients' total annual income does not exceed $25,000 without dependents, or is less than $40,000 with dependents.

**Other Program Information**
Physicians should call the toll-free number to discuss their patient's eligibility with a program representative.

## SANDOZ PHARMACEUTICALS CORPORATION

Sandoz/NORD Drug Cost Share Program
National Organization for Rare Disorders
Sandoz/NORD DCSP
P.O. Box 8923
New Fairfield, CT 06812 (800) 447-6673

**Products Covered by the Program**
Clozaril (clozapine); DynaCirc (isradapine); Eldepryl (selegiline hydrochloride); Lescol (fluvastatin) Sandimmune (cyclosporine); Sandostatin (octreotide acetate); Parlodel (bromocriptine mesylate).

**Eligibility**
Financial need based on information provided by applicant and assessed by Community Advisory Board.

## SANOFI WINTHROP PHARMACEUTICALS

Sanofi Winthrop Pharmaceuticals
Needy Patient Program
c/o Product Information Department
90 Park Avenue
New York, NY 10016 (800) 446-6267

(212) 907-2000
or Your Local Representative

**Products Covered by the Program**
Aralen; Breonesin; Bronkometer; Danocrine; Drisdol; Hytakerol; Isuprel; Mytelase: NegGram: PhisoHex; Primaquine; Plaquenil; Trancopal

## SCHERING LABORATORIES/KEY PHARMACEUTICALS

**Name of Program**
Commitment to Care

Physician Requests Should be Directed to:
For Intron A/Eulexin (800) 521-7157

**For Other Products**
Schering Laboratories/Key Pharmaceuticals
Patient Assistance Program
P.O. Box 52122
Phoenix, AZ 85072 (800) 656-9485

**Products Covered by the Program**
All products.

**Eligibility**
Patient eligibility is determined on a case-by-case basis based upon economic and insurance criteria. The company does not require indigent patients to participate in copayments or costsharing. Eligibility criteria are currently being evaluated and may be subject to change.

**Other Program Information**
Physician and patient complete an application form. Application is reviewed on a case-by-case basis. Repeat requests require a new application form to be completed.

## SEARLE

Patients in Need Foundation
Administrator
5200 Old Orchard Road
Skokie, IL 60077 (800) 542-2526
or Local Searle Sales Representative

**Products Covered by the Program**
*Antihypertensives:* Aldactazide (spironolactone with hydrochlorothiazide); Aldactone (spironolactone); Calan SR (verapamil HCl) sustained-release; Kerlone (betaxolol HCl) *Antihypertensive/Anti-Anginal/Antiarrhythmic:* Calan (verapamil HCl) *Antiarrhythmics:* Norpace (disopyramide phosphate); Norpace CR (disopyramide phosphate) extended-release *Prevention of NSAID-induced gastric ulcers:* Cytotec (misoprostol) *Quinolone Anti-infective:* Maxaquin (lomefloxacin)

**Eligibility**
The physician is the sole determinant of a patient's eligibility for the program based on medical and economic need. Searle provides guidelines for physicians to consider, but they are not requirements. Searle does not review documentation for eligibility.

**Other Program Information**
Patients in Need program certificates for free Searle medications are made available to physicians. The physician gives the patient the prescription for an appropriate Searle medication along with a certificate for the Patients in Need Program. The patient then takes the prescription and the certificate to the pharmacy of his/her choosing, and the pharmacist dispenses the prescription to the patient free of charge. The pharmacist submits the certificate to Searle and is reimbursed by Searle.

## SERONO LABORATORIES, INC.

Serono Laboratories' Helping Hand Program
Gina Cella
Director, Corporate Communications
Serono Laboratories, Inc.
100 Longwater Circle
Norwell, MA 02061 (617) 982-9000

**Products Covered by the Program**
Metrodin (follicle stimulating hormone; urofollitropin for injection, USP)

**Eligibility**
Patient is not covered for outpatient prescription drugs under private insurance or a public program. Patient may or may not be poor, but retail drug purchase would cause hardship. Eligibility is determined by the physician based on company guidelines. No documentation is required.

**Other Product Information**
Referral must be made by the physician.

## SIGMA-TAU PHARMACEUTICALS

Michael McCourt
Carnitor Drug Assistance Program Administrator
National Organization for Rare Diseases (800) 999-6673
P.O. Box 8923 (203) 746-6518
New Fairfield, CT 06812-1783 Fax: (203) 746-6481

## SMITHKLINE BEECHAM PHARMACEUTICALS

**Name of Program**
SB Access to Care Program
SmithKline Beecham Pharmaceuticals
One Franklin Plaza-FP1320(215) 751-5722 (Physician Requests)
Philadelphia, PA 19101 (800) 546-0420 (Patient Requests)

**Products Covered by the Program**
Amoxil (amoxicillin), Augmentin (amoxicillin/clavulanate potassium), Bactroban (mupirocin), Compazine (prochloroperazine), Dyazide (hydrochlorothiazide/trimterene), Famvir (famciclovir), Relafen (nabumetone), Ridaura (auranofin), Tagamet (cimetidine), and most other SmithKline Beecham prescription products.

**Eligibility**
Patient may not be covered for prescription drugs under private insurance or public program. Eligibility is determined by the company based on information provided by the physician.

**Other Program Information**
Individual physicians determine which patients are eligible and would benefit most from the program. Physicians are required to submit forms to enroll patients in the program. A three-month supply is available at any one time. Reapplications are required. The requested product will be sent to the local SB pharmaceutical consultant for delivery to the requesting physician.

**Name of Program**
Paxil Access to Care Program

Physicians can enroll eligible patients in a certificate program by calling (800) 729-4544

**Name of Program**
Emanise/Kytril/Triostat Compassionate Care Programs
SmithKline Beecham Pharmaceuticals
One Franklin Plaza-FP1320
Philadelphia, PA 19101 (800) 866-6273

**Products Covered by the Program**
Eminase (anistreplase); Kytril (granisetron); Triostat (liothyronine sodium injection)

**Other Program Information**
For each eligible patient, hospitals should submit a Hospital Consent Form and an Application Form with any one of the following documents: a copy of the patient's medical record, a pharmacy record, or the patient's bill. Eminase, Kytril or Triostat replacement vials will be shipped directly to the supplying hospital within 30 days after the application has been approved.

## SOLVAY PHARMACEUTICALS, INC.

Patient Assistance Program
Solvay Pharmaceuticals, Inc.
901 Sawyer Road
Marietta, GA 30062

**Eligibility**
Eligibility is determined on a case-by-case basis in consultation with each prescribing physician and is based on a patient's inability to pay, lack of insurance, and ineligibility for Medicaid. Patient must be a resident of the U.S.

**Other Product Information**
Physicians apply on behalf of the patient by submitting a written request on a request form. Blank request forms can be obtained by writing to Solvay Pharmaceuticals, Inc. or by calling the Patient Assistance Program Message Center at (800) 788-9277.

## SYNTEX LABORATORIES

**Name of Program**
Syntex Patient Assistance Program Hotline (800) 822-8255
in Washington, DC (202) 508-6568
Hours: 9 a.m. to 5 p.m. EST, Monday through Friday

**Products Covered by the Program**
All Syntex products other than Cytovene (ganciclovir sodium)

are included in this program. Cytovene is included in the Syntex Provisional Assistance Program for Cytovene.

**Eligibility**
To be eligible, the patient must be medically indigent; and ineligible for any form of third-party outpatient during reimbursement. Medicare patients lacking supplemental insurance covering outpatient prescription drugs are eligible for the program, provided they are medically indigent.

**Other Program Information**
Eligible patients may receive up to a three-month supply of Syntex products. The product may be sent directly to the physician's office or to a pharmacy of the patient's choice.

**Name of Program**
Syntex Provisional Assistance Program for Cytovene

Physician Requests Should be Directed to:
Cytovene Medical Information line (800) 444-4200
Hours: 9 a.m. to 5 p.m. EST, Monday through Friday.

**Products Covered by the Program**
Cytovene 500 mg sterile powder (ganciclovir sodium) 10mL vial (intravenous form)

**Eligibility**
Syntex Laboratories, Inc. will provide cytovene free of charge when it is prescribed for an immunocompromised patient who has been diagnosed as having cytomegalovirus (CMV) retinitis, or when prescribed for prevention of CMV infection in a transplant patient, if that patient does not have the means to purchase the drug and that patient is not eligible for any form of third-party reimbursement to otherwise pay for the drug.

**Other Product Information**
The treating physician should contact the Cytovene Medical Information Line to prequalify a patient who falls under the eligibility guidelines described above. Syntex will then drop ship 25 vials of Cytovene directly to the physician, along with completion forms.

## 3M PHARMACEUTICALS

Indigent Patient Pharmaceutical Program
Medical Services Department
275-3W-01, 3M Center
P.O. Box 33275
St. Paul, MN 55133-3275 (800) 328-0255

**Products Covered by the Program**
Most drug products sold by 3M Pharmaceuticals in the U.S.

**Eligibility**
Patients whose financial and insurance circumstances prevent them from obtaining 3M Pharmaceuticals drug products considered to be necessary by their physician. Consideration is on a case-by-case basis.

## THE UPJOHN COMPANY

Upjohn Patient Assistance Program (800) 242-7014

**Products Covered by the Program**
Call (800) 242-7014 for a listing of eligible products covered under the Upjohn Patient Assistance Program.

**Eligibility**
Program provides up to a maximum of 120 consecutive days of selected Upjohn medication assistance to eligible patients who have special needs due to short-term financial hardship. The patient must be a resident of the U.S. or its territories. All alternative funding sources must be investigated.

**Other Program Information**
The healthcare provider calls the Upjohn Patient Assistance Program to discuss initial patient eligibility. The caller, if not a physician, must have the attending physician's DEA information. The patient provides the necessary information to the physician and/or the Upjohn Patient Assistance Program claims processor to initiate the enrollment process. The patient will be required to pay a $4 co-pay each time a prescription is filled at the pharmacy.

## WYETH-AYERST LABORATORIES

**Name of Program**
Norplant Foundation
P.O. Box 25223
Alexandria, VA 22314 (703) 706-5933

**Products Covered by the Program**
The Norplant (levonorgestrel implants) five-year contraceptive system.

**Eligibility**
Determined on a case-by-case basis and limited to individuals who cannot afford the product and who are ineligible for coverage under private and public sector programs.

**Name of Program**
Wyeth-Ayers Laboratories Indigent Patient Program
John E. James
Professional Services IPP
555 E. Lancaster Avenue
St. Davids, PA 19087 (800) 568-9938

**Products Covered by the Program**
Various products (not including schedule II, III, or IV products)

**Eligibility**
Limited to individuals, on a case-by-case basis, who have been identified by their physicians as "indigent."

## ZENECA PHARMACEUTICALS

Zeneca Pharmaceuticals Foundation
Patient Assistance Program
Yvonne A. Graham
Program Director
P.O. Box 15197
Wilmington, DE 19850-5197 (800) 424-3727

**Products Covered by the Program**
Nolvadex (tamoxifen citrate); Sorbitrate (isorbide dinitrate); Tenoretic (atenolol/chlorthiazide); Tenormin (atenolol); Zestril (lisinopril); Zestoretic (lisinopril/hydrochlorthiazide); Zoladex (goserelin acetate implant)

**Eligibility**
Determination is made by the company based on income level/assets and absence of outpatient private insurance or participation in a public program. There is an allowance for short-term compassionate supplies in the case of unique financial circumstances.

**Other Program Information**
Specific forms are obtained from the sales rep or from Zeneca Pharmaceuticals Foundation. Automatic refills of a one- to three-month supply are made for up to one year. After that time, reapplication is required every 12 months.

# Discount Drug Programs

Help can be just a phone call away. Ten states have special drug programs that give huge discounts to seniors who are ineligible for Medicaid and who don't have private insurance. For example, seniors in New Jersey can get their prescriptions for only $5, and in Maine they can get them for as little as $2.

Often all it takes is a phone call and filling out a simple form. You will have to meet income eligibility, but you can make upwards of $23,000 a year and still be eligible in New York, for example. If your state is not listed below, contact your state Department of Aging, but also check out the free drug programs sponsored by the drug manufacturers themselves. You will find a detailed description of this program on page 188.

## Connecticut

Conn PACE
P.O. Box 5011
Hartford, CT 06102 800-423-5026

**Eligibility Requirements**
- You must be 65 years old or older.
- You must have lived in Connecticut for six months.
- Your income cannot exceed $13,800 if you are single, and $16,600 if you are married.
- You may not have an insurance plan that pays for all or a portion of each prescription, a deductible insurance plan that includes prescriptions, or Medicaid.

**Cost**
- You pay a $15 one time registration fee.
- You pay $12 for each prescription.
- You must get generic drugs whenever possible, unless you are willing to pay the difference in price.

## Delaware

Nemours Health Clinic
915 N. Dupont Blvd.
Milford, DE 19963 — 302-424-5420
800-763-9326

**Eligibility Requirements**

- You must be a Delaware resident.
- You must be U.S. citizen.
- You must be 65 or older.
- Income requirements for single $11,300; for married $15,500.

**Cost**

- You must pay 20% of the prescription drug cost.

## Illinois

Pharmaceutical Assistance Program
Illinois Department of Revenue
P.O. Box 19021
Springfield, IL 62794 — 800-624-2459

**Eligibility Requirements**

- You must be 65 years of age or older, or over 16 and totally disabled, or a widow or widower who turned 63 before spouse's death.
- You must be a resident of Illinois.
- Your income must be less than $14,000.
- You must file a Circuit Breaker claim form.

**Cost**

- Pharmaceutical Assistance card will cost either $40 or $80, depending upon your income.
- Your monthly deductible will be $15 if the cost of your card is $40, and $25 if the cost of your card is $80.

- You must choose the generic brand when available, unless you are willing to pay the difference in price.

## Maine

Elderly Low-Cost Drug Program
Bureau of Taxation
State Office Building
Augusta, ME 04333
800-773-7895
207-626-8475

**Eligibility requirements**

- You must be a Maine resident.
- You may not be receiving SSI payments.
- You must be at least 62 years old or part of a household where one person is 62 years old.
- Your income may not exceed $9,700 if you live alone; $12,1 00 if you are married or have dependents.

**Cost**

- Each drug will cost $2 or 20% of the price allowed by the Department of Human Services, whichever is greater.

## Maryland

Maryland Pharmacy Assistance Program
P.O. Box 386
Baltimore, MD 21203-0386
410-225-5397
800-492-1974

**Eligibility**

- For anyone in the state who cannot afford their medications. Income requirements vary, so it is best to call.

## New Jersey

Pharmaceutical Assistance to the Aged and Disabled (PAAD)
Special Benefit Programs
CN 715
Trenton, NJ 08625
800-792-9745
609-588-7049

**Eligibility**

- You must be a New Jersey resident.
- Your income must be less than $16,171 if you are single, or less than $19,828 if you are married.
- You must be at least 65 years of age.
- Drugs purchased outside the state of New Jersey are not covered, nor any pharmaceutical product whose manufacturer has not agreed to provide rebates to the state of New Jersey.

**Cost**

- You pay $5 for each covered prescription. PAAD collects payments made on your behalf from any other assistance program, insurance, or retirement benefits which may cover prescription drugs.

## New York

Elderly Pharmaceutical Insurance Coverage EPIC
P.O. Box 15018
Albany, NY 12212
800-332-3742
518-452-6828

**Eligibility Requirements**

- You must be 65 or older.
- You must reside in New York State.
- Your income must not exceed $17,500 if you are single; or $23,000 if you are married.
- You are not eligible if you receive Medicaid benefits.

**Cost**

- You pay between $3-$23 per prescription depending upon the prescription cost.
- There are two plans for EPIC. You can pay an annual fee depending upon your income to qualify right away. The annual fee ranges from $20 to over $75, which can be paid in installments. The EPIC Deductible plan is that you pay no fee, but you pay full price for your prescriptions until you spend the deductible amount. The deductible amount also varies by income and starts at $468.

## Pennsylvania

PACE Card
(Pennsylvania Pharmaceutical Assistance Contract For The Elderly)
Pennsylvania Department of Aging
P.O. Box 8806
Harrisburg, PA 17105 717-783-1550
800-225-7223

**Eligibility Requirements**

- You must be 65 or older.
- Your income cannot exceed $13,000 if you are single; $16,200 for married couples.
- You must also live in the state for at least 90 days.

**Cost**

- You pay a $6.00 co-payment for each prescription. You may not purchase drugs out of state.
- PACE limits drug amounts to no more than a 30-day supply or 100 pills. There are no vacation supplies allowed.

## Rhode Island

Rhode Island Pharmaceutical Assistance to the Elderly (RIPAE)
Rhode Island Department of Elderly Affairs

160 Pine St.
Providence, RI 02903 401-277-3330

**Eligibility Requirements**

- You must be a Rhode Island resident.
- You must be 65 years old.
- Your income must not exceed $13,860 if you are single; $17,326 if you are married.
- You can not have any other prescription drug coverage.

**Cost**

- Members pay 40% of the cost of prescription drugs used to treat certain illnesses.

## Vermont

VScript Program
Department of Social Welfare
Medicaid Division
103 South Main St.
Waterbury, VT 05676 802-241-2880
800-827-0589

**Eligibility Requirements**

- You must be a resident of Vermont.
- You must be at least 65.
- You may not have income in excess of 175% of the federal poverty guidelines.
- You may not be in a health insurance plan that pays for all or a portion of the applicant's prescription drugs.

**Cost**

- There will be a co-payment requirement. The amount will be a percentage of the charge for a drug, with the percentage amount determined at the beginning of each fiscal year.

# Free Health Care Publications And Videos

# Your Own Medical Library

All it takes is a phone call to get connected to thousands of free publications, journal articles, and research reports on every health topic imaginable. You can learn about the latest gall bladder surgery, ulcer treatment, or cholesterol advice. We have provided you with over 150 of the top, most requested publications, but remember the possibilities are endless. Want to know about the latest type of angioplasty? The National Heart, Lung, and Blood Institute will send you publications looking at the different types of treatments, to help you decide what is best for you. Is your doctor suggesting an operation for your prostate cancer, but you are not sure what to do? The National Cancer Institute can provide you with publications dealing with this type of cancer. If you don't see what you need from the list below, check in the A-Z section of the book, and contact the office listed under your condition. They can send you publications, and possibly even conduct a literature search to see what other information is out there for you.

**Aging**

National Institute on Aging
P.O. Box 8057
Gaithersburg, MD 20898 800-222-2225

*Who? What? Where? Resources for Women's Health & Aging*
*What's Your Aging IQ?*
*In Search of the Secrets of Aging*

**AIDS**

National AIDS Hotline
Centers for Disease Control
P.O. Box 6003
Rockville, MD 20850 800-342-AIDS

*Understanding AIDS*
*HIV Infection and AIDS: Are You At Risk?*
*AIDS and You*
*Caring For Someone with AIDS*

**Alcoholism**

National Clearinghouse for Alcohol and Drug Information
P.O. Box 2345
Rockville, MD 20847 800-729-6686
*If Someone Close Has A Problem With Alcohol or Other Drugs*
*Parent Training Is Prevention*
*Alcoholism Tends To Run In Families*
*Helping Your Child Say "No" A Parent's Guide*

**Allergies**

National Institute of Allergy and Infectious Diseases
Office of Communications
Building 31, Room 7A50
Bethesda, MD 20892 301-496-5717

*Allergic Diseases: Medicine for the Layman*
*Something in the Air: Airborne Allergens*
*Drug Allergy*

**Alzheimer's Disease**

Alzheimer's Disease Education and Referral Center
P.O. Box 8250
Silver Spring, MD 20907 800-438-4380

*Age Page: Confusion and Memory Loss in Old Age*
*Alzheimer's Disease: Q&A*
*General Information on Alzheimer's Disease*
*Alzheimer's Disease: A Guide To Federal Programs*

**Anorexia**

National Institute of Child Health and Human Development
Bldg. 31, Room 2A32
Bethesda, MD 20892 301-496-5133

*Facts About Anorexia Nervosa*

**Anxiety Attacks**

National Institute of Mental Health
5600 Fishers Lane, Room 7C02
Rockville, MD 20857 301-443-4513

*Panic Disorder*
*Understanding Panic Disorder*

**Arthritis**

National Arthritis and Musculoskeletal and Skin Diseases Information Clearinghouse
1 AMS Way
Bethesda, MD 20892 301-495-4484

*Medicine for the Layman: Arthritis*
*Arthritis, Rheumatic Diseases, and Related Disorders*

**Asthma**

National Asthma Education and Prevention Program
National Heart, Lung, and Blood Institute Information Center
P.O. Box 30105
Bethesda, MD 20824 301-251-1222

*Check Your Asthma I.Q.*
*Facts About Asthma*
*Your Asthma Can Be Controlled: Expect Nothing Less*

**Attention Deficit Disorder**

National Institute of Neurological Disorders and Stroke
P.O. Box 5801
Bethesda, MD 20824 800-352-9424

*Attention Deficit Disorder Information Packet*

**Bell's Palsy**

National Institute of Neurological Disorders and Stroke
P.O. Box 5801
Bethesda, MD 20824 800-352-9424

*Bell's Palsy Information Packet*

**Breast Cancer**

National Cancer Institute
Bldg. 31, Room 10A24
Bethesda, MD 20892 800-4-CANCER

*Breast Cancer: What You Should Know*
*Breast Cancer: Understanding Treatment*
*Questions and Answers about Breast Cancer and Mammography*
*Breast Cancer and Mammography: Facts At A Glance*

**Cancer**

National Cancer Institute
Bldg. 31, Room 10A24
Bethesda, MD 20892 800-4-CANCER

*What You Need To Know About Cancer*
*Good News, Better News, Best News: Cancer Prevention*
*Facing Forward: A Guide For Cancer Survivors*
*What Are Clinical Trials All About*
*Chemotherapy and You: A Guide to Self Help During Treatment*

**Carpal Tunnel Syndrome**

National Institute for Occupational Safety and Health
4676 Columbia Parkway
Cincinnati, OH 45226 800-356-4674

*Carpal Tunnel Syndrome*

**Cataracts**

National Eye Institute
Bldg. 31, Room 6A32
Bethesda, MD 20892 301-496-5248

*Don't Lose Sight of Cataracts*
*Cataracts*

**Cesareans**

National Institute of Child Health and Human Development
Building 31, Room 2A32
Bethesda, MD 20892 301-496-5133

*Facts About Cesarean Childbirth*

**Cerebral Palsy**

National Institute of Neurological Disorders and Stroke
P.O. Box 5801
Bethesda, MD 20824 800-352-9424

*Hope Through Research: Cerebral Palsy*

**Child Abuse**

Clearinghouse on Child Abuse and Neglect Information
P.O. Box 1182
Washington, DC 20013 800-FYI-3366

*Child Abuse and Neglects: A Shared Community Concern*
*Child Sexual Abuse Prevention: Tips to Parents*

## Child Health

National Maternal and Child Health Clearinghouse
8201 Greensboro Dr.
Suite 600
McLean, VA 22102 703-821-8955, ext. 254

*Infant Care*
*Nutrition Resources for Early Childhood - A Resource Guide*

## Cholesterol

National Cholesterol Education Program
National Heart, Lung, and Blood Institute
Information Center
P.O. Box 30105
Bethesda, MD 20824 301-251-1222

*So You Have High Blood Cholesterol*
*Step by Step: Eating to Lower Your High Blood Cholesterol*
*Facts About Blood Cholesterol*
*Recipes: A Low-Fat Diet*

## Chronic Fatigue Syndrome

National Institute of Allergy and Infectious Diseases
Bldg. 31, Room 7A50
Bethesda, MD 20892 301-496-5717

*Chronic Fatigue Syndrome Information Packet*

## Chronic Pain

National Institute of Neurological Disorders and Stroke
P.O. Box 5801
Bethesda, MD 20824 800-352-9424

*Hope Through Research: Chronic Pain*

**Contraception**

Office of Consumer Affairs
5600 Fishers Lane, HFE-88
Rockville, MD 20857 301-443-3170

*Comparing Contraceptives*
*The Pill*

**Deafness**

National Institute on Deafness and
Other Communication Disorders
P.O. Box 37777
Washington, DC 20013 800-241-1044

*Hearing Loss: Hope Through Research*
*Deafness, Hearing, and Hearing Disorders Organizational Resources*

**Dental Disease**

National Institute of Dental Research
Bldg. 31, Room 2C35
9000 Rockville Pike
Bethesda, MD 20892 301-496-4261

*Seal Out Dental Decay*
*What You Need To Know About Periodontal Disease*

**Depression**

National Institute of Mental Health
5600 Fishers Lane, Room 7C02
Rockville, MD 20857 301-443-4513

*Depressive Illnesses: Treatments Bring New Hope*
*Plain Talk About Depression*
*Bipolar Disorder: Manic-Depressive Illness*

## Diabetes

National Diabetes Information Clearinghouse
1 Information Way
Bethesda, MD 20892 301-654-3327

*Diabetes In Adults*
*Insulin Dependent Diabetes*
*Monitoring Your Blood Sugar*
*Pregnancy And Diabetes*

## Digestive Diseases

National Digestive Diseases Information Clearinghouse
2 Information Way
Bethesda, MD 20892 301-654-3810

*Facts and Fallacies About Digestive Diseases*
*Your Digestive System And How It Works*
*Constipation*
*Lactose Intolerance*

## Diverticulosis

National Digestive Diseases Information Clearinghouse
2 Information Way
Bethesda, MD 20892 301-654-3810

*Diverticulosis and Diverticulitis*
*Diverticular Disease*

## Dsylexia

National Institutes of Child Health and
Human Development
Building 31, Room 2A32
Bethesda, MD 20892 301-496-5133

*Facts About Dyslexia*

**Ear Infections**

Agency for Health Care Policy and Research
P.O. Box 8547
Silver Spring, MD 20907 800-358-9295

*Otitis Media with Effusion in Young Children*

**Eating Disorders**

National Institute of Mental Health
5600 Fishers Lane, Room 7C02
Rockville, MD 20857 301-443-451

*Eating Disorders*

**Endometriosis**

National Institutes of Child Health and Human Development
Building 31, Room 2A32
Bethesda, MD 20892 301-496-5133

*Facts About Endometriosis*

**Epilepsy**

National Institute of Neurological Disorders and Stroke
P.O. Box 5801
Bethesda, MD 20824 800-352-9424

*Hope Through Research: Epilepsy*

**Family Planning**

Office of Population Affairs Clearinghouse
P.O. Box 30686
Bethesda, MD 20824 301-654-6190

*Your Contraceptive Choices: For Now, For Later*
*Norplant*
*Many Teens Are Saying No*

**Food**

Office of Consumer Affairs
5600 Fishers Lane, HFE-88
Rockville, MD 20857 301-443-3170

*Dietary Guidelines For Americans*
*The New Food Label*

**Fitness**

President's Council on Physical Fitness and Sports
Suite 250 701 Pennsylvania Ave., NW
Washington, DC 20004 202-272-3421

*Walking for Exercise and Pleasure*
*Exercise and Weight Control*
*Fitness Fundamentals*

**Gall Stones**

National Digestive Diseases Information Clearinghouse
2 Information Way
Bethesda, MD 20892 301-654-3810

*Gall Stones Information Packet*

**Glaucoma**

National Eye Institute, Information Office
Building 31, Room 6A32
Bethesda, MD 20892 301-496-5248

*Don't Lose Sight of Glaucoma*

**Handicapped Children**

National Information Center for Handicapped
Children and Youth
P.O. Box 1492
Washington, DC 20013 800-999-5599

*Parents' Guide to Accessing Programs for Infants, Toddlers, Preschoolers with Handicaps*
*Parents' Guide to Accessing Parent Programs, Community Services, and Record Keeping*
*A Parent's Guide to Doctors, Disabilities, and the Family*

**Headaches**

National Institute of Neurological Disorders and Stroke
P.O. Box 5801
Bethesda, MD 20824 800-352-9424

*Hope Through Research: Headaches*

**Heart**

National Heart, Lung, and Blood Institute
Information Center, P.O. Box 30105
Bethesda, MD 20824 301-251-1222

*The Healthy Heart Handbook for Women*
*Check Your Health Heart IQ*
*Exercise And Your Heart: A Guide To Physical Activity*

**High Blood Pressure**

National High Blood Pressure Education Program
National Heart, Lung, and Blood Institute
Information Center, P.O. Box 30105
Bethesda, MD 20824 301-251-1222

*Eat Right To Help Lower Your High Blood Pressure*
*High Blood Pressure: Treat It For Life*
*Facts About How To Prevent High Blood Pressure*

**Hodgkin's Disease**

National Cancer Institute
Bldg. 31, Room 10A24
Bethesda, MD 20892 800-4-CANCER

*What You Need To Know About Hodgkin's Disease*

**Impotence**

National Kidney and Urologic Diseases
Information Clearinghouse
3 Information Way
Bethesda, MD 20892 — 301-654-4415

*Impotence: Information Packet*

**Incontinence**

National Kidney and Urologic Diseases
Information Clearinghouse
3 Information Way
Bethesda, MD 20892 — 301-654-4415

*Age Page: Urinary Incontinence*
*Urinary Tract Infections in Adults*

**Infant Care**

National Maternal and Child Health Clearinghouse
8201 Greensboro Dr., Suite 600
McLean, VA 22102 — 703-821-8955, ext. 254

*Health Diary: Myself-My Baby*

**Lead Poisoning**

Lead Poisoning Prevention Branch
National Center for Environmental Health and Injury Control
Centers for Disease Control
1600 Clifton Rd., NE
Atlanta, GA 30333 — 404-488-4880

*Preventing Lead Poisoning In Young Children*

**Learning Disabilities**

National Institute of Mental Health
5600 Fishers Lane, Room 7C02
Rockville, MD 20857 — 301-443-4513

*Learning Disabilities*

## Lung Cancer

National Cancer Institute
Bldg. 31, Room 10A24
Bethesda, MD 20892 — 800-4-CANCER

*Cancer of the Lung*
*What You Need To Know About Lung Cancer*

## Lupus

National Arthritis and Musculoskeletal and
Skin Diseases Clearinghouse
1 AMS Way
Bethesda, MD 20892 — 301-495-4484

*What Black Women Should Know About Lupus*
*Lupus Information Packet*

## Lyme Disease

National Institute of Allergy and Infectious Diseases
Office of Communications
Building 31, Room 7A50
Bethesda, MD 20892 — 301-496-5717

*Lyme Disease: The Facts, The Challenges*

## Mammograms

Agency for Health Care Policy and Research
P.O. Box 8547
Silver Spring, MD 20907 — 800-358-9295

*Things To Know About Quality Mammograms*

## Medicare

Medicare Hotline
Health Care Financing Administration
6325 Security Blvd
Baltimore, MD 21207 — 800-638-6833

*Guide to Health Insurance for People with Medicare*
*Medicare Highlights*
*Medicare Questions and Answers*

**Menopause**

National Institute on Aging Information Center
P.O. Box 8057
Gaithersburg, MD 20898 800-222-2225

*Menopause*

**Mental Illness**

National Institute of Mental Health
5600 Fishers Lane, Room 7C02
Rockville, MD 20857 301-443-4513

*A Consumer's Guide to Services*
*Plain Talk About the Stigma of Mental Illness*

**Multiple Sclerosis**

National Institute of Neurological Disorders and Stroke
P.O. Box 5801
Bethesda, MD 20824 800-352-9424

*Hope Through Research: Multiple Sclerosis*

**Muscular Dystrophy**

National Institute of Neurological Disorders and Stroke
P.O. Box 5801
Bethesda, MD 20824 800-352-9424

*Muscular Dystrophy Information Packet*

**Nursing Homes**

National Institute on Aging
Information Center
P.O. Box 8057
Gaithersburg, MD 20898 800-222-2225

*When You Need A Nursing Home*

## Obesity

Obesity Education Initiative
National Heart, Lung, and Blood Institute Information Center
P.O. Box 30105
Bethesda, MD 20824 301-251-1222

*Check Your Weight and Heart Disease IQ*

## Osteoporosis

National Arthritis and Musculoskeletal and Skin Diseases
Information Clearinghouse
1 AMS Way
Bethesda, MD 20892 301-495-4484

*Osteoporosis: Cause, Treatment, and Prevention*
*Medicine for the Layman: Osteoporosis*

## Paget's Disease

National Arthritis and Musculoskeletal and Skin Diseases
Information Clearinghouse
1 AMS Way
Bethesda, MD 20892 301-495-4484

*Understanding Paget's Disease*

## Parkinson's Disease

National Institute of Neurological Disorders and Stroke
P.O. Box 5801
Bethesda, MD 20824 800-352-9424

*Hope Through Research: Parkinson's Disease*

## Pregnancy

National Institute of Child Health and Human Development
Bldg. 31, Room 2A32
Bethesda, MD 20892 301-496-5133

*Pregnancy Basics*
*Understanding Gestational Diabetes*

**Prostate**

National Kidney and Urologic Diseases Information Clearinghouse
3 Information Way
Bethesda, MD 20892 — 301-654-4415

*Prostate Enlargement: Benign Prostatic Hyperplasia*
*Age Page: Prostate Problems*

**Rabies**

National Institute of Allergy and Infectious Diseases
Office of Communications
Building 31, Room 7A50
Bethesda, MD 20892 — 301-496-5717

*Rabies*

**Rehabilitation**

National Rehabilitation Information Center
Suite 935, 8455 Colesville Rd.
Silver Spring, MD 20910 — 800-227-0216

*Traumatic Brain Injury*
*Spinal Cord Injury*

**Schizophrenia**

National Institute of Mental Health
5600 Fishers Lane, Room 7C02
Rockville, MD 20857 — 301-443-4513

*Medications for the Treatment of Schizophrenia: Questions and Answers*
*New Developments in the Pharmacologic Treatment of Schizophrenia*

**Sexually Transmitted Diseases**

National Sexually Transmitted Diseases Hotline
P.O. Box 13827
Research Triangle Park, NC 27709 — 800-227-8922

*Some Questions and Answers About Sexually Transmitted Diseases*
*Some Questions and Answers About Chlamydia*
*Some Questions and Answers About Genital Warts*

**Sleep Disorders**

National Center on Sleep Disorders Research
National Heart, Lung, and Blood Institute Information Center
P.O. Box 30105
Bethesda, MD 20824 301-251-1222

*Breathing Disorders During Sleep*

**Smoking**

Office of Smoking and Health
Centers for Disease Control
Mail Stop K-50
4770 Buford Highway, NE
Atlanta, GA 30341 404-488-5705

*Clearing The Air*
*At A Glance- The Health Benefits of Smoking Cessation*
*Out of the Ashes*
*Chew Or Snuff Is Real Bad Stuff*

**Sterilization**

Office of Population Affairs Clearinghouse
P.O. Box 30686
Bethesda, MD 20824 301-654-6190

*Information for Men: Your Sterilization Operation*
*Information for Women: Your Sterilization Operation*

**Steroids**

National Clearinghouse for Alcohol and Drug Information
P.O. Box 2345
Rockville, MD 20847 800-729-6686

*Anabolic Steroids: A Threat to Body and Mind*

**Stress**

National Institute of Mental Health
5600 Fishers Lane, Room 7C02
Rockville, MD 20857 301-443-4513

*Plain Talk About Handling Stress*

**Stroke**

National Institute of Neurological Disorders and Stroke
P.O. Box 5801
Bethesda, MD 20824 800-352-9424

*Hope Through Research: Stroke*

**Sudden Infant Death Syndrome**

National Sudden Infant Death Syndrome Clearinghouse
8201 Greensboro Dr., Suite 600
McLean, VA 22102 703-821-8955

*SIDS Trying To Understand The Mystery*
*What Is SIDS?*
*After Sudden Infant Death: Handling Anniversaries, Birthdays, And Other Special Occasions*

**Tanning**

Office of Consumer Affairs
5600 Fishers Lane, HFE-88
Rockville, MD 20857 301-443-3170

*The Darker Side of Indoor Tanning*

**Tourette Syndrome**

National Institute of Neurological Disorders and Stroke
P.O. Box 5801
Bethesda, MD 20824 800-352-9424

*Fact Sheet: Tourette Syndrome*

**Ulcers**

National Digestive Diseases Information Clearinghouse
2 Information Way
Bethesda, MD 20892 301-654-3810

*Stomach Ulcers*
*Ulcers: Information Packet*

# Videos And Films

Please note that the organizations under *Free Information and Expertise from A-Z* also provide free videos and films. This section represents additional listings for major sources of audio visual materials for most any health care topic.

The U.S. Government's National Library of Medicine contains approximately 22,000 audiovisuals in a variety of formats including videocassettes, audio-cassettes, 16mm Films, filmstrips, slides, videodiscs and computer software. The best way to identify specific titles is to access a database called AVLINE which is available on the MEDLARS database system. Almost any local university library or hospital library can access this database for you. If you have trouble finding a local source for this database,

☎ Contact:
Reference Section
National Library of Medicine
8600 Rockville Pike
Bethesda, MD 20894
(800) 272-4787

## Borrowing Procedures

These audiovisuals are available to the public but only through interlibrary loans. This means that a library has to act as your middleman for obtaining your Video. The library that performs your AVLINE database search or even your local public library can perform the middleman service for you. The loan period is four weeks, including transit time, and no renewals are granted. The only fee involved is a $7 charge to the library for processing an interlibrary loan request. Your local public library may pass along this charge to you.

## Next On Oprah

You can get a video on any medical condition, problem or procedure you can imagine. Below is a sampling of the kinds of titles that are available. You can easily see that you are not likely to find these at your local video store (even in the back room section). But, after this book is printed, you may start seeing some of these videos on the daytime talk shows like Donahue, Oprah and Geraldo. The database shows that you can even get the following videos:

- *Male Transsexual Case #4 Before Surgery.*
  An interview between a psychiatrist and a transsexual patient shortly before surgery to remove the testicles and penis, a vagina constructed and silastic implantation in both breasts.

- *Male Transsexual Case #4 After Surgery.*
  An interview between a psychiatrist and a male transsexual who recently had the surgery mentioned above.

- *Mother of Male Transsexual.*
  Mother discusses her reaction to the surgery scheduled for the next day in which her son will have his testicles and penis removed and a vaginoplasty performed.

- *Easy To Get* and *Penicillin and Venereal Disease.*
  These two WWII era, U.S. Army training films portray stories of how military men pick up girls at drug stores and night clubs and have to suffer the consequences of venereal disease.

## Sampling Of Available Videos

**Chemotherapy**

*Radiation Therapy: Cancer And You*
*Recent Advances In Drug Therapy*
*Safety Issues In Handling Cancer Chemotherapy*
*General Principles Of Cancer Chemotherapy*
*Chemotherapy*
*Chemotherapy Side-Effects*
*Chemotherapy Administration: Current Methods*
*Cancer Treatment Issues*

**Cholesterol**

*Controlling Cholesterol: American Heart Association*
*Cholesterol, Diet And Heart Disease*

**Circumcision**

*Newborn Circumcision: Retracting Old Myths And Managing New Problems*
*Circumcision*

**Death**

*Dealing With Death And Dying*
*When The Time Comes*
*Hospice: The Special Touch*
*Facing Death*

**Headaches**

*Recurrent Headache*
*Pitfalls And Pointers In The Management Of Chronic Headaches*
*The Burdened Shoulder, Diagnosing Joint Pain*
*Medical Treatment Of Headache*
*Diagnosis & Treatment Of Headache*
*Headache (Mechanisms, Causes, Evaluation, and Treatment)*

## Holistic Health

*Holistic Health: Treating The Whole Person*
*Mind Over Medicine*
*Holistic Medicine In Primary Care*
*Dr. Deepak Chopra: Witnessing Spontaneous Cures To Seemingly Terminal Illnesses*
*Recovering The Soul: A Scientific And Spiritual Search*
*Stress And The Family: A Holistic Approach*
*Health, Mind And Behavior: In Space, Toward Peace*
*Well & Strong: A Story of Vera Henderson Who Cured Her Illness By Using A Holistic Medical Center Instead Of Surgery Recommended By Her Doctor*
*The Primary Prevention Of Coronary Heart Disease (A Holistic Approach To Managing The Condition)*
*Other Lives/Other Selves (The Therapeutic Power Of Past Life Regression)*
*Medicine Woman, Medicine Man: Traditional Holistic Medicine In Middle America*

## Infertility

*Laparoscopic Infertility Surgery*
*Six Phases Of Infertility Treatment: Medical And Emotional Aspects*
*Hazardous Inheritance: Workplace Dangers To Reproductive Health*
*Diagnostic Imaging In Fertility Disorders*
*Hi-Tech Babies*
*Infertility*
*In Search Of A Child*
*Investigation Of The Infertile Couple*
*Male Infertility*
*Medical Assistance In Procreation; Should Doctors Impose*
*Non-Medical Restrictions*

## Malpractice

*Ten Procedures For Avoiding Medical Malpractice*
*Malpractice*

*Understanding Emergency Room Medical Malpractice*
*Anatomy Of A Nursing Negligence Case*
*Analysis Of Dental Malpractice*
*Negligence: Legal Aspects Of Negligence*
*Psychological Impact of Malpractice On Physicians*
*The Malpractice Suit: A Survival Guide For Physicians And Their Families*
*Medical Risk Management: How To Reduce Your Chances Of Being Sued*
*Even The Good Guys Get Sued*
*Understanding Obstetric Malpractice*
*Help With Your Deposition*

**Masturbation**

*Child And Adolescent Behavior*
*Sexuality: Its Implications For Nursing Practice*

**Menopause**

*A Clinical Approach To Estrogen Replacement Therapy*

**Penile Implants**

*Impotency: Prosthetic Approach To Impotency*
*Implantation Of An Inflatable Penile Prosthesis In The Treatment Of Erectile Impotence*
*Implantation Of A Penile Prosthesis*
*Transscrotal Approach For Penile Prosthesis Insertion*
*Evaluation And Treatment Of Impotence With The Jonas Penile Prosthesis*
*Diagnosing Erectile Problems*

**Premenstrual Syndrome**

*Menstrual Cycle Related Mood Disorders*

**Prostate**

*Cancer Of The Prostate: An Overview Of Therapies*
*Screening For Carcinoma Of The Prostate*
*The Prostate: Ultrasound With MRI Confirmation*

*Ultrasonically Guided Prostate Biopsy*
*Anatomy And Pathology Of The Prostate*
*Cancer Screening (Complete Screening Examination For Skin, Lung, Breast, Cervical, Ovarian, Prostate, And Colorectal Cancers)*
*Hormonal Treatment For Prostate Cancer*
*Male Reproductive System*
*Male Genitalia, Rectum, And Hernias*

**Stress Management**

*Time And Stress Management*
*Less Stress In 5 Easy Steps* (With Ed Asner)
*Stress Ulcer Disease*
*Neck Pain: Etiology, Diagnosis, and Management*
*Occupational Disorders Of Musicians*
*Lifestyle Modification And Stress Management Objectives*
*Smokeless Tobacco*
*Stress-Related Disorders And Their Management Through Biofeedback And Relaxation Training*
*Managing Stress*
*Managing Job Related Stress*

**Vasectomy**

*Vasectomy (The Five Minute Vasectomy And The Mini Vasectomy)*
*Vasovasostomy: Vasectomy Reversal*
*Bob's Vasectomy*
*Pre-Vasectomy Family Consultation*
*Vasectomy Operating Procedure*
*Technique For Office Vasectomy*

# Free Medical Information And Expertise From A to Z

This chapter brings together the hundreds of different resources on health care throughout the government into one, easy-to-use format. Subjects are listed A to Z alphabetically under topic headings, followed by the best places to contact. If the topic you're interested in doesn't have a subject heading listed in this chapter, you can try one of the following options:

- Page through the topics and contact an office under a similar topic and ask if they know an office that will help. For example, if your child has red spots on the back of his neck, you won't find a listing under red spots but it may be helpful to contact the sources under Child Health or Skin Conditions.

- Contact the main information center at the National Institute of Health (NIH). They will be able to tell you who at NIH is studying your particular problem and provide you with a name and telephone number of the contact person.

Information Office
National Institute of Health
Bethesda, MD 20892
(301) 496-4000

- Contact the National Health Information Center. They can direct you to specialized clearinghouses, as well as health organizations and foundations on virtually any disease or health issue. Through its resource files and database (DIRLINE), they can respond to questions regarding health concerns and can send publications, bibliographies, and other materials. A library focusing on health topics is open to the public, and the Center also produces many different directories and resource guides, which are available for a minimal cost. A publications catalog is available free of charge. Two of the publications include a list of *Selected Federal Health Information Clearinghouses* and *Information Centers and Toll-Free Numbers for Health Information*.

National Health Information Center
P.O. Box 1133
Washington, DC 20013
(800) 336-4797
(301) 565-4167 (in MD)

## What to Expect When You Call

The sources listed in this chapter can provide you with all kinds of information on a topic. They have been established to help callers with their information requests usually provide all or some of the following:

**1) Free Expert Advice**
Many of the people working in these offices are very familiar with their subject areas and often they can provide you with answers you need by simply talking with you for a few minutes on the telephone.

**2) Free Books and Publications**
Most all these offices have free publications they can send to you which can give you more detailed information on the problem you are having.

**3) Database Searches**
These offices will often do custom searches of their computer data bases to find up-to-date articles that are written by the best experts in the world. They will send you these articles free of charge.

**4) Free Videos**
It is not uncommon for these offices to have free videos on your health problem which can be sent to you on a free loan basis. This means you can look at them for free but you have to send

them back. Just look under the appropriate topic in this chapter, contact the office and request information about the videos that are available on that topic. If you are really interested in videos you can look under the *Videos and Films* Section in the *Free Health Care Publications and Videos* Chapter.

**5) Referrals To Other Experts And Organizations**

One of the best uses of these offices is their ability to refer you to others who may be able to help. Like local self-help groups or hospitals in your neighborhood who are familiar with your problem. National organizations, associations or hospitals who offer free advice or help with your conditions. Or famous doctors who are getting grants to study your conditions for free.

The most important point you should remember in contacting these offices is that you may or may not get all the information you need by just contacting one source. Getting help and information in our information society is a game of numbers. The help you need is probably out there, and the more people you contact the more likely you are going to find it. It may take you one, five, ten or even fifteen telephone calls. But who cares if it takes you 20 or 30 minutes to find it. If you need help you should find it. Here's another important tip to remember. If the office you call from this book can't help you, be sure to ask them for a telephone number of someone else who possibly can.

# - A -

## ABETALIPOPROTEINEMIA

National Heart, Lung and Blood Institute
Information Center
P.O. Box 30105
Bethesda, MD 20824-0105 (301) 251-1222

## ABORTION

National Institute of Child Health and Human Development
Bldg. 31, Room 2A32
Bethesda, MD 20892 (301) 496-5133

## ABSTINENCE

Family Life Information Exchange
P.O. Box 30146
Bethesda, MD 20814 (301) 654-6190

## ACCIDENT PREVENTION

National Center for Injury Prevention and Control
Division of Unintentional Injury Prevention
Centers for Disease Control
4770 Buford Hwy., MS K-63
Atlanta, GA 30341-3725 (404) 488-4652

## ACETAMINOPHEN

Food & Drug Administration
(HFE-88), 5600 Fishers Lane
Rockville, MD 20857 (301) 443-3170

## ACHONDROPLASIA

National Institute of Child Health and Human Development
Bldg. 31, Room 2A32
Bethesda, MD 20892 (301) 496-5133

## ACIDOSIS

National Institute of Child Health and Human Development
Bldg. 31, Room 2A32
Bethesda, MD 20892 (301) 496-5133

## ACNE

National Institute of Arthritis and Musculoskeletal and Skin Diseases
1 AMS Way
Bethesda, MD 20892 (301) 495-4484

## ACOUSTIC NEUROMA

National Institute on Deafness and Other Communication Disorders
1 Communication Avenue (800) 241-1044
Bethesda, MD 20892-3456 (800) 241-1055 (TDD)

## ACQUIRED IMMUNE DEFICIENCY DISORDER

*See AIDS*

## ACROMEGALY

National Institute of Diabetes and Digestive and Kidney Diseases
Building 31, Room 9A04
Bethesda, MD 20892 (301) 496-3583

## ACTH

National Heart, Lung and Blood Institute
Information Center
P.O. Box 30105
Bethesda, MD 20824-0105 (301) 251-1222

## ACUPUNCTURE

National Institute of Neurological Disorders and Stroke
Bldg. 31, Room 8A16
Bethesda, MD 20892 (301) 496-5751
(800) 352-9424

## ACUTE HEMORRHAGIC CONJUNCTIVITIS

National Eye Institute
Bldg. 31, Room 6A32
Bethesda, MD 20892 (301) 496-5248

## ACUTE LEUKEMIA

National Cancer Institute
Bldg. 31, Room 10A16
Bethesda, MD 20892 (800) 4-CANCER

## ACUTE MYOCARDIAL INFARCTION

National Heart, Lung and Blood Institute
Information Center
P.O. Box 30105
Bethesda, MD 20824-0105 (301) 251-1222

## ADDISON'S DISEASE

The National Institute of Diabetes and Digestive and Kidney Diseases
Building 31, Room 9A04
Bethesda, MD 20892 (301) 496-3583

## ADENOMA OF THE THYROID

The National Institute of Diabetes and Digestive and Kidney Diseases
Bldg. 31, Room 9A04
Bethesda, MD 20892 (301) 496-3583

## ADOLESCENT DRUG ABUSE

National Clearinghouse for Alcohol and Drug Information
P.O. Box 2345
Rockville, MD 20852 (800) 729-6686

## ADOLESCENT HEALTH

*See also Acne; Puberty; Teenagers*

National Maternal and Child Health Clearinghouse
8201 Greensboro Drive, Suite 600
McLean, VA 22102-3810 (703) 821-8955, ext. 254

## ADOPTION

Family Life Information Exchange
P.O. Box 37299
Washington, DC 20013 (301) 585-6636

## ADRENAL GLAND DISORDERS

National Institute of Diabetes and Digestive
and Kidney Diseases
Building 31, Room 9A04
Bethesda, MD 20892 (301) 496-3583

## ADRENOLEUKODYSTROPHY

National Institute of Neurological Disorders and Stroke
Building 31, Room 8A16
Bethesda, MD 20892 (301) 496-5751
(800) 352-9424

## ADYNAMIA

National Institute of Neurological Disorders and Stroke
Building 31, Room 8A16
Bethesda, MD 20892 (301) 496-5751
(800) 352-9424

## AGAMMAGLOBULINEMIA

National Institute of Allergy and Infectious Diseases
Bldg. 31, Room 7A50
Bethesda, MD 20892 (301) 496-5717

## AGE-RELATED MACULAR DEGENERATION

The National Eye Institute
Bldg. 31, Room 6A32
Bethesda, MD 20892 (301) 496-5248

## AGENESIS

National Institute of Neurological Disorders and Stroke
Bldg. 31, Room 8A16
Bethesda, MD 20892 — (301) 496-5751
(800) 352-9424

## AGENT ORANGE

Your U.S. Senator's Office
U.S. Capitol
Washington, DC 20510 — (202) 224-3121

## AGING

*See also Gerontology; Living Wills; Long Term Care; Nursing Homes*

National Institute on Aging
Information Center
P.O. Box 8057
Gaithersburg, MD 20898-8057 — (800) 222-2225

## AGRANULOCYTOSIS

National Heart, Lung and Blood Institute
Information Center
P.O. Box 30105
Bethesda, MD 20824-0105 — (301) 251-1222

## AIDS

Office of AIDS Coordination
Office of the Commissioner
HF-12, 5600 Fishers Lane
Rockville, MD 20857 — (301) 443-0104

National AIDS Information Clearinghouse (800) 458-5231
(800) 342-AIDS
(800) 344-7432 (Servicio en Espanol)
(800) 243-7012 (TTY-Deaf Access)

AIDS Clinical Trials Information Services (800) 874-2572

## AIR POLLUTION

Public Information Center
Environmental Protection Agency
401 M Street, SW
Washington, DC 20460 (202) 260-7751

## ALBINISM

National Eye Institute
Bldg. 31, Room 6A32
Bethesda, MD 20892 (301) 496-5248

## ALBRIGHT'S SYNDROME

National Institute of Arthritis and Musculoskeletal and Skin Diseases
1 AMS Way
Bethesda, MD 20892 (301) 495-4484

## ALCOHOLISM

*See also Drug Abuse; Pregnancy and Alcohol; Workplace Drug Abuse*

National Clearinghouse for Alcohol and Drug Information
P.O. Box 2345
Rockville MD 20852 (301) 468-2600
(800) 729-6686

National Institute on Alcohol Abuse and Alcoholism
National Institutes of Health
6000 Executive Boulevard, Suite 409
Bethesda, MD 20892-7003 (301) 443-3860

## ALDOSTERONISM

National Heart, Lung and Blood Institute Information Center
P.O. Box 30105
Bethesda, MD 20824-0105 (301) 251-1222

## ALEXANDER'S SYNDROME

National Institute of Neurological Disorders and Stroke
Building 31, Room 8A16
Bethesda, MD 20892 (301) 496-5751
(800) 352-9424

## ALKAPTONURIA

National Heart, Lung and Blood Institute Information Center
P.O. Box 30105
Bethesda, MD 20824-0105 (301) 251-1222

## ALKYLATING AGENTS

National Cancer Institute
Building 31, Room 10A16
Bethesda, MD 20892 (800) 4-CANCER

## ALLERGENICS

Center for Biologics Evaluation and Research
Congressional Public Affairs Branch
Woodmont Office Center

Suite 200 North
1401 Rockville Pike
Rockville, MD 20852-1448 (301) 594-1800

## ALLERGIC RHINITIS

National Institute of Allergy and Infectious Diseases
Building 31, Room 7A50
Bethesda, MD 20892 (301) 496-5717

## ALLERGIES

National Institute of Allergy and Infectious Diseases
Building 31, Room 7A50
Bethesda, MD 20892 (301) 496-5717

## ALOPECIA

National Institute of Arthritis and Musculoskeletal and Skin Diseases
1 AMS Way
Bethesda, MD 20892 (301) 495-4484

## ALPERS SYNDROME

National Institute of Neurological Disorders and Stroke
Bldg. 31, Room 8A16
Bethesda, MD 20892 (301) 496-5751
(800) 352-9424

## ALPHA-1-ANTITRYPSIN DEFICIENCY

National Institute of Diabetes and Digestive and Kidney Diseases
Bldg. 31, Room 9A04
Bethesda, MD 20892 (301) 496-3583

## ALTERNATIVE MEDICINE PRACTICES

Office for the Study of Alternative Medicine
National Institutes of Health
Executive Plaza South, Suite 450
6120 Executive Boulevard
Rockville, MD 20892 (301) 402-2466

## ALVEOLAR BONE

National Institute of Dental Research
Building 31, Room 2C35
31 Center Drive, MSC-2290
Bethesda, MD 20892-2290 (301) 496-4261

## ALVEOLAR MICROLITHIASIS

National Heart, Lung and Blood Institute Information Center
P.O. Box 30105
Bethesda, MD 20824-0105 (301) 251-1222

## ALVEOLAR PROTEINOSIS

National Heart, Lung and Blood Institute
Information Center
P.O. Box 30105
Bethesda, MD 20824-0105 (301) 251-1222

## ALZHEIMER'S DISEASE

*See also Aging; Dementia; Presenile Dementia*

Alzheimer's Disease Education and Referral Center
P.O. Box 8250 (301) 495-3311
Silver Spring, MD 20907 (800) 438-4380

## AMAUROTIC IDIOCY

National Institute of Neurological Disorders and Stroke
Bldg. 31, Room 8A16
Bethesda, MD 20892 (301) 496-5751
(800) 352-9424

## AMBIGUOUS GENITALIA

National Institute of Child Health and
Human Development
Bldg. 31, Room 2A32
Bethesda, MD 20892 (301) 496-5133

## AMBLYOPIA

National Eye Institute
Building 31
Room 6A32
Bethesda, MD 20892 (301) 496-5248

## AMEBIASIS

National Institute of Allergy and Infectious Diseases
Building 31
Room 7A50
Bethesda, MD 20892 (301) 496-5717

## AMINO ACID DISORDERS

National Institute of Child Health and
Human Development
Bldg. 31, Room 2A32
Bethesda, MD 20892 (301) 496-5133

## AMNIOCENTESIS

*See also Pregnancy*

National Institute of Child Health and Human Development
Bldg. 31, Room 2A32
Bethesda, MD 20892 (301) 496-5133

## AMYLOID POLYNEUROPATHY

National Institute of Neurological Disorders and Stroke
Bldg. 31, Room 8A16
Bethesda, MD 20892 (301) 496-5751
(800) 352-9424

## AMYLOIDOSIS

National Institute of Arthritis and Musculoskeletal and Skin Diseases
1 AMS Way
Bethesda, MD 20892 (301) 495-4484

## AMYOTONIA CONGENITA

National Institute of Neurological Disorders and Stroke
Bldg. 31, Room 8A16
Bethesda, MD 20892 (301) 496-5751
(800) 352-9424

## AMYOTROPHIC LATERAL SCLEROSIS

National Institute of Diabetes and Digestive and Kidney Diseases
Bldg. 31, Room 9A04
Bethesda, MD 20892 (301) 496-3583

## ANALGESIC-ASSOCIATED NEPHROPATHY

National Institute of Diabetes and Digestive
and Kidney Diseases
Building 31, Room 9A04
Bethesda, MD 20892 (301) 496-3583

## ANAPHORESIS

National Arthritis and Musculoskeletal and Skin Diseases
Information Clearinghouse
1 AMS Way
Bethesda, MD 20892 (301) 495-4484

## ANAPLASIS

National Cancer Institute
Building 31, Room 10A16
Bethesda, MD 20892 (800) 4-CANCER

## ANEMIA

National Institute of Diabetes and Digestive
and Kidney Diseases
Bldg. 31, Room 9A04
Bethesda, MD 20892 (301) 496-3583

## ANENCEPHALY

National Institute of Neurological Disorders and Stroke
Bldg. 31, Room 8A16
Bethesda, MD 20892 (301) 496-5751
(800) 352-9424

## ANEURYSMS

National Heart, Lung and Blood Institute
Information Center
P.O. Box 30105
Bethesda, MD 20824-0105 (301) 251-1222

## ANGELMAN'S DISEASE

National Institute of Neurological Disorders and Stroke
Bldg. 31, Room 8A16
Bethesda, MD 20892 (301) 496-5751
(800) 352-9424

## ANGINA PECTORIS

National Heart, Lung and Blood Institute
Information Center
P.O. Box 30105
Bethesda, MD 20824-0105 (301) 251-1222

## ANGIOEDEMA

National Institute of Allergy and Infectious Diseases
Building 31, Room 7A50
Bethesda, MD 20892 (301) 496-5717

## ANGIOGRAPHY

National Heart, Lung and Blood Institute
Information Center
P.O. Box 30105
Bethesda, MD 20824-0105 (301) 251-1222

## ANGIOPLASTY

National Heart, Lung and Blood Institute
Information Center
P.O. Box 30105
Bethesda, MD 20824-0105 (301) 251-1222

## ANILINE DYES

National Cancer Institute
Building 31
Room 10A16
Bethesda, MD 20892 (800) 4-CANCER

## ANIMAL RESEARCH

National Institute of Mental Health
Information Resources and Inquiries
Room 7C-02
Rockville, MD 20857 (301) 443-4515

## ANIRIDIA

National Eye Institute
Building 31
Room 6A32
Bethesda, MD 20892 (301) 496-5248

## ANKLOGLASSIA

*See Tongue-Tied*

## ANKYLOSIS SPONDYLITIS

National Institute of Arthritis and Musculoskeletal and Skin Diseases
1 AMS Way
Bethesda, MD 20892 (301) 495-4484

## ANOREXIA

*See also Eating Disorders*

National Institute of Diabetes and Digestive and Kidney Diseases
National Institutes of Health
Bldg. 31, Room 9A04
Bethesda, MD 20892 (301) 496-3583

## ANOSMIA

National Institute of Neurological Disorders and Stroke
Bldg. 31, Room 8A16
Bethesda, MD 20892 (301) 496-5751
(800) 352-9424

## ANOXIA

National Heart, Lung and Blood Institute
Information Center
P.O. Box 30105
Bethesda, MD 20824-0105 (301) 251-1222

## ANTENATAL DIAGNOSIS

National Institute of Child Health and Human Development
Building 31, Room 2A32
Bethesda, MD 20892 (301) 496-5133

## ANTHRAX

National Institute of Allergy and Infectious Diseases
Bldg. 31, Room 7A50
Bethesda, MD 20892 (301) 496-5717

## ANTIALPHATRYPSIN

National Institute of Diabetes and Digestive and Kidney Diseases
Bldg. 31, Room 9A04
Bethesda, MD 20892 (301) 496-3583

## ANTIBIOTICS

National Institute of Allergy and Infectious Diseases
Bldg. 31, Room 7A50
Bethesda, MD 20892 (301) 496-5717

## ANTI-CANCER DRUGS

*See also Cancer*

National Cancer Institute
Bldg. 31, Room 10A16
Bethesda, MD 20892 (800) 4-CANCER

## ANTICOAGULANTS

National Heart, Lung and Blood Institute
Information Center
P.O. Box 30105
Bethesda, MD 20824-0105 (301) 251-1222

## ANTIDIURETIC HORMONE

National Institute of Diabetes and Digestive and Kidney Diseases
Bldg. 31, Room 9A04
Bethesda, MD 20892 (301) 496-3583

## ANTIHISTAMINES

Food & Drug Administration
5600 Fishers Lane (HFE-88)
Rockville, MD 20857 (301) 443-3170

## ANTIMETABOLITES

National Cancer Institute
Bldg. 31, Room 10A16
Bethesda, MD 20892 (800) 4-CANCER

## ANTI-INFLAMMATORY DRUGS

Food & Drug Administration
(HFE-88), 5600 Fishers Lane
Rockville, MD 20857 (301) 443-3170

## ANTINEOPLASTIC

National Cancer Institute
Bldg. 31, Room 10A16
Bethesda, MD 20892 (800) 4-CANCER

## ANTISOCIAL BEHAVIOR

National Institute of Mental Health
5600 Fishers Lane

Room 7C-02
Rockville, MD 20857 (301) 443-4515

## ANTIVIRAL SUBSTANCES

National Institute of Allergy and Infectious Diseases
Building 31, Room 7A50
Bethesda, MD 20892 (301) 496-5717

## ANXIETY ATTACKS

National Institute of Mental Health
5600 Fishers Lane, Room 7C-02
Rockville, MD 20857 (301) 443-4515

## AORTIC INSUFFICIENCY/STENOSIS

National Heart, Lung and Blood Institute
Information Center
P.O. Box 30105
Bethesda, MD 20824-0105 (301) 251-1222

## AORTITIS

National Heart, Lung and Blood Institute
Information Center
P.O. Box 30105
Bethesda, MD 20824-0105 (301) 251-1222

## APHAKIA

National Eye Institute
Bldg. 31, Room 6A32
Bethesda, MD 20892 (301) 496-5248

## APHASIA

National Institute on Deafness and Other Communication Disorders
1 Communication Avenue
Bethesda, MD 20892-3456
(301) 496-7243
(800) 241-1044
(800) 241-1055 (TDD)

## APHTHOUS STOMATITIS

National Institute of Dental Research
Bldg. 31, Room 2C35
31 Center Drive, MSC-2290
Bethesda, MD 20892-2290
(301) 496-4261

## APLASTIC ANEMIA

National Heart, Lung and Blood Institute
Information Center
P.O. Box 30105
Bethesda, MD 20824-0105
(301) 251-1222

## APNEA

*See Sudden Infant Death Syndrome*

## APRAXIA

National Institute of Neurological Disorders and Stroke
Bldg. 31, Room 8A16
Bethesda, MD 20892
(301) 496-5751
(800) 352-9424

## ARACHNOIDITIS

National Institute of Neurological Disorders and Stroke
Bldg. 31, Room 8A16
Bethesda, MD 20892
(301) 496-5751
(800) 352-9424

## ARAN DUCHENNE SPINALMUSCULAR DYSTROPHY

National Institute of Neurological Disorders and Stroke
Bldg. 31, Room 8A16
Bethesda, MD 20892
(301) 496-5751
(800) 352-9424

## ARNOLD-CHIARI MALFORMATIONS

National Institute of Neurological Disorders and Stroke
Bldg. 31, Room 8A16
Bethesda, MD 20892
(301) 496-5751
(800) 352-9424

## ARRHYTHMIAS

National Heart, Lung and Blood Institute
Information Center
P.O. Box 30105
Bethesda, MD 20824-0105
(301) 251-1222

## ARTERIOSCLEROSIS

National Heart, Lung and Blood Institute
Information Center
P.O. Box 30105
Bethesda, MD 20824-0105
(301) 251-1222

## ARTERIOVENOUS MALFORMATIONS

National Institute of Neurological Disorders and Stroke
Bldg. 31, Room 8A16
Bethesda, MD 20892 (301) 496-5751
(800) 352-9424

## ARTERITIS

National Eye Institute
Bldg. 31, Room 6A32
Bethesda, MD 20892 (301) 496-5248

## ARTHRITIS

National Institute of Arthritis and Musculoskeletal and Skin Diseases
1 AMS Way
Bethesda, MD 20892 (301) 495-4484

## ARTHROGRYPOSIS MULTIPLEX CONGENITA

National Institute of Arthritis and Musculoskeletal and Skin Diseases
1 AMS Way
Bethesda, MD 20892 (301) 495-4484

## ARTHROPLASTY

National Arthritis and Musculoskeletal and Skin Diseases
Information Clearinghouse
1 AMS Way
Bethesda, MD 20892 (301) 495-4484

## ARTHROSCOPY

National Arthritis and Musculoskeletal and Skin Diseases
Information Clearinghouse
1 AMS Way
Bethesda, MD 20892 (301) 495-4484

## ARTIFICIAL BLOOD VESSELS

National Heart, Lung and Blood Institute
Information Center
P.O. Box 30105
Bethesda, MD 20824-0105 (301) 251-1222

## ARTIFICIAL HEARTS

National Heart, Lung and Blood Institute
Information Center
P.O. Box 30105
Bethesda, MD 20824-0105 (301) 251-1222

## ARTIFICIAL INSEMINATION

*See also In Vitro Fertilization*

National Institute of Child Health and Human Development
Building 31, Room 2A32
Bethesda, MD 20892 (301) 496-5133

## ARTIFICIAL JOINTS

National Institute of Arthritis and Musculoskeletal and Skin Diseases
1 AMS Way
Bethesda, MD 20892 (301) 495-4484

## ARTIFICIAL LUNG

National Heart, Lung and Blood Institute
Information Center
P.O. Box 30105
Bethesda, MD 20824-0105 (301) 251-1222

## ASBESTOS

*See also Asbestosis*

Environmental Protection Agency
401 M St., SW
Washington, DC 20460 (703) 305-5938
(800) 368-5888

## ASBESTOSIS

*See also Asbestos*

National Heart, Lung and Blood Institute
Information Center
P.O. Box 30105
Bethesda, MD 20824-0105 (301) 251-1222

## ASIATIC FLU

*See Flu*

## ASPARAGINASE

National Cancer Institute
Bldg. 31, Room 10A16
Bethesda, MD 20892 (800) 4-CANCER

## ASPARTAME

National Institute of Neurological Disorders and Stroke
Building 31, Room 8A16
Bethesda, MD 20892
(301) 496-5751
(800) 352-9424

## ASPERGER'S SYNDROME

National Institute of Neurological Disorders and Stroke
Building 31, Room 8A16
Bethesda, MD 20892
(301) 496-5751
(800) 352-9424

## ASPERGILLOSIS

National Institute of Allergy and Infectious Diseases
Bldg. 31, Room 7A50
Bethesda, MD 20892
(301) 496-5717

## ASPHYXIA

National Institute of Neurological Disorders and Stroke
Bldg. 31, Room 8A16
Bethesda, MD 20892
(301) 496-5751
(800) 352-9424

## ASPIRIN ALLERGY

National Institute of Allergy and Infectious Diseases
Bldg. 31, Room 7A50
Bethesda, MD 20892
(301) 496-5717

## ASTHMA

National Heart, Lung and Blood Institute
P.O. Box 30105
Bethesda, MD 20824-0105 (301) 251-1222

National Institute of Allergy and Infectious Diseases
Bldg. 31, Room 7A50
Bethesda, MD 20892 (301) 496-5717

## ASTIGMATISM

National Eye Institute
Bldg. 31, Room 6A32
Bethesda, MD 20892 (301) 496-5248

## ASYMMETRIC SEPTAL HYPERTROPHY

National Heart, Lung and Blood Institute
Information Center
P.O. Box 30105
Bethesda, MD 20824-0105 (301) 251-1222

## ATAXIA

National Institute of Neurological Disorders and Stroke
Bldg. 31, Room 8A16
Bethesda, MD 20892 (301) 496-5751
(800) 352-9424

## ATAXIA TELANGIECTASIA

National Cancer Institute
Bldg. 31, Room 10A16
Bethesda, MD 20892 (800) 4-CANCER

## ATELECTASIS

National Heart, Lung and Blood Institute Information Center
P.O. Box 30105
Bethesda, MD 20824-0105 (301) 251-1222

## ATHERECTOMY

National Heart, Lung and Blood Institute Information Center
P.O. Box 30105
Bethesda, MD 20824-0105 (301) 251-1222

## ATHEROSCLEROSIS

National Heart, Lung and Blood Institute
Information Center
P.O. Box 30105
Bethesda, MD 20824-0105 (301) 251-1222

National Institute of Neurological Disorders and Stroke
Bldg. 31, Room 8A16
Bethesda, MD 20892 (301) 496-5751
(800) 352-9424

## ATHETOSIS

National Institute of Neurological Disorders and Stroke
Bldg. 31, Room 8A16
Bethesda, MD 20892 (301) 496-5751
(800) 352-9424

## ATHLETE'S FOOT

*See Fungal Infections*

## ATOPIC DERMATITIS

National Institute of Arthritis and Musculoskeletal and Skin Diseases
1 AMS Way
Bethesda, MD 20892 (301) 495-4484

## ATRIAL FIBRILLATION

National Heart, Lung and Blood Institute Information Center
P.O. Box 30105
Bethesda, MD 20824-0105 (301) 251-1222

## ATTENTION DEFICIT DISORDER

National Institute of Neurological Disorders and Stroke
Bldg. 31, Room 8A16
Bethesda, MD 20892 (301) 496-5751
(800) 352-9424

## AUTISM

National Institute of Child Health and Human Development
Bldg. 31, Room 2A32
Bethesda, MD 20892 (301) 496-5133

## AUTOIMMUNE DISEASE

National Institute of Arthritis and Musculoskeletal and Skin Diseases
1 AMS Way
Bethesda, MD 20892 (301) 495-4484

## AUTOSOMAL DOMINANT DISEASE

*See Huntington's Chorea*

# - B -

## B-19 INFECTION

National Institute of Child Health and Human Development
Bldg. 31, Room 2A32
Bethesda, MD 20892 (301) 496-5133

## BABY BOTTLE TOOTH DECAY

National Institute of Dental Research
31 Center Drive, MSC-2290
Bethesda, MD 20892-2290 (301) 496-4261

## BACILLUS CALMETTE-GUERIN (BCG)

National Cancer Institute
Bldg. 31, Room 10A16
Bethesda, MD 20892 (800) 4-CANCER

## BACK PROBLEMS

National Institute of Arthritis and Musculoskeletal and Skin Diseases
1 AMS Way
Bethesda, MD 20892 (301) 495-4484

## BACTERIAL MENINGITIS

National Institute of Allergy and Infectious Diseases
Building 31, Room 7A50
Bethesda, MD 20892 (301) 496-5717

## BACTERIOLOGY

National Institute of Allergy and Infectious Diseases
Bldg. 31, Room 7A50
Bethesda, MD 20892 (301) 496-5717

## BAD BREATH

*See Halitosis*

## BAGASSOSIS

National Institute of Occupational Safety and Health
4676 Columbia Parkway, MS C-13
Cincinnati, OH 45226 (800) 35-NIOSH

## BARLOW'S SYNDROME

National Heart, Lung, and Blood Institute Information Center
P.O. Box 30105
Bethesda, MD 20824-0105 (301) 251-1222

## BARTTER'S SYNDROME

National Heart, Lung, and Blood Institute Information Center
P.O. Box 30105
Bethesda, MD 20824-0105 (301) 251-1222

## BASAL CELL CARCINOMA

National Cancer Institute
Bldg. 31, Room 10A16
Bethesda, MD 20892 (800) 4-CANCER

## BATTEN'S DISEASE

National Institute of Neurological Disorders and Stroke
Bldg. 31, Room 8A16 (301) 496-5751
Bethesda, MD 20892 (800) 352-9424

## BATTERED CHILD

*See Child Abuse*

## BATTERED ELDERLY

*See Aging; Elder Abuse*

## BATTERED SPOUSES

National Institute of Mental Health
5600 Fishers Ln., Room 7C-02
Rockville, MD 20857 (301) 443-4515

National Resource Center on Domestic Violence
6400 Flank Drive, Suite 1300
Harrisburg, PA 17112 (800) 537-2238

## BED WETTING

National Institute of Child Health and Human Development
Bldg. 31, Room 2A32
Bethesda, MD 20892 (301) 496-5133

## BEDSONIA

National Institute of Diabetes and Digestive and Kidney Diseases

Bldg. 31, Room 9A04
Bethesda, MD 20892 (301) 496-3583

## BEHAVIOR AND HEALTH

National Institute of Child Health and Human Development
Bldg. 31, Room 2A32
Bethesda, MD 20892 (301) 496-5133

## BEHAVIOR DEVELOPMENT

National Institute of Child Health and Human Development
Human Learning and Behavior Branch
National Institutes of Health
Bethesda, MD 20892 (301) 496-6591

## BEHCET'S DISEASE

National Eye Institute
Bldg. 31, Room 6A32
Bethesda, MD 20892 (301) 496-5248

## BEJEL

National Sexually Transmitted Diseases Hotline
P.O. Box 13827
Research Triangle Park, NC 27709 (800) 227-8922

## BELL'S PALSY

National Institute of Neurological Disorders and Stroke
Bldg. 31, Room 8A06 (301) 496-5751
Bethesda, MD 20892 (800) 352-9424

## BENIGN CONGENITAL HYPOTONIA

National Institute of Neurological Disorders and Stroke
Bldg. 31, Room 8A16 (301) 496-5751
Bethesda, MD 20892 (800) 352-9424

## BENIGN MUCOSAL PEMPHIGOID

National Cancer Institute
Bldg. 31, Room 10A16
Bethesda, MD 20892 (800) 4-CANCER

## BENIGN PROSTATIC HYPERPLASIA

National Institute of Diabetes and Digestive and Kidney Diseases
Bldg. 31, Room 9A04
Bethesda, MD 20892 (301) 496-3583

## BENZO(A)PYRENE

National Cancer Institute
Bldg. 31, Room 10A16
Bethesda, MD 20892 (800) 4-CANCER

## BERGER'S DISEASE

National Institute of Diabetes and Digestive and Kidney Diseases
Bldg. 31, Room 9A04
Bethesda, MD 20892 (301) 496-3583

## BERIBERI

National Institute of Diabetes and Digestive and Kidney Diseases

Bldg. 31, Room 9A04
Bethesda, MD 20892 (301) 496-3583

## BERNARD-SOULIER SYNDROME

National Institute of Diabetes and Digestive and Kidney Diseases
Building 31, Room 9A04
Bethesda, MD 20892 (301) 496-3583

## BETA BLOCKER DRUGS

Food & Drug Administration
(HFE-88), 5600 Fishers Lane
Rockville, MD 20857 (301) 443-3170

## BETA-THALASSEMIA

National Heart, Lung, and Blood Institute
Information Center
P.O. Box 30105
Bethesda, MD 20824-0105 (301) 251-1222

## BILIARY CIRRHOSIS

National Institute of Diabetes and Digestive and Kidney Diseases
Bldg. 31, Room 9A04
Bethesda, MD 20892 (301) 496-3583

## BILIRUBINEMIA

National Institute of Child Health and Human Development
Bldg. 31, Room 2A32
Bethesda, MD 20892 (301) 496-5133

## BINOCULAR VISION

National Eye Institute
Building 31, Room 6A32
Bethesda, MD 20892 (301) 496-5248

## BINSWANGER'S DISEASE

National Institute of Neurological Disorders and Stroke
Building 31, Room 8A16 (301) 496-5751
Bethesda, MD 20892 (800) 352-9424

## BIOFEEDBACK

National Institute of Mental Health
5600 Fishers Lane, Room 7C-02
Rockville, MD 20857 (301) 443-4515

## BIOMEDICAL ENGINEERING

National Institute of General Medical Sciences
Building 31, Room 4A52
Bethesda, MD 20892 (301) 496-7301

## BIOMEDICAL RESEARCH

Office of Science and Health Reports
National Center for Research Resources
National Institutes of Health
Bethesda, MD 20892 (301) 496-5545

## BIOPHYSICS

National Institutes of Health

Building 31, Room 4A52
Bethesda, MD 20892 (301) 496-7301

## BIOPSIES

National Cancer Institute
Bldg. 31, Room 10A16
Bethesda, MD 20892 (800) 4-CANCER

## BIOTECHNOLOGY

National Agricultural Library Building
10301 Baltimore Boulevard, 4th Floor
Beltsville, MD 20705 (301) 504-5947

## BIRTH

National Institute of Child Health and Human Development
Bldg. 31, Room 2A32
Bethesda, MD 20892 (301) 496-5133

## BIRTH CONTROL

*See Contraception; Family Planning; Oral Contraceptives*

## BIRTH DEFECTS

*See also Congenital Abnormalities; Neural Tube Defects*

National Institute of Child Health and Human Development
Bldg. 31, Room 2A32
Bethesda, MD 20892 (301) 496-5133

## BIRTH WEIGHT

*See also Child Health*

National Institute of Child Health and Human Development
Bldg. 31, Room 2A32
Bethesda, MD 20892 (301) 496-5133

## BLACK LUNG DISEASE

National Heart, Lung, and Blood Institute
Information Center
P.O. Box 30105
Bethesda, MD 20824-0105 (301) 251-1222

## BLACK TONGUE

National Institute of Dental Research
Bldg. 31, Room 2C35
31 Center Drive, MSC-2290
Bethesda, MD 20892-2290 (301) 496-4261

## BLADDER CANCER

National Cancer Institute
Building 31, Room 10A16
Bethesda, MD 20892 (800) 4-CANCER

## BLASTOMYCOSIS

National Institute of Allergy and Infectious Diseases
Bldg. 31, Room 7A50
Bethesda, MD 20892 (301) 496-5717

## BLEOMYCIN

National Cancer Institute
Building 31
Room 10A16
Bethesda, MD 20892 (800) 4-CANCER

## BLEPHARITIS

National Eye Institute
Building 31
Room 6A32
Bethesda, MD 20892 (301) 496-5248

## BLEPHAROSPASM

National Institute of Neurological Disorders and Stroke
Bldg. 31, Room 8A16
Bethesda, MD 20892 (301) 496-5751
(800) 352-9424

## BLINDNESS

National Eye Institute
Building 31
Room 6A32
Bethesda, MD 20892 (301) 496-5248

## BLISTERING DISORDERS

National Arthritis and Musculoskeletal and Skin Diseases
Information Clearinghouse
1 AMS Way
Bethesda, MD 20892 (301) 495-4484

## BLOCH-SULZBERGER SYNDROME

National Institute of Neurological Disorders and Stroke
Bldg. 31, Room 8A16
Bethesda, MD 20892 (301) 496-5751
(800) 352-9424

## BLOOD

National Heart, Lung, and Blood Institute
Information Center
P.O. Box 30105
Bethesda, MD 20824-0105 (301) 251-1222

## BLOOD BRAIN BARRIER

National Institute of Neurological Disorders and Stroke
Bldg. 31, Room 8A16
Bethesda, MD 20892 (301) 496-5751
(800) 352-9424

## BLOOD COAGULATION

National Heart, Lung, and Blood Institute
Information Center
P.O. Box 30105
Bethesda, MD 20824-0105 (301) 251-1222

## BLOOD DISEASES

National Heart, Lung, and Blood Institute
Information Center
P.O. Box 30105
Bethesda, MD 20824-0105 (301) 251-1222

## BLOOD PRODUCTS

Center for Biologics Evaluation and Research
Food and Drug Administration
1401 Rockville Pike
Suite 200 N.
Rockville, MD 20857 (301) 594-1800

## BLOOD SUBSTITUTES

National Heart, Lung, and Blood Institute
Information Center
P.O. Box 30105
Bethesda, MD 20824-0105 (301) 251-1222

## BLOOD TESTING

*See Blood Products*

## BLUE BABY

National Institute of Child Health and Human Development
Building 31
Room 2A32
Bethesda, MD 20892 (301) 496-5133

## BODY WEIGHT

National Institute of Diabetes and Digestive and Kidney Diseases
Building 31
Room 9A04
Bethesda, MD 20892 (301) 496-3583

## BOLIVIAN HEMORRHAGIC FEVER

National Institute of Allergy and Infectious Diseases
Bldg. 31, Room 7A50
Bethesda, MD 20892 (301) 496-5717

## BONE CANCER

*See also Cancer*

National Cancer Institute
Bldg. 31, Room 10A16
Bethesda, MD 20892 (800) 4-CANCER

## BONE DISORDERS

National Institute of Arthritis and Musculoskeletal and Skin Diseases
1 AMS Way
Bethesda, MD 20892 (301) 495-4484

## BONE MARROW FAILURE

National Heart, Lung, and Blood Institute
Information Center
P.O. Box 30105
Bethesda, MD 20824-0105 (301) 251-1222

## BONE MARROW TRANSPLANTS

National Cancer Institute
Bldg. 31, Room 10A16
Bethesda, MD 20892 (800) 4-CANCER

## BOTULISM

National Institute of Allergy and Infectious Diseases
Building 31
Room 7A50
Bethesda, MD 20892 (301) 496-5717

## BOWEL DISEASE

National Institute of Diabetes and Digestive and Kidney Diseases
Building 31
Room 9A04
Bethesda, MD 20892 (301) 496-3583

## BOWEN'S DISEASE

National Cancer Institute
Building 31
Room 10A16
Bethesda, MD 20892 (800) 4-CANCER

## BRACHIAL PLEXUS INJURIES

National Institute of Neurological Disorders and Stroke
Bldg. 31, Room 8A16
Bethesda, MD 20892 (301) 496-5751
(800) 352-9424

## BRADYCARDIA

National Heart, Lung, and Blood Institute
Information Center
P.O. Box 30105
Bethesda, MD 20824-0105 (301) 251-1222

## BRAIN

National Institute of Neurological Disorders and Stroke
Bldg. 31, Room 8A16 (301) 496-5751
Bethesda, MD 20892 (800) 352-9424

## BRAIN CANCER

*See also Cancer*

National Cancer Institute
Bldg. 31, Room 10A16
Bethesda, MD 20892 (800) 4-CANCER

## BRAIN DEATH

National Institute of Neurological Disorders and Stroke
Bldg. 31, Room 8A16 (301) 496-5751
Bethesda, MD 20892 (800) 352-9424

## BRAIN INJURIES

National Rehabilitation Information Center
8455 Colesville Road, Suite 935 (301) 588-9284
Silver Spring, MD 20910 (800) 346-2742 (Voice and TDD)

National Institute of Neurological Disorders and Stroke
Bldg. 31, Room 8A16 (301) 496-5751
Bethesda, MD 20892 (800) 352-9424

## BRAIN TUMORS

National Cancer Institute
Bldg. 31, Room 10A16
Bethesda, MD 20892 (800) 4-CANCER

## BREAST CANCER

*See also Cancer*

National Cancer Institute
Bldg. 31, Room 10A16
Bethesda, MD 20892 (800) 4-CANCER

## BREASTFEEDING

National Institute of Child Health and Human Development
Bldg. 31, Room 2A32
Bethesda, MD 20892 (301) 496-5133

## BREAST IMPLANTS

Division of Consumer Affairs (HFZ-210)
Center for Devices and Radiological Health
Food and Drug Administration
Rockville, MD 20857 (301) 443-4190

## BRONCHIECTASIS

National Heart, Lung, and Blood Institute
Information Center
P.O. Box 30105
Bethesda, MD 20824-0105 (301) 251-1222

## BRONCHITIS

National Heart, Lung, and Blood Institute
Information Center
P.O. Box 30105
Bethesda, MD 20824-0105 (301) 251-1222

## BRUCELLOSIS

National Institute of Allergy and Infectious Diseases
Building 31, Room 7A50
Bethesda, MD 20892 (301) 496-5717

## BRUXISM

National Institute of Dental Research
Bldg. 31, Room 2C35
31 Center Drive, MSC-2290
Bethesda, MD 20892 (301) 496-4261

## BUBONIC PLAGUE

National Institute of Allergy and Infectious Diseases
Bldg. 31, Room 7A50
Bethesda, MD 20892 (301) 496-5717

## BUERGER'S DISEASE

National Heart, Lung, and Blood Institute
Information Center
P.O. Box 30105
Bethesda, MD 20824-0105 (301) 251-1222

## BULBAR PALSY

National Institute of Neurological Disorders and Stroke
Bldg. 31, Room 8A16
Bethesda, MD 20892 (301) 496-5751
(800) 352-9424

## BULIMIA

*See also Anorexia; Eating Disorders*

National Institute of Diabetes and Digestive and Kidney Diseases
National Institutes of Health
Bldg. 31, Room 3A18B
Bethesda, MD 20892 (301) 496-7823

## BULLOUS PEMPHIGOID

National Institute of Arthritis and Musculoskeletal
and Skin Diseases
1 AMS Way
Bethesda, MD 20892 (301) 495-4484

## BURKITT'S LYMPHOMA

National Cancer Institute
Bldg. 31, Room 10A16
Bethesda, MD 20892 (800) 4-CANCER

## BURN RESEARCH

National Institute of General Medical Sciences
Bldg. 31, Room 4A52
Bethesda, MD 20892 (301) 496-7301

## BURNING MOUTH SYNDROME

National Institute of Dental Research
Building 31, Room 2C35
31 Center Drive, MSC-2290
Bethesda, MD 20892 (301) 496-4261

## BURSITIS

National Institute of Arthritis and Musculoskeletal and Skin Diseases
1 AMS Way
Bethesda, MD 20892 (301) 495-4484

## BUSULFAN

National Cancer Institute
Bldg. 31, Room 10A16
Bethesda, MD 20892 (800) 4-CANCER

## BYSSINOSIS

National Heart, Lung, and Blood Institute
Information Center
P.O. Box 30105
Bethesda, MD 20824-0105 (301) 251-1222

# - C -

## CAFFEINE

Food & Drug Administration
(HFE-88), 5600 Fishers Lane
Rockville, MD 20857 (301) 443-3170

## CANAVAN'S DISEASE

National Institute of Neurological Disorders and Stroke
Bldg. 31, Room 8A16
Bethesda, MD 20892 (301) 496-5751
(800) 352-9424

## CANCER

*See also Anti-Cancer Drugs; Radiation; specific type of Cancer*

National Cancer Institute
Building 31, Room 10A18
9000 Rockville Pike
Bethesda, MD 20892 (800) 4-CANCER

## CANDIDA

National Institute of Allergy and Infectious Diseases
Bldg. 31, Room 7A50
Bethesda, MD 20892 (301) 496-5717

## CANKER SORES

National Institute of Dental Research
Bldg. 31, Room 2C35
31 Center Drive, MSC-2290
Bethesda, MD 20892 (301) 496-4261

## CARBOHYDRATES

Food & Drug Administration
(HFE-88), 5600 Fishers Lane
Rockville, MD 20857 (301) 443-3170

## CARCALON

National Cancer Institute
Bldg. 31, Room 10A16
Bethesda, MD 20892 (800) 4-CANCER

## CARCINOGENS

National Institute of Occupational Safety and Health
4676 Columbia Parkway
Cincinnati, OH 45226 (800) 35-NIOSH
(513) 533-8326

National Cancer Institute
Bldg. 31, Room 10A16
Bethesda, MD 20892 (800) 4-CANCER

## CARCINOMA

National Cancer Institute
Bldg. 31, Room 10A16
Bethesda, MD 20892 (800) 4-CANCER

## CARDIOMEGALY

National Heart, Lung, and Blood Institute
Information Center
P.O. Box 30105
Bethesda, MD 20824-0105 (301) 251-1222

## CARDIOMYOPATHY

National Heart, Lung, and Blood Institute
Information Center
P.O. Box 30105
Bethesda, MD 20824-0105 (301) 251-1222

## CARDIOPULMONARY RESUSCITATION

National Heart, Lung, and Blood Institute
Information Center

P.O. Box 30105
Bethesda, MD 20824-0105 (301) 251-1222

## CARDIOVASCULAR DISEASE

*See also Heart Disease*

National Heart, Lung, and Blood Institute Information Center
P.O. Box 30105
Bethesda, MD 20824-0105 (301) 251-1222

## CARDITIS

National Heart, Lung, and Blood Institute Information Center
P.O. Box 30105
Bethesda, MD 20824-0105 (301) 251-1222

## CARIES

National Institute of Dental Research
Building 31, Room 2C35
31 Center Drive, Room 2C35
Bethesda, MD 20892 (301) 496-4261

## CARMUSTINE

National Cancer Institute
Bldg. 31, Room 10A16
Bethesda, MD 20892 (800) 4-CANCER

## CAROTID ENDARTERECTOMY

National Institute of Neurological Disorders and Stroke
Bldg. 31, Room 8A16 (301) 496-5751
Bethesda, MD 20892 (800) 352-9424

## CARPAL TUNNEL SYNDROME

National Institute of Arthritis and Musculoskeletal and Skin Diseases
1 AMS Way
Bethesda, MD 20892 (301) 495-4484

## CARPET FUMES

Consumer Information Center
P.O. Box 100
Pueblo, CO 81002

## CATAPHASIA

National Institute of Neurological Disorders and Stroke
Bldg. 31, Room 8A16 (301) 496-5751
Bethesda, MD 20892 (800) 352-9424

## CATAPLEXY

National Institute of Neurological Disorders and Stroke
Bldg. 31, Room 8A16 (301) 496-5751
Bethesda, MD 20892 (800) 352-9424

## CATARACTS

National Eye Institute
Bldg. 31, Room 6A32
Bethesda, MD 20892 (301) 496-5248

## CAT CRY SYNDROME

National Institute of Child Health and Human Development

Bldg. 31, Room 2A32
Bethesda, MD 20892 (301) 496-5133

## CAT SCRATCH FEVER

National Institute of Allergy and Infectious Diseases
Bldg. 31, Room 7A50
Bethesda, MD 20892 (301) 496-5717

## CATHETERIZATION

National Heart, Lung, and Blood Institute
Information Center
P.O. Box 30105
Bethesda, MD 20824-0105 (301) 251-1222

## CEA

National Cancer Institute
Bldg. 31, Room 10A16
Bethesda, MD 20892 (800) 4-CANCER

## CELIAC DISEASE

National Institute of Diabetes and Digestive and Kidney Diseases
Bldg. 31, Room 9A04
Bethesda, MD 20892 (301) 496-3583

## CELLULITE

Food & Drug Administration
(HFE-88), 5600 Fishers Ln.
Rockville, MD 20857 (301) 443-3170

## CENTENARIANS

National Institute on Aging
Information Center
P.O. Box 8057
Gaithersburg, MD 20898-8057

(800) 222-2225

## CENTRAL CORE DISEASE

National Institute of Neurological Disorders and Stroke
Bldg. 31, Room 8A16
Bethesda, MD 20892

(301) 496-5751
(800) 352-9424

## CEREBELLAR ARTERIOSCLEROSIS

National Institute of Neurological Disorders and Stroke
Bldg. 31, Room 8A16
Bethesda, MD 20892

(301) 496-5751
(800) 352-9424

## CEREBELLAR ATAXIA

National Institute of Neurological Disorders and Stroke
Bldg. 31, Room 8A16
Bethesda, MD 20892

(301) 496-5751
(800) 352-9424

## CEREBELLAR LESIONS

National Institute of Neurological Disorders and Stroke
Bldg. 31, Room 8A16
Bethesda, MD 20892

(301) 496-5751
(800) 352-9424

## CEREBRAL ARTERIOVENOUS MALFORMATIONS

National Institute of Neurological Disorders and Stroke
Bldg. 31, Room 8A16
Bethesda, MD 20892
(301) 496-5751
(800) 352-9424

## CEREBRAL ATROPHY

National Institute of Neurological Disorders and Stroke
Bldg. 31, Room 8A16
Bethesda, MD 20892
(301) 496-5751
(800) 352-9424

## CEREBRAL PALSY

National Institute of Neurological Disorders and Stroke
Bldg. 31, Room 8A16
Bethesda, MD 20892
(301) 496-5751
(800) 352-9424

## CEREBROTENDIOUS XANTHOMATOSIS

National Institute of Neurological Disorders and Stroke
Bldg. 31, Room 8A16
Bethesda, MD 20892
(301) 496-5751
(800) 352-9424

## CEREBROVASCULAR DISEASE

National Institute of Neurological Disorders and Stroke
Bldg. 31, Room 8A16
Bethesda, MD 20892
(301) 496-5751
(800) 352-9424

## CEROID LIPOFUSCINOSIS

National Institute of Neurological Disorders and Stroke
Bldg. 31, Room 8A16 (301) 496-5751
Bethesda, MD 20892 (800) 352-9424

## CERVICAL CANCER

*See also Cancer*

National Cancer Institute
Bldg. 31, Room 10A16
Bethesda, MD 20892 (800) 4-CANCER

## CERVICAL CAP

*See also Contraception*

Food and Drug Administration
(HFE-88), 5600 Fishers Lane
Rockville, MD 20857 (301) 443-3170

## CERVICAL DISORDERS

*See also Cervical Cancer*

National Institute of Child Health and Human Development
Building 31, Room 2A32
Bethesda, MD 20892 (301) 496-5133

## CESAREANS

National Institute of Child Health and Human Development
Building 31, Room 2A32
Bethesda, MD 20892 (301) 496-5133

## CESTODE

*See Tapeworm*

## CHAGAS' DISEASE

National Institute of Allergy and Infectious Diseases
Bldg. 31, Room 7A50
Bethesda, MD 20892 (301) 496-5717

## CHALAZION

National Eye Institute
Bldg. 31, Room 6A32
Bethesda, MD 20892 (301) 496-5248

## CHANCROID

National Sexually Transmitted Diseases Hotline
P.O. Box 13827
Research Triangle Park, NC 27709 (800) 227-8922

## CHANGE OF LIFE

*See Menopause*

## CHAPARRAL TEA

National Cancer Institute
Bldg. 31, Room 10A16
Bethesda, MD 20892 (800) 4-CANCER

## CHARCOAL BROILING OF MEAT

National Cancer Institute
Building 31, Room 10A16
Bethesda, MD 20892 (800) 4-CANCER

## CHARCOT-MARIE-TOOTH DISEASE

National Institute of Neurological Disorders and Stroke
Building 31, Room 8A16 (301) 496-5751
Bethesda, MD 20892 (800) 352-9424

## CHARGE SYNDROME

National Institute of Child Health and Human Development
Bldg. 31, Room 2A32
Bethesda, MD 20892 (301) 496-5133

## CHEDIAK-HIGASHI SYNDROME

National Institute of Allergy and Infectious Diseases
Bldg. 31, Room 7A50
Bethesda, MD 20892 (301) 496-5717

## CHEILOSCHISIS

*See Harelip*

## CHELATION THERAPY

National Heart, Lung, and Blood Institute
Information Center

P.O. Box 30105
Bethesda, MD 20824-0105 (301) 251-1222

## CHEMICAL SPILLS

Environmental Protection Agency
401 M Street, SW
Washington, DC 20460
(800) 426-4791

## CHEMOTHERAPY

National Cancer Institute
Bldg. 31, Room 10A16
Bethesda, MD 20892 (800) 4-CANCER

## CHEWING TOBACCO AND SNUFF

*See Smoking; Smokeless Tobacco*

## CHICKEN POX

National Institute of Allergy and Infectious Diseases
Bldg. 31, Room 7A50
Bethesda, MD 20892 (301) 496-5717

## CHILBLAIN

National Arthritis and Musculoskeletal and Skin Diseases Information Clearinghouse
1 AMS Way
Bethesda, MD 20892 (301) 495-4484

## CHILD ABUSE AND FAMILY VIOLENCE

National Resource Center on Domestic Violence
6400 Flank Drive, Suite 1300
Harrisburg, PA 17112 (800) 537-2238

## CHILD DEVELOPMENT

National Institute of Child Health and Human Development
Bldg. 31, Room 2A32
Bethesda, MD 20892 (301) 496-5133

## CHILD HEALTH

*See also Lead Poisoning*

National Institute of Child Health and Human Development
Bldg. 31, Room 2A32
Bethesda, MD 20892 (301) 496-5133

National Maternal and Child Health Clearinghouse
8201 Greensboro Drive, Suite 600
McLean, VA 22102-3810 (703) 821-8955, ext. 254

## CHILD REARING

National Institute of Mental Health
5600 Fishers Ln., Room 7C-02
Rockville, MD 20857 (301) 443-4515

## CHILDBIRTH

*See also Postnatal Care*

National Institute of Child Health and Human Development

Bldg. 31, Room 2A32
Bethesda, MD 20892 (301) 496-5133

## CHILDHOOD ARTHRITIS

National Arthritis and Musculoskeletal and Skin Diseases
Information Clearinghouse
1 AMS Way
Bethesda, MD 20892 (301) 495-4484

## CHILDHOOD ASTHMA

*See Asthma*

## CHILDHOOD MENTAL DISORDERS

National Institute of Mental Health
5600 Fishers Lane, Room 7C-02
Rockville, MD 20857 (301) 443-4515

## CHILDHOOD NUTRITION

National Institute of Child Health and Human Development
Bldg. 31, Room 2A32
Bethesda, MD 20892 (301) 496-5133

National Maternal and Child Health Clearinghouse
8201 Greensboro Drive, Suite 600
McLean, VA 22101-3810 (703) 821-8955, ext. 254

## CHILDREN OF ALCOHOLICS

National Clearinghouse for Alcohol and Drug Information
P.O. Box 2345
Rockville, MD 20847-2345 (800) 729-6686

## CHINESE RESTAURANT SYNDROME

Food and Nutrition Information Center
National Agricultural Library, Room 304
Beltsville, MD 20705 (301) 504-5719

## CHLAMYDIA

National Sexually Transmitted Diseases Hotline
P.O. Box 13827
Research Triangle Park, NC 27709 (800) 227-8922

## CHLOASMA

National Institute of Child Health and Human Development
Bldg. 31, Room 2A32
Bethesda, MD 20892 (301) 496-5133

## CHLORAMBUCIL

National Cancer Institute
Bldg. 31, Room 10A16
Bethesda, MD 20892 (800) 4-CANCER

## CHOLECYSTECTOMY

*See Gallbladder*

## CHOLELITHOTOMY

*See Gallstones*

## CHOLERA

National Institute of Allergy and Infectious Diseases
Bldg. 31, Room 7A50
Bethesda, MD 20892 (301) 496-5717

## CHOLESTEROL

National Heart, Lung, and Blood Institute
Information Center
P.O. Box 30105
Bethesda, MD 20824-0105 (301) 251-1222

National Cholesterol Education Program
Information Center
P.O. Box 30105
Bethesda, MD 20824-0105 (301) 251-1222

## CHONDROCALCINOSIS

National Institute of Arthritis and Musculoskeletal and Skin Diseases
1 AMS Way
Bethesda, MD 20892 (301) 495-4484

## CHONDROMALACIA

National Arthritis and Musculoskeletal and Skin Diseases Clearinghouse
1 AMS Way
Bethesda, MD 20892 (301) 495-4484

## CHONDROSARCOMA

National Cancer Institute
Building 31, Room 10A16
Bethesda, MD 20892 (800) 4-CANCER

## CHORDOMA

National Cancer Institute
Building 31, Room 10A16
Bethesda, MD 20892 (800) 4-CANCER

## CHORIOCARCINOMA

National Cancer Institute
Building 31, Room 10A16
Bethesda, MD 20892 (800) 4-CANCER

## CHORIONIC VILLUS SAMPLING

National Institute of Child Health and Human Development
Building 31, Room 2A32
Bethesda, MD 20892 (301) 496-5133

## CHOROIDITIS

National Eye Institute
Building 31, Room 6A32
Bethesda, MD 20892 (301) 496-5248

## CHRONIC BRONCHITIS

National Heart, Lung, and Blood Institute Information Center
P.O. Box 30105
Bethesda, MD 20824-0105 (301) 251-1222

## CHRONIC COUGH

National Heart, Lung, and Blood Institute
Information Center

P.O. Box 30105
Bethesda, MD 20824-0105 (301) 251-1222

## CHRONIC EBV

National Institute of Allergy and Infectious Diseases
Bldg. 31, Room 7A50
Bethesda, MD 20892 (301) 496-5717

## CHRONIC FATIGUE SYNDROME

National Institute of Allergy and Infectious Diseases
Bldg. 31, Room 7A50
Bethesda, MD 20892 (301) 496-5717

## CHRONIC GRANULOMATOUS DISEASE

National Institute of Allergy and Infectious Diseases
Bldg. 31, Room 7A50
Bethesda, MD 20892 (301) 496-5717

## CHRONIC INFECTIONS

National Institute of Allergy and Infectious Diseases
Bldg. 31, Room 7A50
Bethesda, MD 20892 (301) 496-5717

## CHRONIC MYELOGENOUS LEUKEMIA

National Cancer Institute
Bldg. 31, Room 10A16
Bethesda, MD 20892 (800) 4-CANCER

## CHRONIC OBSTRUCTIVE LUNG DISEASE

National Heart, Lung, and Blood Institute Information Center
P.O. Box 30105
Bethesda, MD 20824-0105 (301) 251-1222

## CHRONIC PAIN

National Institute of Neurological Disorders and Stroke
Bldg. 31, Room 8A16 (301) 496-5751
Bethesda, MD 20892 (800) 352-9424

## CHRYSOTHERAPY

National Arthritis and Musculoskeletal and Skin Diseases Clearinghouse
1 AMS Way
Bethesda, MD 20892 (301) 495-4484

## CHURG-STRAUSS SYNDROME

National Institute of Allergy and Infectious Diseases
Bldg. 31, Room 7A50
Bethesda, MD 20892 (301) 496-5717

## CICATRICIAL PEMPHIGOID

National Eye Institute
Bldg. 31, Room 6A32
Bethesda, MD 20892 (301) 496-5248

## CIGARETTES

*See Smoking*

## CIRCULATION DISORDERS

National Heart, Lung, and Blood Institute
Information Center
P.O. Box 30105
Bethesda, MD 20824-0105 (301) 251-1222

## CIRCUMCISION

National Institute of Child Health and
Human Development
Bldg. 31, Room 2A32
Bethesda, MD 20892 (301) 496-5133

## CIRRHOSIS

National Institute of Diabetes and Digestive
and Kidney Diseases
Bldg. 31, Room 9A04
Bethesda, MD 20892 (301) 496-3583

## CISPLATIN

National Cancer Institute
Bldg. 31, Room 10A16
Bethesda, MD 20892 (800) 4-CANCER

## CLAUDICATION

National Heart, Lung, and Blood Institute
Information Center
P.O. Box 30105
Bethesda, MD 20824-0105 (301) 251-1222

## CLAUSTROPHOBIA

National Institute of Mental Health
5600 Fishers Lane, Room 7C-02
Rockville, MD 20857 (301) 443-4515

## CLEFT PALATE

National Institute of Dental Research
Building 31, Room 2C35
31 Center Dr., MSC-2290
Bethesda, MD 20892 (301) 496-4261

## CLIMACTERIC

*See Menopause*

## CLONING

National Institute of Child Health and Human Development
Bldg. 31, Room 2A32
Bethesda, MD 20892 (301) 496-5133

## CLOTTING DISORDERS

National Heart, Lung, and Blood Institute
Information Center
P.O. Box 30105
Bethesda, MD 20824-0105 (301) 251-1222

## CLUSTER HEADACHE

*See Histamine Headache*

## CMV

*See Cytomegalovirus*

## COAL WORKER'S PNEUMOCONIOSIS

*See Black Lung*

## COAT'S DISEASE

National Eye Institute
Bldg. 31, Room 6A32
Bethesda, MD 20892 (301) 496-5248

## COBALT

National Cancer Institute
Bldg. 31, Room 10A16
Bethesda, MD 20892 (800) 4-CANCER

## COCAINE

*See also Drug Abuse*

National Clearinghouse for Alcohol and Drug Information
P.O. Box 2345
Rockville, MD 20847-2345 (800) 729-6686

## COCKAYNE'S SYNDROME

National Institute on Aging Information Center
P.O. Box 8057
Gaithersburg, MD 20898-8057 (800) 222-2225

## CODEINE

Food and Drug Administration
(HFE-88), 5600 Fishers Lane
Rockville, MD 20857 (301) 443-3170

## COFFEE

*See Caffeine*

## COGAN'S SYNDROME

National Eye Institute
Building 31, Room 6A32
Bethesda, MD 20892 (301) 496-5248

## COGNITION

National Institute of Child Health and Human Development
Building 31, Room 2A32
Bethesda, MD 20892 (301) 496-5133

## COLD SORES

*See Fever Blisters*

## COLEY'S MIXED TOXINS

National Cancer Institute
Building 31, Room 10A16
Bethesda, MD 20892 (800) 4-CANCER

## COLIC

National Institute of Child Health and Human Development
Building 31, Room 2A32
Bethesda, MD 20892 (301) 496-5133

National Maternal and Child Health Clearinghouse
8201 Greensboro Dr., Suite 600
McLean, VA 22102-3810 (703) 821-8955, ext. 254

## COLITIS

National Institute of Diabetes and Digestive and Kidney Diseases
Bldg. 31, Room 9A04
Bethesda, MD 20892 (301) 496-3583

## COLLAGEN DISEASE

National Institute of Arthritis and Musculoskeletal
and Skin Diseases
1 AMS Way
Bethesda, MD 20892 (301) 495-4484

## COLLAPSED LUNGS

National Heart, Lung, and Blood Institute
Information Center
P.O. Box 30105
Bethesda, MD 20824-0105 (301) 251-1222

## COLON PROBLEMS

National Digestive Diseases Information Clearinghouse
2 Information Way
Bethesda, MD 20892 (301) 654-3810

## COLOR BLINDNESS

National Eye Institute
Bldg. 31, Room 6A32
Bethesda, MD 20892 (301) 496-5248

## COLORECTAL NEOPLASMS

National Cancer Institute
Bldg. 31, Room 10A16
Bethesda, MD 20892 (800) 4-CANCER

## COLOSTOMY

National Institute of Diabetes and Digestive and Kidney Diseases
Bldg. 31, Room 9A04
Bethesda, MD 20892 (301) 496-3583

National Cancer Institute
Bldg. 31, Room 10A16
Bethesda, MD 20892 (800) 4-CANCER

## COLPOCYSTITIS

National Kidney and Urologic Diseases
Information Clearinghouse
3 Information Way
Bethesda, MD 20892 (301) 654-4415

## COMAS

National Institute of Neurological Disorders and Stroke
Bldg. 31, Room 8A16
Bethesda, MD 20892 (301) 496-5751
(800) 352-9424

## COMEDO (Blackheads)

*See Acne*

## COMMON COLD

National Institute of Allergy and Infectious Diseases
Bldg. 31, Room 7A50
Bethesda, MD 20892 (301) 496-5717

## COMMUNICABLE & INFECTIOUS DISEASES

National Institute of Allergy and Infectious Diseases
Bldg. 31, Room 7A50
Bethesda, MD 20892 (301) 496-5717

Centers for Disease Control; Disease Hotline
4770 Buford Hwy., NE
Atlanta, GA 30341 (404) 332-4555

## COMMUNICATION DISORDERS

*See also Deafness*

National Institute on Deafness and Other Communication Disorders
1 Communication Ave.
Bethesda, MD 20892-3456 (800) 241-1044
(800) 241-1055 (TDD)

## COMPULSION

National Institute of Mental Health
5600 Fishers Lane, Room 7C-02
Rockville, MD 20857 (301) 443-4515

## COMPUTER ACCESS

National Library of Medicine
Bldg. 38, Room 2S10
Bethesda, MD 20892 (301) 496-6308

## CONDOMS

Center for Devices and Radiological Health
Food and Drug Administration
5600 Fishers Lane, HF2-210
Rockville, MD 20857 (301) 443-4690

## CONGENITAL ABNORMALITIES

*See also Birth Defects*

National Eye Institute
Bldg. 31, Room 6A32
Bethesda, MD 20892 (301) 496-5248

## CONGENITAL ADRENAL HYPERPLASIA

National Institute of Diabetes and Digestive and Kidney Diseases
Bldg. 31, Room 9A04
Bethesda, MD 20892 (301) 496-3583

## CONGENITAL HEART DISEASE

National Heart, Lung, and Blood Institute
Information Center
P.O. Box 30105
Bethesda, MD 20824-0105 (301) 251-1222

## CONGENITAL INFECTIONS

National Institute of Allergy and Infectious Diseases
Bldg. 31, Room 7A50
Bethesda, MD 20892 (301) 496-5717

## CONGESTIVE HEART FAILURE

National Heart, Lung, and Blood Institute
Information Center
P.O. Box 30105
Bethesda, MD 20824-0105 (301) 251-1222

## CONJUNCTIVITIS

National Eye Institute
Bldg. 31, Room 6A32
Bethesda, MD 20892 (301) 496-5248

## CONNECTIVE TISSUE DISEASES

National Institute of Arthritis and Musculoskeletal
and Skin Diseases
1 AMS Way
Bethesda, MD 20892 (301) 495-4484

## CONSTIPATION

National Institute of Diabetes and Digestive
and Kidney Diseases
Bldg. 31, Room 9A04
Bethesda, MD 20892 (301) 496-3583

## CONSUMER PRODUCT INJURIES

Consumer Product Safety Commission
4330 East West Hwy.
Bethesda, MD 20814 (301) 504-0424

## CONTACT DERMATITIS

Food and Drug Administration
(HFE-88), 5600 Fishers Lane
Rockville, MD 20857 (301) 443-3170

## CONTACT LENSES

National Eye Institute
Building 31, Room 6A32
Bethesda, MD 20892 (301) 496-5248

## CONTRACEPTION

*See also Family Planning; Oral Contraceptives*

Contraception Evaluation Branch
6100 Executive Boulevard
Bethesda, MD 20892 (301) 496-4924

Family Life Information Exchange
P.O. Box 37299
Washington, DC 20013 (301) 585-6636

## COOKWARE

Food and Drug Administration
(HFE-88), 5600 Fishers Lane
Rockville, MD 20857 (301) 443-3170

## COOLEY'S ANEMIA

National Heart, Lung, and Blood Institute
Information Center
P.O. Box 30105
Bethesda, MD 20824-0105 (301) 251-1222

## COR PULMONALE

National Heart, Lung, and Blood Institute
Information Center
P.O. Box 30105
Bethesda, MD 20824-0105 (301) 251-1222

## CORNEAL DISORDERS AND TRANSPLANTS

National Eye Institute
Bldg. 31, Room 6A32
Bethesda, MD 20892 (301) 496-5248

## CORNELIA deLANGE SYNDROME

National Institute of Child Health and Human Development
Bldg. 31, Room 2A32
Bethesda, MD 20892 (301) 496-5133

## CORONARY ANGIOPLASTY

National Heart, Lung, and Blood Institute
Information Center
P.O. Box 30105
Bethesda, MD 20824-0105 (301) 251-1222

## CORONARY DISEASE

*See Cardiovascular Disease; Heart Disease*

## COSMETIC ALLERGY

Office of Cosmetics and Colors
Food and Drug Administration
200 C Street, SW
Washington, DC 20204 (202) 205-4094

## COSMETIC SURGERY

*See Face Lifts*

## COSTOCHONDRITIS

National Institute of Arthritis and Musculoskeletal and Skin Diseases
1 AMS Way
Bethesda, MD 20892 (301) 495-4484

## COT DEATH

*See Sudden Infant Death Syndrome*

## COUGHING

National Heart, Lung and Blood Institute
Information Center
P.O. Box 30105
Bethesda, MD 20824-0105 (301) 251-1222

## COWPOX

National Arthritis and Musculoskeletal and
Skin Diseases Clearinghouse
1 AMS Way
Bethesda, MD 20892 (301) 495-4484

## COXSACKIE VIRUS

National Institute of Allergy and Infectious Diseases
Bldg. 31, Room 7A50
Bethesda, MD 20892 (301) 496-5717

## CPR

*See Cardiopulmonary Resuscitation*

## CRACK COCAINE

*See also Drug Abuse*

National Clearinghouse for Alcohol and Drug Information
P.O. Box 2345
Rockville, MD 20852 (301) 468-2600
(800) 729-6686

## CRANIAL ABNORMALITIES

National Institute of Dental Research
Bldg. 31, Room 2C35
31 Center Drive, MSC-2290
Bethesda, MD 20892-2290 (301) 496-4261

## CRANIOFACIAL MALFORMATIONS

National Institute of Dental Research
Bldg. 31, Room 2C35
31 Center Drive, MSC-2290
Bethesda, MD 20892-2290 (301) 496-4261

## CRETINISM

National Institute of Diabetes and Digestive
and Kidney Diseases
Bldg. 31, Room 9A04
Bethesda, MD 20892 (301) 496-3583

## CREUTZFELDT-JAKOB DISEASE

National Institute of Neurological Disorders and Stroke
Bldg. 31, Room 8A16
Bethesda, MD 20892 (301) 496-5751
(800) 352-9424

## CRIB DEATH

*See Sudden Infant Death Syndrome*

## CRIGLER-NAJAR SYNDROME

National Institute of Diabetes and Digestive
and Kidney Diseases
Bldg. 31, Room 9A04
Bethesda, MD 20892 (301) 496-3583

## CRITICAL CARE

Office of the Director
National Institutes of Health
Bldg. 31, Room 2B03
Bethesda, MD 20892 (301) 496-4143

## CROHN'S DISEASE

National Institute of Diabetes
and Digestive and Kidney Diseases
Bldg. 31, Room 9A04
Bethesda, MD 20892 (301) 496-3583

National Digestive Diseases Information Clearinghouse
2 Information Way
Bethesda, MD 20892 (301) 654-3810

## CROSS-EYE

National Eye Institute
Bldg. 31, Room 6A32
Bethesda, MD 20892 (301) 496-5248

## CRYOSURGERY

National Eye Institute
Bldg. 31, Room 6A32
Bethesda, MD 20892 (301) 496-5248

## CRYPTOCOCCOSES

National Institute of Allergy and Infectious Diseases
Bldg. 31, Room 7A50
Bethesda, MD 20892 (301) 496-5717

## CRYPTOSPORIDIOSIS

National Institute of Allergy and Infectious Diseases
Bldg. 31, Room 7A50
Bethesda, MD 20892 (301) 496-5717

## CUSHING'S DISEASE

*See Cushing's Syndrome*

## CUSHING'S SYNDROME

National Institute of Diabetes and Digestive and Kidney Diseases
Bldg. 31, Room 9A04
Bethesda, MD 20892 (301) 496-3583

## CUTIS LAXA

National Heart, Lung, and Blood Institute Information Center
P.O. Box 30105
Bethesda, MD 20824-0105 (301) 251-1222

## CYCLIC IDIOPATHIC EDEMA

National Heart, Lung, and Blood Institute Information Center
P.O. Box 30105
Bethesda, MD 20824-0105 (301) 251-1222

## CYCLITIS

National Eye Institute
Bldg. 31, Room 6A32
Bethesda, MD 20892 (301) 496-5248

## CYCLOPHOSPHAMIDE

National Cancer Institute
Bldg. 31, Room 10A16
Bethesda, MD 20892 (800) 4-CANCER

## CYCLOSPORINE-ASSOCIATED HYPERTENSION

National Cancer Institute Information Center
P.O. Box 30105
Bethesda, MD 20824-0105 (301) 251-1222

## CYSTIC ACNE

National Institute of Arthritis and Musculoskeletal and Skin Diseases
1 AMS Way
Bethesda, MD 20892 (301) 495-4484

## CYSTIC FIBROSIS

National Institute of Diabetes and Digestive and Kidney Diseases
Bldg. 31, Room 9A04
Bethesda, MD 20892 (301) 496-3583

## CYSTIC MASTITIS

*See Fibrocystic Breast Disease*

## CYSTINOSIS

National Institute of Child Health and Human Development
Building 31, Room 2A32
Bethesda, MD 20892 (301) 496-5133

## CYSTINURIA

National Institute of Diabetes and Digestive and Kidney Diseases
Bldg. 31, Room 9A04
Bethesda, MD 20892 (301) 496-3583

## CYSTITIS

National Institute of Diabetes and Digestive and Kidney Diseases
Bldg. 31, Room 9A04
Bethesda, MD 20892 (301) 496-3583

## CYTARABINE

National Cancer Institute
Bldg. 31, Room 10A16
Bethesda, MD 20892 (800) 4-CANCER

## CYTOMEGALIC INCLUSION BODY DISEASE

National Institute of Neurological Disorders and Stroke
Bldg. 31, Room 8A16 (301) 496-5751
Bethesda, MD 20892 (800) 352-9424

## CYTOMEGALOVIRUS (CMV)

National Heart, Lung, and Blood Institute
Information Center
P.O. Box 30105
Bethesda, MD 20824-0105 (301) 251-1222

Centers for Disease Control
Information Resources Management Office
1600 Clifton Drive
Atlanta, GA 30333 (404) 332-4555

# - D -

## DACTINOMYCIN

National Cancer Institute
Bldg. 31, Room 10A16
Bethesda, MD 20892 (800) 4-CANCER

## DALTONISM

*See Color Blindness*

## DANDY-WALKER SYNDROME

National Institute of Neurological Disorders and Stroke
Bldg. 31, Room 8A16
Bethesda, MD 20892 (301) 496-5751
(800) 352-9424

## DARIER'S DISEASE

National Institute of Arthritis and Musculoskeletal
and Skin Diseases
1 AMS Way
Bethesda, MD 20892 (301) 495-4484

## DAUNORUBICIN

National Cancer Institute
Bldg. 31, Room 10A16
Bethesda, MD 20892 (800) 4-CANCER

## DAY CARE

Clearinghouse on Child Abuse and Neglect Information
P.O. Box 1182
Washington, DC 20013
(800) FYI-3366
(800) 394-3366

## DEAFNESS

*See also Communication Disorders*

National Institute on Deafness and Other Communication Disorders Clearinghouse
1 Communication Avenue
Bethesda, MD 20892-3456
(301) 496-7243
(800) 241-1044
(301) 241-1055 (TDD)

## DEATH

*See also Living Wills*

National Institute on Aging
Information Center
P.O. Box 8057
Bethesda, MD 20898-80507
(800) 222-2225

National Institute of Mental Health
5600 Fishers Ln.
Room 7C-02
Rockville, MD 20857
(301) 443-4515

Division of Vital Statistics
National Center for Health Statistics
6525 Belcrest Road
Hyattsville, MD 20782
(301) 436-8952

## DECARBAZINE

National Cancer Institute
Bldg. 31, Room 10A16
Bethesda, MD 20892 (800) 4-CANCER

## DECUBITUS ULCERS

National Institute of Arthritis and Musculoskeletal and Skin Diseases
1 AMS Way
Bethesda, MD 20892 (301) 495-4484

## DEGENERATIVE BASAL GANGLIA DISEASE

National Institute of Neurological Disorders and Stroke
Bldg. 31, Room 8A16
Bethesda, MD 20892 (301) 496-5751
(800) 352-9424

## DEGENERATIVE JOINT DISEASE

National Institute of Arthritis and Musculoskeletal and Skin Diseases
1 AMS Way
Bethesda, MD 20892 (301) 495-4484

## DEGLUTITION

National Institute of Dental Research
Bldg. 31, Room 2C35
31 Center Drive, MSC-2290
Bethesda, MD 20892-2290 (301) 496-4261

## DEJERINE-SOTTAS DISEASE

National Institute of Neurological Disorders and Stroke
Bldg. 31, Room 8A16 (301) 496-5751
Bethesda, MD 20892 (800) 352-9424

## DEMENTIA

*See also Mental Illness; Alzheimer's Disease; Presenile Dementia*

National Institute on Aging
Information Center
P.O. Box 8057
Gaithersburg, MD 20898-8057 (800) 222-2225

National Institute of Neurological Disorders and Stroke
Building 31, Room 8A06 (301) 496-5751
Bethesda, MD 20892 (800) 352-9424

## DEMYELINATING DISEASES

National Institute of Neurological Disorders and Stroke
Building 31, Room 8A06 (301) 496-5751
Bethesda, MD 20892 (800) 352-9424

## DENGUE

National Institute of Allergy and Infectious Diseases
Building 31. Room 7A50
Bethesda, MD 20892 (301) 496-5717

## DENTAL DISEASE

National Institute of Dental Research
Bldg. 31, Room 2C35

31 Center Drive, MSC-2290
Bethesda, MD 20892-2290 (301) 496-4261

## DENTAL PROCEDURES AND AIDS

Centers for Disease Control
National AIDS Clearinghouse
P.O. Box 6003
Rockville, MD 20849-6003 (800) 458-5231

## DENTAL RESTORATIVE MATERIALS

National Institute of Dental Research
Bldg. 31, Room 2C35
Bethesda, MD 20892 (301) 496-4261

## DENTAL SEALANTS

National Institute of Dental Research
Bldg. 31, Room 2C35
31 Center Drive, MSC-2290
Bethesda, MD 20892 (301) 496-4261

## DENTAL X-RAYS

National Institute of Dental Research
Bldg. 31, Room 2C35
31 Center Drive, MSC-2290
Bethesda, MD 20892 (301) 496-4261

## DENTOBACTERIAL PLAQUE INFECTION

National Institute of Dental Research
Bldg. 31, Room 2C35
31 Center Dr., MSC-2290
Bethesda, MD 20892-2290 (301) 496-4261

## DENTURES

National Institute of Dental Research
31 Center Dr., MSC-2290
Bethesda, MD 20892-2290 (301) 496-4261

## DEPRESSION

National Institute of Mental Health
5600 Fishers Ln., Room 7C-02
Rockville, MD 20857 (301) 443-4515

## DEPTH PERCEPTION

National Eye Institute
Bldg. 31, Room 6A32
Bethesda, MD 20892 (301) 496-5248

## DERMAGRAPHISMS

National Institute of Allergy and Infectious Diseases
Bldg. 31, Room 7A50
Bethesda, MD 20892 (301) 496-5717

## DERMATITIS HERPETIFORMIS

National Institute of Arthritis and Musculoskeletal and Skin Diseases
1 AMS Way
Bethesda, MD 20892 (301) 495-4484

## DERMATOGRAPHISM

National Institute of Allergy and Infectious Diseases

Building 31, Room 7A50
Bethesda, MD 20892 (301) 496-5717

## DERMATOLOGY

National Institute of Arthritis and Musculoskeletal and Skin Diseases
1 AMS Way
Bethesda, MD 20892 (301) 495-4484

## DERMATOMYOSITIS

National Institute of Arthritis and Musculoskeletal and Skin Diseases
1 AMS Way
Bethesda, MD 20892 (301) 495-4484

## DES

National Cancer Institute
Building 31, Room 10A18
Bethesda, MD 20892 (800) 4-CANCER

## DEVELOPMENTAL DISABILITIES

Center for Developmental Disabilities
Benson Building, First Floor
Columbia, SC 29208 (800) 922-9234, Ext. 201

## DEVIC'S SYNDROME

National Institute of Neurological Disorders and Stroke
Bldg. 31, Room 8A16
Bethesda, MD 20892 (301) 496-5751
(800) 352-9424

## DEXTRANASE

National Institute of Dental Research
Bldg. 31, Room 2C35
31 Center Dr., MSC-2290
Bethesda, MD 20892-2290 (301) 496-4261

## DHOBIE ITCH

National Arthritis and Musculoskeletal and
Skin Diseases Clearinghouse
1 AMS Way
Bethesda, MD 20892 (301) 495-4484

## DIABETES

National Diabetes Information Clearinghouse
1 Information Way
Bethesda, MD 20892 (301) 654-3810

## DIABETIC NEUROPATHY

National Institute of Neurological Disorders and Stroke
Bldg. 31, Room 8A16
Bethesda, MD 20892 (301) 496-5751
(800) 352-9424

## DIABETIC RETINOPATHY

National Eye Institute
Bldg. 31, Room 6A32
Bethesda, MD 20892 (301) 496-5248

## DIAGNOSTIC IMAGING

National Cancer Institute
6100 Executive Blvd., Room 800
Rockville, MD 20892 (800) 4-CANCER

## DIALYSIS

National Kidney and Urologic Diseases Information Clearinghouse
3 Information Way
Bethesda, MD 20892 (301) 654-4415

## DIAPER RASH

Over-the-Counter Drug Evaluation Division
Food and Drug Administration
5600 Fishers Lane
Rockville, MD 20857 (301) 594-1924

## DIARRHEA

National Institute of Diabetes and Digestive and Kidney Diseases
Bldg. 31, Room 9A04
Bethesda, MD 20892 (301) 496-3583

National Institute of Allergy and Infectious Diseases
Building 31, Room 7A50
Bethesda, MD 20892 (301) 496-5717

## DIET

*See Nutrition; Food*

## DIETARY SUPPLEMENTS

National Institute on Aging
Information Center
P.O. Box 8057
Gaithersburg, MD 20898-8057 (800) 222-2225

## DIETHYLSTILBESTROL (DES)

*See DES*

## DIETING

Food and Drug Administration
(HFE-88), 5600 Fishers Lane
Rockville, MD 20857 (301) 443-3170

## DIFFUSE SCLEROSIS

National Institute of Neurological Disorders and Stroke
Bldg. 31, Room 8A16 (301) 496-5751
Bethesda, MD 20892 (800) 352-9424

## DIGESTIVE DISEASES

National Digestive Diseases Information Clearinghouse
2 Information Way
Bethesda, MD 20892 (301) 654-3810

## DIOXIN

Toxic Substances Control Act Hotline

401 M St., SW
Washington, DC 20024 (202) 554-1404

## DIPHTHERIA

National Institute of Allergy and Infectious Diseases
Building 31, Room 7A50
Bethesda, MD 20892 (301) 496-5717

## DISABILITIES

*See also Rehabilitation*

National Rehabilitation Information Center
8455 Colesville Rd.
Suite 935
Silver Spring, MD 20910
(800) 346-2742

## DISABLED INFANTS

National Information Clearinghouse for Infants with
Disabilities and Life-Threatening Conditions (NICIDLC)
Benson Building, First Floor
Columbia, SC 29208 (800) 922-9234
(800) 922-1107 (in SC)

## DISASTERS

National Institute of Mental Health
5600 Fishers Lane, Room 7C-02
Rockville, MD 20857 (301) 443-4515

Federal Emergency Management Agency
500 C St., SW
Washington, DC 20472 (202) 646-4600

## DISCOID LUPUS ERYTHEMATOSUS

National Institute of Arthritis and Musculoskeletal and Skin Diseases
1 AMS Way
Bethesda, MD 20892 (301) 495-4484

## DISEASE HOTLINE

Centers for Disease Control
Disease Hotline
4770 Buford Hwy., NE
Atlanta, GA 30341 (404) 332-4555

## DIURETICS

National Heart, Lung, and Blood Institute
Information Center
P.O. Box 30105
Bethesda, MD 20824-0105 (301) 251-1222

## DIURNALDYSTONIA

National Institute of Neurological Disorders and Stroke
Building 31, Room 8A16
Bethesda, MD 20892 (301) 496-5751
(800) 352-9424

## DIVERTICULITIS

National Institute of Diabetes and Digestive and Kidney Diseases
Bldg. 31, Room 9A04
Bethesda, MD 20892 (301) 496-3583

## DIVORCE

National Institute of Mental Health
5600 Fishers Ln.
Room 7C-02
Rockville, MD 20857 (301) 443-4515

## DIZYGOTIC TWINS (Fraternal Twins)

*See Twins*

## DIZZINESS

National Institute of Neurological Disorders and Stroke
Bldg. 31, Room 8A16
Bethesda, MD 20892 (301) 496-5751
(800) 352-9424

## DNA

*See also Genetics; Genetic Testing*

National Cancer Institute
Bldg. 31, Room 10A16
Bethesda, MD 20892 (800) 4-CANCER

## DOWN'S SYNDROME

National Institute of Child Health and Human Development
Bldg. 31, Room 2A32
Bethesda, MD 20892 (301) 496-5133

## DOXORRUBICIN

National Cancer Institute
Bldg. 31, Room 10A24
Bethesda, MD 20892 (800) 4-CANCER

## DPT VACCINE (Diphtheria-Pertussis-Tetanus)

*See Immunizations*

## DRINKING AND CANCER

National Cancer Institute
Bldg. 31, Room 10A16
Bethesda, MD 20892 (800) 4-CANCER

## DRINKING WATER

Environmental Protection Agency
401 M St., SW
Washington, DC 20460 (800) 426-4791

## DROPSY

*See Edema*

## DRUG ABUSE

*See also Alcoholism; specific drug; Workplace Drug Abuse*

National Drug Abuse Information and Treatment Hotline
c/o Phoenix House Foundation

164 W 74th St. (800) 662-HELP
New York, NY 10023 (800) 66-AYUNDA (Spanish speakers)

National Clearinghouse for Alcohol and Drug Information
P.O. Box 2345
Rockville, MD 20852 (301) 468-2600
(800) 729-6686

## DRUG ALLERGY

National Institute of Allergy and Infectious Diseases
Bldg. 31, Room 7A50
Bethesda, MD 20892 (301) 496-5717

## DRUG DEVELOPMENT

Food and Drug Administration
(HFE-88), 5600 Fishers Lane
Rockville, MD 20857 (301) 443-3170

## DRUG EVALUATION

Center for Drug Evaluation and Research
Food and Drug Administration
5600 Fishers Lane
Rockville, MD 20857 (301) 295-1012

## DRUG HEMOLYTIC ANEMIA

National Institute of Diabetes and Digestive
and Kidney Diseases
Bldg. 31, Room 9A04
Bethesda, MD 20892 (301) 496-3583

## DRUG INTERACTIONS

Food and Drug Administration
(HFE-88), 5600 Fishers Lane
Rockville, MD 20857 (301) 443-3170

## DRUG LABELING

Food and Drug Administration
(HFE-88), 5600 Fishers Lane
Rockville, MD 20857 (301) 443-3170

## DRUG PURPURA

National Institute of Diabetes and Digestive
and Kidney Diseases
Bldg. 31, Room 9A04
Bethesda, MD 20892 (301) 496-3583

## DRUG RESISTANCE

National Institute of Allergy and Infectious Diseases
Bldg. 31, Room 7A50
Bethesda, MD 20892 (301) 496-5717

## DRUG TESTING

National Institute of Justice
U.S. Department of Justice
P.O. Box 6000
Rockville, MD 20850 (800) 851-3420

## DRUG TREATMENT

*See also Drug Abuse*

National Clearinghouse for Alcohol and Drug Information
P.O. Box 2345
Rockville, MD 20852 (800) 729-6686

## DRUNK DRIVING

National Center for Statistics and Analysis
National Highway Traffic Safety Administration
400 7th Street SW
Washington, DC 20590 (202) 366-1470

## DRY EYES

National Eye Institute
Building 31, Room 6A32
Bethesda, MD 20892 (301) 496-5248

## DRY MOUTH

National Institute of Dental Research
Building 31, Room 2C35
31 Center Dr., MSC-2290
Bethesda, MD 20892-2290 (301) 496-4261

## DUCHENNE MUSCULAR DYSTROPHY

National Institute of Arthritis and Musculoskeletal and Skin Diseases
1 AMS Way
Bethesda, MD 20892 (301) 495-4484

## DUPUYTREN'S CONTRACTURE

National Institute of Arthritis and Musculoskeletal and Skin Diseases
1 AMS Way
Bethesda, MD 20892 (301) 495-4484

## DUST INHALATION DISEASES

National Heart, Lung, and Blood Institute
Information Center
P.O. Box 30105
Bethesda, MD 20824-0105 (301) 251-1222

National Institute of Occupational Safety and Health
4676 Columbia Parkway
Cincinnati OH 45226 (800) 35-NIOSH

## DWARFISM

National Institute of Child Health and Human Development
Bldg. 31, Room 2A32
Bethesda, MD 20892 (301) 496-5133

## DYSAUTONOMIA

National Institute of Neurological Disorders and Stroke
Bldg. 31, Room 8A16
Bethesda, MD 20892 (301) 496-5751
(800) 352-9424

## DYSENTERY

National Institute of Allergy and Infectious Diseases
Bldg. 31, Room 7A50
Bethesda, MD 20892 (301) 496-5717

## DYSKINESIA

National Institute of Neurological Disorders and Stroke
Bldg. 31, Room 8A16
Bethesda, MD 20892 (301) 496-5751
(800) 352-9424

## DYSLEXIA

National Institute of Child Health and Human Development
Bldg. 31, Room 2A32
Bethesda, MD 20892 (301) 496-5133

National Institute on Deafness and Other Communication Disorders
1 Communication Ave.
Bethesda, MD 20892-3456 (800) 241-1044
(800) 241-1055 (TDD)

National Institute of Neurological Disorders and Stroke
Bldg. 31, Room 8A16
Bethesda, MD 20892 (301) 496-5751
(800) 352-9424

## DYSMENORRHEA

National Institute of Child Health and Human Development
Bldg. 31, Room 2A32
Bethesda, MD 20892 (301) 496-5133

## DYSPEPSIA

National Digestive Diseases Information Clearinghouse
2 Information Way
Bethesda, MD 20892 (301) 654-3810

## DYSTONIA

National Institute of Neurological Disorders and Stroke
Bldg. 31, Room 8A16
Bethesda, MD 20892 (301) 496-5751
(800) 352-9424

# - E -

## EAR INFECTIONS

National Institute on Deafness and Other Communication Disorders
1 Communication Ave.
Bethesda, MD 20892-3456 (800) 241-1044
(800) 241-1055 (TDD)

## EATING DISORDERS

*See also Anorexia*

National Institute of Diabetes and Digestive and Kidney Diseases
Bldg. 31, Room 3A18B
Bethesda, MD 20892 (301) 496-7823

## EATON-LAMBERT MYASTHENIC SYNDROME

National Institute of Neurological Disorders and Stroke
Bldg. 31, Room 8A16
Bethesda, MD 20892 (301) 496-5751
(800) 352-9424

## ECHOCARDIOGRAPHY

National Heart, Lung, and Blood Institute
Information Center
P.O. Box 30105
Bethesda, MD 20824-0105 (301) 251-1222

## ECLAMPSIA

*See also Pregnancy*

National Institute of Child Health and Human Development
Bldg. 31, Room 2A32
Bethesda, MD 20892 (301) 496-5133

## ECTODERMAL DYSPLASIAS

National Institute of Arthritis and Musculoskeletal and Skin Diseases
1 AMS Way
Bethesda, MD 20892 (301) 495-4484

## ECTOPIC HORMONES

National Institute of Diabetes and Digestive and Kidney Diseases
Building 31, Room 9A04
Bethesda, MD 20892 (301) 496-3583

## ECTOPIC PREGNANCY

National Institute of Child Health and Human Development
Building 31, Room 2A32
Bethesda, MD 20892 (301) 496-5133

## ECZEMA

National Institute of Arthritis and Musculoskeletal and Skin Diseases
1 AMS Way
Bethesda, MD 20892 (301) 495-4484

National Institute of Allergy and Infectious Diseases
Bldg. 31, Room 7A50
Bethesda, MD 20892 (301) 496-5717

## EDEMA

National Heart, Lung, and Blood Institute
Information Center
P.O. Box 30105
Bethesda, MD 20824-0105 (301) 251-1222

## EGGS

*See also Food*

Food and Drug Administration
(HFE-88), 5600 Fishers Lane
Rockville, MD 20857 (301) 443-3170

## EHLERS-DANLOS SYNDROME

National Institute of Arthritis and Musculoskeletal and Skin Diseases
1 AMS Way
Bethesda, MD 20892 (301) 495-4484

## EISENMENGER'S SYNDROME

National Heart, Lung, and Blood Institute
Information Center

P.O. Box 30105
Bethesda, MD 20824-0105 (301) 251-1222

## EKGs

National Heart, Lung, and Blood Institute
Information Center
P.O. Box 30105
Bethesda, MD 20824-0105 (301) 251-1222

## ELDER ABUSE

*See also Aging*

National Resource on Domestic Violence
6400 Flank Drive, Suite 1300
Harrisburg, PA 17112 (800) 537-2238

## ELDERLY

*See Aging*

## ELECTRICAL STIMULATION

Center for Devices and Radiological Health
12721 Twinbrook Parkway
Rockville, MD 20857 (301) 443-3840

## ELECTRIC BLANKETS

Center for Devices and Radiological Health
(HFZ-210), Food and Drug Administration
5600 Fishers Lane
Rockville, MD 20857 (301) 443-6597

## ELECTROCARDIOGRAM

National Heart, Lung, and Blood Institute
Information Center
P.O. Box 30105
Bethesda, MD 20824-0105 (301) 251-1222

## ELECTROMAGNETIC FIELDS

Center for Devices and Radiological Health
(HFZ-210)
Food and Drug Administration
5600 Fishers Lane
Rockville, MD 20857 (301) 443-6597

## ELECTRO-SHOCK TREATMENT

National Institute of Mental Health
5600 Fishers Lane
Room 7C-02
Rockville, MD 20857 (301) 443-4515

## ELEPHANTIASIS

National Institute of Allergy and Infectious Diseases
Bldg. 31, Room 7A50
Bethesda, MD 20892 (301) 496-5717

## EMBOLISMS

National Heart, Lung, and Blood Institute
Information Center
P.O. Box 30105
Bethesda, MD 20824-0105 (301) 251-1222

## EMPHYSEMA

National Heart, Lung, and Blood Institute
Information Center
P.O. Box 30105
Bethesda, MD 20824-0105 (301) 251-1222

## ENAMEL

National Institute of Dental Research
Building 31, Room 2C35
31 Center Drive, MSC-2290
Bethesda, MD 20892-2290 (301) 496-4261

## ENCEPHALITIS

National Institute of Allergy and Infectious Diseases
Building 31, Room 7A50
Bethesda, MD 20892 (301) 496-5717

Centers for Disease Control Information Resources Management Office
4770 Buford Hwy., NE
Atlanta, GA 30341 (404) 332-4555

## ENCEPHALITIS LETHARGICA

National Institute of Neurological Disorders and Stroke
Bldg. 31, Room 8A16 (301) 496-5751
Bethesda, MD 20892 (800) 352-9424

## ENCEPHALOMYELITIS

National Institute of Neurological Disorders and Stroke
Bldg. 31, Room 8A16 (301) 496-5751
Bethesda, MD 20892 (800) 352-9424

## ENCOPRESIS

National Institute of Child Health and Human Development
Building 31, Room 2A32
Bethesda, MD 20824 (301) 496-5133

## ENDOCARDITIS

National Heart, Lung, and Blood Institute
Information Center
P.O. Box 30105
Bethesda, MD 20824-0105 (301) 251-1222

## ENDOCRINE GLANDS

National Institute of Child Health and Human Development
Bldg. 31, Room 2A32
Bethesda, MD 20892 (301) 496-5133

## ENDOCRINOLOGIC MUSCLE DISEASE

National Institute of Neurological Disorders and Stroke
Bldg. 31, Room 8A16
Bethesda, MD 20892 (301) 496-5751
(800) 352-9424

## ENDODONTICS

National Institute of Dental Research
Bldg. 31, Room 2C35
31 Center Drive, MSC-2290
Bethesda, MD 20892-2290 (301) 496-4261

## ENDOGENOUS DEPRESSION

*See Depression*

## ENDOMETRIOSIS

National Institute of Child Health and Human Development
Bldg. 31, Room 2A32
Bethesda, MD 20892 (301) 496-5133

## ENIGMATIC BLISTERING DISORDERS

National Institute of Arthritis and Musculoskeletal and Skin Diseases
1 AMS Way
Bethesda, MD 20892 (301) 495-4484

## ENTERIC DISEASES

Centers for Disease Control
Information Resources Management Office
Mail Stop C-15, 1600 Clifton Rd., NE
Atlanta, GA 30333 (404) 332-4555

National Institute of Diabetes and Digestive and Kidney Diseases
Bldg. 31, Room 9A04
Bethesda, MD 20892 (301) 496-3583

## ENVIRONMENTAL HEALTH

National Institute of Environmental Health Sciences
P.O. Box 12233
Research Triangle Park, NC 27709 (919) 541-3345

## ENVIRONMENTAL ISSUES

Environmental Protection Agency
Public Information Center
401 M St., SW
Mail Code 3404
Washington, DC 20460 (202) 260-7751

## EOSINOPHILIC GRANULOMA

National Heart, Lung, and Blood Institute
Information Center
P.O. Box 30105
Bethesda, MD 20824-0105 (301) 251-1222

## EPICONDYLITIS

*See Tennis Elbow*

## EPIDEMIOLOGY

National Heart, Lung and Blood Institute
Information Center
P.O. Box 30105
Bethesda, MD 20824-0105 (301) 251-1222

## EPIDERMODYSPLASIA VERRUCIFORMIS

National Institute of Arthritis and Musculoskeletal
and Skin Diseases
1 AMS Way
Bethesda, MD 20892 (301) 495-4484

## EPIDERMOLYSIS BULLOSA

National Institute of Arthritis and Musculoskeletal and Skin Diseases
1 AMS Way
Bethesda, MD 20892 (301) 495-4484

## EPIGLOTTITIS

National Institute of Allergy and Infectious Diseases
Bldg. 31, Room 7A50
Bethesda, MD 20892 (301) 496-5717

## EPIKERATOPHAKIA

National Eye Institute
Bldg. 31, Room 6A32
Bethesda, MD 20892 (301) 496-5248

## EPILEPSY

National Institute of Neurological Disorders and Stroke
Bldg. 31, Room 8A16 (301) 496-5751
Bethesda, MD 20892 (800) 352-9424

## EPISTAXIS

*See Nosebleeds*

## EPSTEIN-BARR SYNDROME

National Institute of Allergy and Infectious Diseases
Bldg. 31, Room 7A50
Bethesda, MD 20892 (301) 496-5717

## EQUINE ENCEPHALITIS

National Institute of Allergy and Infectious Diseases
Bldg. 31, Room 7A50
Bethesda, MD 20892 (301) 496-5717

## ERYTHEMA ELEVATUM DIUTINUM

National Institute of Arthritis and Musculoskeletal and Skin Diseases
1 AMS Way
Bethesda, MD 20892 (301) 495-4484

## ERYTHEMA MULTIFORME

National Institute of Allergy and Infectious Diseases
Building 31, Room 7A50
Bethesda, MD 20892 (301) 496-5717

## ERYTHEMA NODOSUM

National Institute of Allergy and Infectious Diseases
Building 31, Room 7A50
Bethesda, MD 20892 (301) 496-5717

## ERYTHROBLASTOSIS FETALIS

National Institute of Child Health and Human Development
Building 31, Room 2A32
Bethesda, MD 20892 (301) 496-5133

## ERYTHROCYTES

*See Blood*

## ESOPHAGEAL DISORDERS

National Institute of Diabetes and Digestive
and Kidney Diseases
Building 31, Room 9A04
Bethesda, MD 20892 (301) 496-3583

National Cancer Institute
Bldg. 31, Room 10A16
Bethesda, MD 20892 (800) 4-CANCER

## ESOTROPIA

*See Cross-Eye*

## ESTRAMUSTINE

National Cancer Institute
Bldg. 31, Room 10A16
Bethesda, MD 20892 (800) 4-CANCER

## ESTREPTOZOCINA

National Cancer Institute
Bldg. 31, Room 10A16
Bethesda, MD 20892 (800) 4-CANCER

## ESTROGEN

National Institute of Child Health and Human Development
Bldg. 31, Room 2A32
Bethesda, MD 20892 (301) 496-5133

National Institute on Aging
Information Center
P.O. Box 8057
Gaithersburg, MD 20898-8057 (800) 222-2225

## EUTHANASIA

*See Living Wills*

## EWING'S SARCOMA

National Cancer Institute
Bldg. 31, Room 10A16
Bethesda, MD 20892 (800) 4-CANCER

## EXERCISE

*See also Worksite Health and Safety*

National Institute of Arthritis and Musculoskeletal and Skin Diseases
1 AMS Way
Bethesda, MD 20892 (301) 495-4484

President's Council on Physical Fitness and Sports
701 Pennsylvania Avenue, NW
Suite 250
Washington, DC 20004 (202) 272-3421

## EXOTROPIA

National Eye Institute
Bldg. 31, Room 6A32
Bethesda, MD 20892 (301) 496-5248

## EXPERIMENTAL ALLERGIC ENCEPHALOMYELITIS

National Institute of Neurological Disorders and Stroke
Bldg. 31, Room 8A16
Bethesda, MD 20892
(301) 496-5751
(800) 352-9424

## EXTENDED CARE FACILITY

*See Long Term Care; Nursing Homes*

## EXTRACORPOREAL SHOCK-WAVE LITHOTRIPSY

National Institute of Diabetes and Digestive and Kidney Diseases
Bldg. 31, Room 9A04
Bethesda, MD 20892
(301) 496-3583

## EXTRAPYRAMIDAL DISORDERS

National Institute of Neurological Disorders and Stroke
Bldg. 31, Room 8A16
Bethesda, MD 20892
(301) 496-5751
(800) 352-9424

## EYE BANKS

National Eye Institute
Bldg. 31, Room 6A32
Bethesda, MD 20892
(301) 496-5248

## EYE CARE

*See also Vision; Contact Lenses*

National Eye Institute
Building 31, Room 6A32
Bethesda, MD 20892 (301) 496-5248

## EYE EXERCISES

National Eye Institute
Building 31, Room 6A32
Bethesda, MD 20892 (301) 496-5248

## EYE TUMORS

National Eye Institute
Building 31, Room 6A32
Bethesda, MD 20892 (301) 496-5248

# - F -

## FABRY'S DISEASE

National Institute of Neurological Disorders and Stroke
Building 31, Room 8A16 (301) 496-5751
Bethesda, MD 20892 (800) 352-9424

## FACE LIFTS

Center for Devices and Radiological Health
Food and Drug Administration, HFZ-210
Rockville, MD 20857 (301) 443-4190

## FACIAL TICS

National Institute of Neurological Disorders and Stroke
Bldg. 31, Room 8A16 (301) 496-5751
Bethesda, MD 20892 (800) 352-9424

## FAINTING

National Heart, Lung, and Blood Institute Information Center
P.O. Box 30105
Bethesda, MD 20824-0105 (301) 251-1222

## FALLS AND FRAILTY

*See also Aging*

National Institute on Aging Information Center
P.O. Box 8057
Gaithersburg, MD 20898-8057 (800) 222-2225

## FAMILIAL ATAXIA TELANGIECTASIA

National Institute of Neurological Disorders and Stroke
Building 31, Room 8A16 (301) 496-5751
Bethesda, MD 20892 (800) 352-9424

National Cancer Institute
Bldg. 31, Room 10A16
Bethesda, MD 20892 (800) 4-CANCER

## FAMILIAL MULTIPLE ENDOCRINE NEOPLASIA

National Institute of Diabetes and Digestive and Kidney Diseases
Bldg. 31, Room 9A04
Bethesda, MD 20892 (301) 496-3583

## FAMILIAL SPASTIC PARAPARESIS

National Institute of Neurological Disorders and Stroke
Bldg. 31, Room 8A16 (301) 496-5751
Bethesda, MD 20892 (800) 352-9424

## FAMILY PLANNING

*See also Contraception*

National Institute of Child Health and Human Development
Bldg. 31, Room 2A32
Bethesda, MD 20892 (301) 496-5133

Family Life Information Exchange
P.O. Box 37299
Washington, DC 20013 (301) 585-6636

## FAMILY VIOLENCE

National Resource Center on Domestic Violence
6400 Flank Dr., Suite 1300
Harrisburg, PA 17112 (800) 537-2238

## FANCONI'S ANEMIA

National Heart, Lung, and Blood Institute Information Center
P.O. Box 30105
Bethesda, MD 20824-0105 (301) 251-1222

## FARMERS LUNG

National Institute of Occupational Safety and Health
4676 Columbia Parkway, MS C-13
Cincinnati, OH 45226 (800) 35-NIOSH

## FARSIGHTEDNESS

National Eye Institute
Bldg. 31, Room 6A32
Bethesda, MD 20892 (301) 496-5248

## FASCIOLIASIS

National Institute of Allergy and Infectious Diseases
Bldg. 31, Room 7A50
Bethesda, MD 20892 (301) 496-5717

## FAST FOOD

*See also Food*

Food and Drug Administration
HFE-88, 5600 Fishers Lane
Rockville, MD 20857 (301) 443-3170

## FASTING

Food and Nutrition Information Center
National Agricultural Library, Room 304
Beltsville, MD 20705 (301) 504-5719

## FATHERHOOD

National Institute of Child Health
and Human Development
Bldg. 31, Room 2A32
Bethesda, MD 20892 (301) 496-5133

## FAT SUBSTITUTES

*See also Food; Nutrition*

Food and Drug Administration
(HFE-88), 5600 Fishers Lane
Rockville, MD 20857 (301) 443-3170

## FEBRILE CONVULSIONS

National Institute of Neurological Disorders and Stroke
Bldg. 31, Room 8A16
Bethesda, MD 20892 (301) 496-5751
(800) 352-9424

## FEBRILE SEIZURES

National Institute of Child Health and Human Development
Building 31, Room 2A32
Bethesda, MD 20892 (301) 496-5133

## FEEDING IMPAIRMENTS

National Institute of Dental Research
Building 31, Room 2C35
31 Center Dr., MSC-2290
Bethesda, MD 20892 (301) 496-4261

## FEET

National Institute of Arthritis and Musculoskeletal and Skin Diseases
1 AMS Way
Bethesda, MD 20892 (301) 495-4484

## FERTILITY

National Institute of Child Health and Human Development
Building 31, Room 2A32
Bethesda, MD 20892 (301) 496-5133

## FETAL ALCOHOL SYNDROME

National Institute of Child Health and Human Development
Bldg. 31, Room 2A32
Bethesda, MD 20892 (301) 496-5133

National Clearinghouse for Alcohol and Drug Information
P.O. Box 2345
Rockville, MD 20852 (800) 729-6686

## FETAL MONITORING

*See also Sudden Infant Death Syndrome*

National Institute of Child Health and Human Development
Bldg. 31, Room 2A32
Bethesda, MD 20892 (301) 496-5133

## FEVERS

National Institute of Allergy and Infectious Diseases
Bldg. 31, Room 7A50
Bethesda, MD 20892 (301) 496-5717

## FEVER BLISTERS

National Institute of Dental Research
Bldg. 31, Room 2C35
31 Center Dr., MSC-2290
Bethesda, MD 20892-2290 (301) 496-4261

## FIBER

Food and Drug Administration
(HFE-88), 5600 Fishers Lane
Rockville, MD 20857 (301) 443-3170

## FIBRILLATION

National Heart, Lung, and Blood Institute
Information Center
P.O. Box 30105
Bethesda, MD 20824-0105 (301) 251-1222

## FIBRINOLYSIS

National Heart, Lung, and Blood Institute
Information Center
P.O. Box 30105
Bethesda, MD 20824-0105 (301) 251-1222

## FIBROCYSTIC DISEASE OF THE BREAST

National Cancer Institute
Bldg. 31, Room 10A16
Bethesda, MD 20892 (800) 4-CANCER

## FIBROID TUMORS

National Institute of Child Health
and Human Development
Bldg. 31, Room 2A32
Bethesda, MD 20892 (301) 496-5133

## FIBROMUSCULAR HYPERPLASIA

National Institute of Arthritis and Musculoskeletal
and Skin Diseases
1 AMS Way
Bethesda, MD 20892 (301) 495-4484

## FIBROMYALGIA

National Institute of Arthritis and Musculoskeletal
and Skin Diseases
1 AMS Way
Bethesda, MD 20892 (301) 495-4484

## FIBROSITIS

National Institute of Arthritis and Musculoskeletal
and Skin Diseases
1 AMS Way
Bethesda, MD 20892 (301) 495-4484

## FIBROTIC LUNG DISEASES

National Heart, Lung, and Blood Institute
Information Center
P.O. Box 30105
Bethesda, MD 20824-0105 (301) 251-1222

## FIBROUS DYSPLASIA

National Institute of Neurological Disorders and Stroke
Bldg. 31, Room 8A16
Bethesda, MD 20892 (301) 496-5751
(800) 352-9424

## FIFTH DISEASE

National Institute of Allergy and Infectious Diseases
Bldg. 31, Room 7A50
Bethesda, MD 20892 (301) 496-5717

## FILARIASIS

National Institute of Allergy and Infectious Diseases
Bldg. 31, Room 7A50
Bethesda, MD 20892 (301) 496-5717

## FLOATERS

National Eye Institute
Bldg. 31, Room 6A32
Bethesda, MD 20892 (301) 496-5248

## FLOPPY BABY

National Institute of Neurological Disorders and Stroke
Bldg. 31, Room 8A16 (301) 496-5751
Bethesda, MD 20892 (800) 352-9424

## FLOXIRIDINE

National Cancer Institute
Bldg. 31, Room 10A16
Bethesda, MD 20892 (800) 4-CANCER

## FLU

National Institute of Allergy and Infectious Diseases

Building 31, Room 7A50
Bethesda, MD 20892 (301) 496-5717

Centers for Disease Control
1600 Clifton Rd., NE
Atlanta, GA 30333
Disease Hotline (404) 332-4555

## FLUORESCEIN ANGIOGRAPHY

National Eye Institute
Bldg. 31, Room 6A32
Bethesda, MD 20892 (301) 496-5248

## FLUORESCENT LAMPS

Center for Devices and Radiological Health
(HFZ-210), Food and Drug Administration
5600 Fishers Lane
Rockville, MD 20857 (301) 443-4690

## FLUORIDATION

National Institute of Dental Research
Bldg. 31, Room 2C35
31 Center Dr., MSC-2290
Bethesda, MD 20892-2290 (301) 496-4261

## FLUOROSCOPY

Center for Devices and Radiological Health
(HFZ-210), Food and Drug Administration
5600 Fishers Lane
Rockville, MD 20857 (301) 443-4690

## FLUOROSIS

National Institute of Dental Research
Bldg. 31, Room 2C35
31 Center Dr., MSC-2290
Bethesda, MD 20892-2290 (301) 496-4261

## FLUOROURACIL

National Cancer Institute
Bldg. 31, Room 10A16
Bethesda, MD 20892 (800) 4-CANCER

## FOOD

*See also Nutrition*

Center for Nutrition Policy and Promotion
USDA
Suite 200 North Lobby
1120 20th St, NW
Washington, DC 20036 (202) 418-2312

Agricultural Research Service
U.S. Department of Agriculture
Room 363
6505 Belcrest Rd
Hyattsville, MD 20782 (301) 436-8617

Food and Nutrition Information Center
National Agricultural Library
Room 304
Beltsville, MD 20705 (301) 504-5719

Center for Food Safety and Applied Nutrition
200 C Street SW
Washington, DC 20204 (202) 205-4317

Food and Nutrition Service
Park Office Bldg.
3101 Park Center Dr.
Alexandria, VA 22302 (703) 305-2554

## FOOD ADDITIVES

Center for Food Safety and Applied Nutrition
Food and Drug Administration
Office of Constituents
200 C Street, SW, HFF-11
Washington, DC 20204 (202) 205-4317

## FOOD ALLERGIES

*See Allergies*

## FOOD AND DRUG INTERACTIONS

Food and Drug Administration
(HFE-88), 5600 Fishers Lane
Rockville, MD 20857 (301) 443-3170

## FOOD IRRADIATION

Center for Food Safety and Applied Nutrition
Food and Drug Administration
Office of Constituents
200 C Street, SW, HFF-11
Washington, DC 20204 (202) 205-4317

## FOOD LABELING

Food Labeling Education Information Center
National Exchange for Food Labeling Education

Food and Nutrition Information Center
National Agricultural Library
10301 Baltimore Blvd., Room 304
Beltsville, MD 20704 (301) 504-5472

## FOOD POISONING

National Institute of Allergy and Infectious Diseases
Bldg. 31, Room 7A50
Bethesda, MD 20892 (301) 496-5717

## FOOD PRESERVATIVES

Food and Drug Administration
(HFE-88), 5600 Fishers Lane
Rockville, MD 20857 (301) 443-3170

## FOOD SAFETY

Center for Food Safety and Applied Nutrition
Food and Drug Administration
Office of Constituents
200 C Street, SW, HFF-11
Washington, DC 20204 (202) 205-4317

## FORMALDEHYDE EXPOSURE

Public Information Center
Environmental Protection Agency
401 M St., SW
Washington, DC 20460 (202) 260-7751

## FRACTURE HEALING

National Institute of Arthritis and Musculoskeletal and Skin Diseases

1 AMS Way
Bethesda, MD 20892 (301) 495-4484

## FRAGILE X SYNDROME

National Institute of Child Health and Human Development
Bldg. 31, Room 2A32
Bethesda, MD 20892 (301) 496-5133

## FRIEDREICH'S ATAXIA

National Institute of Neurological Disorders and Stroke
Bldg. 31, Room 8A16
Bethesda, MD 20892 (301) 496-5751
(800) 352-9424

## FROEHLICH'S SYNDROME

National Institute of Diabetes and Digestive and Kidney Diseases
Bldg. 31, Room 9A04
Bethesda, MD 20892 (301) 496-3583

## FRUITS AND VEGETABLES

*See also Food*

Food and Drug Administration
(HFE-88), 5600 Fishers Lane
Rockville, MD 20857 (301) 443-3170

## FUCH'S DYSTROPHY

National Eye Institute
Bldg. 31, Room 6A32
Bethesda, MD 20892 (301) 496-5248

## FUNGAL DISEASES OF THE EYE

National Eye Institute
Building 31, Room 6A32
Bethesda, MD 20892 (301) 496-5248

## FUNGAL INFECTIONS

National Institute of Allergy and Infectious Diseases
Bldg. 31, Room 7A50
Bethesda, MD 20892 (301) 496-5717

## FUNNEL CHEST

National Heart, Lung, and Blood Institute
Information Center
P.O. Box 30105
Bethesda, MD 20824-0105 (301) 251-1222

## FURRY TONGUE

*See Black Tongue*

# - G -

## G6PD DEFICIENCY

National Heart, Lung, and Blood Institute
Information Center
P.O. Box 30105
Bethesda, MD 20824-0105 (301) 251-1222

## GALACTORRHEA

National Institute of Diabetes and Digestive
and Kidney Diseases
Building 31, Room 9A04
Bethesda, MD 20892 (301) 496-3583

## GALACTOSEMIA

National Institute of Diabetes and Digestive
and Kidney Diseases
Bldg. 31, Room 9A04
Bethesda, MD 20892 (301) 496-3583

## GALLBLADDER

National Institute of Diabetes and Digestive
and Kidney Diseases
Bldg. 31, Room 9A04
Bethesda, MD 20892 (301) 496-3583

## GALLSTONES

National Institute of Diabetes and Digestive
and Kidney Diseases
Bldg. 31, Room 9A04
Bethesda, MD 20892 (301) 496-3583

## GAS

National Digestive Diseases Information Clearinghouse
2 Information Way
Bethesda, MD 20892 (301) 654-3810

## GASTRIC HYPERSECRETION

National Institute of Diabetes and Digestive
and Kidney Diseases
Bldg. 31, Room 9A04
Bethesda, MD 20892 (301) 496-3583

## GASTRINOMA

National Institute of Diabetes and Digestive
and Kidney Diseases
Building 31, Room 9A04
Bethesda, MD 20892 (301) 496-3583

## GASTRITIS

National Institute of Diabetes and Digestive
and Kidney Diseases
Building 31, Room 9A04
Bethesda, MD 20892 (301) 496-3583

## GAUCHER'S DISEASE

National Institute of Neurological Disorders and Stroke
Bldg. 31, Room 8A16
Bethesda, MD 20892 (301) 496-5751
(800) 352-9424

## GENERIC DRUGS

Center for Drug Evaluation and Research
Food and Drug Administration
HFD 8, Room 14B45
5600 Fishers Lane
Rockville, MD 20857 (301) 594-1012

## GENETIC PANCREA

National Institute of Diabetes and Digestive and Kidney Diseases
Bldg. 31, Room 9A04
Bethesda, MD 20892 (301) 496-3583

## GENETICS

*See also DNA*

National Maternal and Child Health Clearinghouse
38th & R Sts., NW
Washington, DC 20057 (703) 821-8955, ext. 254

## GENETIC TESTING AND COUNSELING

National Maternal and Child Health Clearinghouse
8201 Greensboro Dr., Suite 600
McLean, VA 22101-3810 (703) 821-8955, ext. 254

## GENITAL HERPES

National Institute of Allergy and Infectious Diseases
Bldg. 31, Room 7A50
Bethesda, MD 20892 (301) 496-5717

National Sexually Transmitted Diseases Hotline
P.O. Box 13827
Research Triangle Park, NC 27709 (800) 227-8922

## GENITAL WARTS

National Institute of Allergy and Infectious Diseases
Building 31, Room 7A50
Bethesda, MD 20892 (301) 496-5717

National Sexually Transmitted Diseases Hotline
P.O. Box 13827
Research Triangle Park, NC 27709 (800) 227-8922

## GERIATRICS

*See Aging; Gerontology*

## GERMAN MEASLES

National Institute of Allergy and Infectious Diseases
Bldg. 31, Room 7A50
Bethesda, MD 20892 (301) 496-5717

## GERONTOLOGY

*See also Aging; Long-Term Care*

Gerontology Research Center
Francis Scott Key Medical Center
4940 Eastern Ave.
Baltimore, MD 21224 (301) 558-8114

National Institute on Aging
P.O. Box 8057
Gaithersburg, MD 20898-8057 (800) 222-2225

## GERSON METHOD

National Cancer Institute
Bldg. 31, Room 10A16
Bethesda, MD 20892 (800) 4-CANCER

## GERSTMANN'S SYNDROME

National Institute of Neurological Disorders and Stroke
Building 31, Room 8A16
Bethesda, MD 20892 (301) 496-5751
(800) 352-9424

## GESTATION

National Institute of Child Health
and Human Development
Building 31, Room 2A32
Bethesda, MD 20892 (301) 496-5133

## GESTATIONAL DIABETES

National Institute of Child Health
and Human Development
Building 31, Room 2A32
Bethesda, MD 20892 (301) 496-5133

## GIARDIASIS

National Institute of Allergy and Infectious Diseases
Bldg. 31, Room 7A50
Bethesda, MD 20892 (301) 496-5717

## GIGANTISM

National Institute of Diabetes and Digestive
and Kidney Diseases
Bldg. 31, Room 9A04
Bethesda, MD 20892 (301) 496-3583

## GILBERT'S SYNDROME

National Institute of Diabetes and Digestive
and Kidney Diseases
Bldg. 31, Room 9A04
Bethesda, MD 20892 (301) 496-3583

## GILLES DE LA TOURETTE'S DISEASE

National Institute of Neurological Disorders and Stroke
Bldg. 31, Room 8A16
Bethesda, MD 20892 (301) 496-5751
(800) 352-9424

## GINGIVITIS

National Institute of Dental Research
Bldg. 31, Room 2C35
31 Center Dr., MSC-2290
Bethesda, MD 20892-2290 (301) 496-4261

## GLAUCOMA

National Eye Institute
Bldg. 31, Room 6A32
Bethesda, MD 20892 (301) 496-5248

## GLIOMAS

National Institute of Neurological Disorders and Stroke
Bldg. 31, Room 8A16
Bethesda, MD 20892 (301) 496-5751
(800) 352-9424

## GLOBOID CELL LEUKODYSTROPHY

National Institute of Neurological Disorders and Stroke
Bldg. 31, Room 8A16
Bethesda, MD 20892 (301) 496-5751
(800) 352-9424

## GLOMERULONEPHRITIS

National Institute of Diabetes and Digestive
and Kidney Diseases
Bldg. 31, Room 9A04
Bethesda, MD 20892 (301) 496-3583

## GLUCOSE INTOLERANCE

National Institute of Diabetes and Digestive
and Kidney Diseases
Bldg. 31, Room 9A04
Bethesda, MD 20892 (301) 496-3583

## GLUTEN INTOLERANCE

National Institute of Diabetes and Digestive
and Kidney Diseases
Bldg. 31, Room 9A04
Bethesda, MD 20892 (301) 496-3583

## GLYCOGEN STORAGE DISEASE

National Institute of Diabetes and Digestive
and Kidney Diseases
Bldg. 31, Room 9A04
Bethesda, MD 20892 (301) 496-3583

## GOITER

National Institute of Diabetes and Digestive and Kidney Diseases
Bldg. 31, Room 9A04
Bethesda, MD 20892 (301) 496-3583

## GONADS

National Institute of Child Health and Human Development
Bldg. 31, Room 2A32
Bethesda, MD 20892 (301) 496-5133

## GONORRHEA

National Institute of Allergy and Infectious Diseases
Bldg. 31, Room 7A50
Bethesda, MD 20892 (301) 496-5717

National Sexually Transmitted Diseases Hotline
P.O. Box 13827
Research Triangle Park, NC 27709 (800) 227-8922

## GOODPASTURE'S SYNDROME

National Heart, Lung, and Blood Institute Information Center
P.O. Box 30105
Bethesda, MD 20824-0105 (301) 251-1222

National Institute of Diabetes and Digestive and Kidney Diseases
Bldg. 31, Room 9A04
Bethesda, MD 20892 (301) 496-3583

## GOUT

National Institute of Arthritis and Musculoskeletal
and Skin Diseases

1 AMS Way
Bethesda, MD 20892 (301) 495-4484

## GRAINS

Food and Nutrition Information Center
National Agricultural Library
Room 304
Beltsville, MD 20705-2351 (301) 504-5719

## GRANULOCYTOPENIA

National Institute of Arthritis and Musculoskeletal
and Skin Diseases
1 AMS Way
Bethesda, MD 20892 (301) 495-4484

## GRANULOMATOUS DISEASE

National Institute of Allergy and Infectious Diseases
Bldg. 31, Room 7A50
Bethesda, MD 20892 (301) 496-5717

## GRAPE CURE

National Cancer Institute
Bldg. 31, Room 10A16
Bethesda, MD 20892 (800) 4-CANCER

## GRAVE'S DISEASE

National Eye Institute
Bldg. 31, Room 6A32
Bethesda, MD 20892 (301) 496-5248

National Institute of Diabetes and Digestive and Kidney Diseases
Bldg. 31, Room 9A04
Bethesda, MD 20892 (301) 496-3583

## GRIEF

National Institute of Mental Health
5600 Fishers Lane, Room 7C-02
Rockville, MD 20857 (301) 443-4515

## GRIPPE

*See Flu*

## GROWTH HORMONE DEFICIENCY

National Institute of Diabetes and Digestive and Kidney Diseases
Bldg. 31, Room 9A04
Bethesda, MD 20892 (301) 496-3583

## GUILLAIN-BARRE SYNDROME

National Institute of Neurological Disorders and Stroke
Bldg. 31, Room 8A16
Bethesda, MD 20892 (301) 496-5751
(800) 352-9424

## GUM DISEASE

National Institute of Dental Research
Bldg. 31, Room 2C35
31 Center Dr., MSC-2290
Bethesda, MD 20892-2290 (301) 496-4261

## GYNECOMASTIA

National Institute of Child Health and Human Development
Bldg. 31, Room 2A32
Bethesda, MD 20892 (301) 496-5133

## GYRATE ATROPHY

National Eye Institute
Bldg. 31, Room 6A32
Bethesda, MD 20892 (301) 496-5248

# - H -

## HAILEY'S DISEASE

National Institute of Diabetes and Digestive and Kidney Diseases
Bldg. 31, Room 9A04
Bethesda, MD 20892 (301) 496-3583

## HAIR LOSS

National Institute of Arthritis and Musculoskeletal and Skin Diseases
1 AMS Way
Bethesda, MD 20892 (301) 495-4484

## HAIR REMOVAL

Center for Devices and Radiological Health
Food and Drug Administration (HFZ-210)
5600 Fishers Lane
Rockville, MD 20857 (301) 443-4690

## HAIR SPRAY

Office of Cosmetics and Colors
Food and Drug Administration
200 C St., SW
Washington, DC 20204 (202) 205-4530

## HAIRY TONGUE

*See Black Tongue*

## HALITOSIS

National Institute of Dental Research
Bldg. 31, Room 2C35
31 Center Dr., MSC-2290
Bethesda, MD 20892-2290 (301) 496-4261

## HALLERVORDEN-SPATZ DISEASE

National Institute of Neurological Disorders and Stroke
Bldg. 31, Room 8A16 (301) 496-5751
Bethesda, MD 20892 (800) 352-9424

## HAND, FOOT AND MOUTH DISEASE

National Institute of Allergy and Infectious Diseases
Bldg. 31, Room 7A50
Bethesda, MD 20892 (301) 496-5717

## HANDICAPPED

*See also Disabilities*

Clearinghouse on Disabilities
Switzer Building, 330 C Street SW
Washington, DC 20202 (202) 205-8241

ERIC Clearinghouse on Handicapped and Gifted Children
Council for Exceptional Children
1920 Association Drive
Reston, VA 22091 (703) 264-9474

The National Information Center for Children and
Youth with Disabilities
P.O. Box 1492
Washington, DC 20013-1492 (800) 695-0285

The National Institute on Disability and Rehabilitation Research
Switzer Building, 330 C Street, SW
Washington, DC 20202 (202) 205-8134

## HANDICAPPED CHILDREN

The National Information Center for Children and
Youth with Disabilities
P.O. Box 1492
Washington, DC 20013 (800) 695-0285

## HANSEN'S DISEASE

National Institute of Allergy and Infectious Diseases
Bldg. 31, Room 7A50
Bethesda, MD 20892 (301) 496-5717

## HAPPY PUPPET SYNDROME

National Institute of Neurological Disorders and Stroke
Bldg. 31, Room 8A16
Bethesda, MD 20892 (301) 496-5751
(800) 352-9424

## HARADA'S DISEASE

National Eye Institute
Building 31, Room 6A32
Bethesda, MD 20892 (301) 496-5248

## HARDENING OF THE ARTERIES

National Heart, Lung, and Blood Institute
Information Center
P.O. Box 30105
Bethesda, MD 20824-0105 (301) 251-1222

## HARELIP

National Institute on Deafness and Other
Communication Disorders Clearinghouse
1 Communication Avenue
Bethesda, MD 20892-3456 (800) 241-1044
(800) 241-1055 (TDD)

## HASHIMOTO'S DISEASE

National Institute of Diabetes and Digestive
and Kidney Diseases
Bldg. 31, Room 9A04
Bethesda, MD 20892 (301) 496-3583

## HAVERHILL FEVER (Rat Bite Fever)

National Institute of Allergy and Infectious Diseases
Bldg. 31, Room 7A50
Bethesda, MD 20892 (301) 496-5717

## HAY FEVER

National Institute of Allergy and Infectious Diseases
Bldg. 31, Room 7A50
Bethesda, MD 20892 (301) 496-5717

## HAZARDOUS SUBSTANCES

Agency for Toxic Substances and Disease Registry
1600 Clifton Rd., NE
Atlanta, GA 30333 (404) 639-0600

Public Information Center
Environmental Protection Agency
401 M Street, SW
Washington, DC 20460 (202) 260-7751

## HEADACHES

National Institute of Neurological Disorders and Stroke
Building 31, Room 8A16 (301) 496-5751
Bethesda, MD 20892 (800) 352-9424

## HEAD INJURIES

National Institute of Neurological Disorders and Stroke
Bldg. 31, Room 8A16
Bethesda, MD 20892 (301) 496-5751
(800) 352-9424

## HEAD LICE

National Institute of Allergy and Infectious Diseases
Bldg. 31, Room 7A50
Bethesda, MD 20892 (301) 496-5717

## HEALTH CARE COSTS

Health Care Financing Administration
ORD-ES
Room 2230-OM
6325 Security Blvd.
Baltimore, MD 21207 (410) 966-6584

## HEALTH CARE POLICY

Agency for Health Care Policy and Research
2101 E. Jefferson Street
Rockville, MD 20852 (301) 594-1357

## HEALTH FOODS

*See also Food; Nutrition*

Food and Nutrition Information Center
National Agricultural Library, Room 304
Beltsville, MD 20705 (301) 504-5719

## HEALTH FRAUD

Center for Devices and Radiological Health
(HFZ-210), Food and Drug Administration
5600 Fishers Lane
Rockville, MD 20857 (301) 443-4690

## HEALTH INSURANCE

National Institute on Alcohol Abuse and Alcoholism
6000 Executive Boulevard, Suite 409
MSC-7003
Bethesda, MD 20892-7003 (301) 443-3860

## HEALTH SPAS

Federal Trade Commission
Washington, DC 20580 (202) 326-2222

## HEALTH STATISTICS

National Center for Health Statistics
6525 Belcrest Rd., Room 1064
Hyattsville, MD 20782 (301) 436-8500

*Morbidity and Mortality Weekly Report*
Centers for Disease Control
1600 Clifton Rd., NE
Atlanta, GA 30333 (404) 639-2104

## HEARING AIDS

National Institute on Deafness and Other
Communication Disorders Clearinghouse
1 Communication Avenue
Bethesda, MD 20892-3456 (800) 241-1044
(800) 241-1055 (TDD)

## HEARING LOSS

National Institute of Neurological Disorders and Stroke
Bldg. 31, Room 8A16
Bethesda, MD 20892 (301) 496-5751
(800) 352-9424

National Institute on Deafness and Other
Communication Disorders
1 Communication Avenue
Bethesda, MD 20892-3456 (800) 241-1044
(800) 241-1055 (TDD)

## HEART ATTACKS

National Heart, Lung, and Blood Institute
Information Center
P.O. Box 30105
Bethesda, MD 20824-0105 (301) 251-1222

## HEARTBURN

National Digestive Diseases Information Clearinghouse
2 Information Way
Bethesda, MD 20892 (301) 654-3810

## HEART DISEASE

*See also Cardiovascular Disease*

National Heart, Lung and Blood Institute
Information Center
P.O. Box 30105
Bethesda, MD 20824-0105 (301) 251-1222

## HEART-LUNG MACHINES

National Heart, Lung, and Blood Institute
Information Center
P.O. Box 30105
Bethesda, MD 20824-0105 (301) 251-1222

## HEART MURMURS

National Heart, Lung, and Blood Institute
Information Center
P.O. Box 30105
Bethesda, MD 20824-0105 (301) 251-1222

## HEART TRANSPLANTS

National Heart, Lung, and Blood Institute
Information Center
P.O. Box 30105
Bethesda, MD 20824-0105 (301) 251-1222

## HEAT STROKE

National Institute on Aging
Information Center
P.O. Box 8057
Gaithersburg, MD 20898-8057 (800) 222-2225

## HEBEPHRENIA

National Institute of Mental Health
5600 Fishers Lane
Room 7C-02
Rockville, MD 20857 (301) 443-4515

## HEMIPLEGIA

National Institute of Neurological Disorders and Stroke
Building 31, Room 8A16
Bethesda, MD 20892 (301) 496-5751
(800) 352-9424

## HEMODIALYSIS

National Institute of Diabetes and Digestive and Kidney Diseases
Building 31, Room 9A04
Bethesda, MD 20892 (301) 496-3583

## HEMOGLOBIN GENETICS

National Institute of Diabetes and Digestive
and Kidney Diseases
Building 31, Room 9A04
Bethesda, MD 20892 (301) 496-3583

## HEMOGLOBINOPATHIES

National Institute of Diabetes and Digestive
and Kidney Diseases
Building 31, Room 9A04
Bethesda, MD 20892 (301) 496-3583

## HEMOLYTIC ANEMIA

National Institute of Diabetes and Digestive
and Kidney Diseases
Bldg. 31, Room 9A04
Bethesda, MD 20892 (301) 496-3583

National Institute of Allergy and Infectious Diseases
Bldg. 31, Room 7A50
Bethesda, MD 20892 (301) 496-5717

## HEMOLYTIC DISEASE

National Institute of Child Health and Human Development
Bldg. 31, Room 2A32
Bethesda, MD 20892 (301) 496-5133

National Heart, Lung, and Blood Institute
Information Center
P.O. Box 30105
Bethesda, MD 20824-0105 (301) 251-1222

## HEMOPHILIA

National Heart, Lung, and Blood Institute
Information Center
P.O. Box 30105
Bethesda, MD 20824-0105 (301) 251-1222

## HEMOPHILUS INFLUENZA

National Institute of Allergy and Infectious Diseases
Bldg. 31, Room 7A50
Bethesda, MD 20892 (301) 496-5717

## HEMORRHAGIC DIATHESIS

National Institute of Diabetes and Digestive
and Kidney Diseases
Bldg. 31, Room 9A04
Bethesda, MD 20892 (301) 496-3583

National Heart, Lung, and Blood Institute
Information Center
P.O. Box 30105
Bethesda, MD 20824-0105 (301) 251-1222

## HEMORRHOIDS

National Institute of Diabetes and Digestive
and Kidney Diseases
Bldg. 31, Room 9A04
Bethesda, MD 20892 (301) 496-3583

National Heart, Lung, and Blood Institute
Information Center
P.O. Box 30105
Bethesda, MD 20824-0105 (301) 251-1222

## HEMOSIDEROSIS

National Heart, Lung, and Blood Institute
Information Center
P.O. Box 30105
Bethesda, MD 20824-0105 (301) 251-1222

## HENOCH-SCHONLEIN PURPURA

National Institute of Allergy and Infectious Diseases
Bldg. 31, Room 7A50
Bethesda, MD 20892 (301) 496-5717

## HEPATITIS

National Institute of Allergy and Infectious Diseases
Bldg. 31, Room 7A50
Bethesda, MD 20892 (301) 496-5717

National Digestive Diseases Information Clearinghouse
2 Information Way
Bethesda, MD 20892 (301) 654-3810

Centers for Disease Control
Information Resources Management Office
Mail Stop C-13
1600 Clifton Road, NE
Atlanta, GA 30333 (404) 332-4555

## HERNIAS

National Digestive Diseases Information Clearinghouse
2 Information Way
Bethesda, MD 20892 (301) 654-3810

## HERNIATED DISCS

*See also Back Problems*

National Institute of Arthritis and Musculoskeletal and Skin Diseases
1 AMS Way
Bethesda, MD 20892 (301) 495-4484

## HEROIN

*See also Drug Abuse*

National Clearinghouse for Alcohol and Drug Information
P.O. Box 2345
Rockville, MD 20852 (301) 468-2600
(800) 729-6686

## HERPES

National Sexually Transmitted Diseases Hotline
P.O. Box 13827
Research Triangle Park, NC 27709 (800) 227-8922

## HERPES ZOSTER (SHINGLES)

National Institute of Allergy and Infectious Diseases
Bldg. 31, Room 7A50
Bethesda, MD 20892 (301) 496-5717

## HIATAL HERNIAS

National Institute of Diabetes and Digestive and Kidney Diseases
Bldg. 31, Room 9A04
Bethesda, MD 20892 (301) 496-3583

## HICCUPS

National Heart, Lung, and Blood Institute
Information Center
P.O. Box 30105
Bethesda, MD 20824-0105 (301) 251-1222

## HIGH BLOOD PRESSURE

National Heart, Lung and Blood Institute
Information Center
P.O. Box 30105
Bethesda, MD 20824-0105 (301) 251-1222

## HIGH-DENSITY LIPOPROTEINS

*See also Cholesterol*

National Heart, Lung and Blood Institute
Information Center
P.O. Box 30105
Bethesda, MD 20824-0105 (301) 251-1222

## HIRSCHSPRUNG'S DISEASE

National Institute of Diabetes and Digestive and Kidney Diseases
Bldg. 31, Room 9A04
Bethesda, MD 20892 (301) 496-3583

## HIRSUTISM

National Institute of Arthritis and Musculoskeletal and Skin Diseases
1 AMS Way
Bethesda, MD 20892 (301) 495-4484

## HISTIOCYTOSIS

National Cancer Institute
Bldg. 31, Room 10A16
Bethesda, MD 20892 — (800) 4-CANCER

National Heart, Lung, and Blood Institute
Information Center
P.O. Box 30105
Bethesda, MD 20824-0105 — (301) 251-1222

## HISTOPLASMOSIS

National Institute of Allergy and Infectious Diseases
Bldg. 31, Room 7A50
Bethesda, MD 20892 — (301) 496-5717

## HIVES

National Institute of Allergy and Infectious Diseases
Bldg. 31, Room 7A50
Bethesda, MD 20892 — (301) 496-5717

## HIV INFECTION

*See also AIDS*

National Sexually Transmitted Diseases Hotline
P.O. Box 13827
Research Triangle Park, NC 27709 — (800) 227-8922

National AIDS Information Clearinghouse
P.O. Box 6003 — (800) 458-5231
Rockville, MD 20850 — (800) 342-AIDS
(800) 344-7432 (Servicio en Espanol)
(800) 243-7889 (TTY-Deaf Access)

## HODEOLUM

*See Stye*

## HODGKIN'S DISEASE

National Cancer Institute
Bldg. 31, Room 10A16
Bethesda, MD 20892 (800) 4-CANCER

## HOLISTIC MEDICINE

*See Alternative Medicine*

## HOMELESSNESS

Policy Research Associates, Inc.
262 Delaware Ave.
Delmar, NY 12054 (800) 444-7415

## HOMEOPATHY

*See Alternative Medicine*

## HOMOCYSTINURIA

National Institute of Child Health and Human Development
Bldg. 31, Room 2A32
Bethesda, MD 20892 (301) 496-5133

## HOMOSEXUALITY

National Institute of Child Health and Human Development
Building 31, Room 2A32
Bethesda, MD 20892 (301) 496-5133

## HOME TEST KITS

Center for Devices and Radiological Health
Food and Drug Administration (HFZ-210)
5600 Fishers Lane
Rockville, MD 20857 (301) 443-4690

## HOOKWORM DISEASE

National Institute of Allergy and Infectious Diseases
Bldg. 31, Room 7A50
Bethesda, MD 20892 (301) 496-5717

## HORMONES

*See also Menopause*

National Institute of Diabetes and Digestive and Kidney Diseases
Bldg. 31, Room 9A04
Bethesda, MD 20892 (301) 496-3583

National Institute of Child Health and Human Development
Bldg. 31, Room 2A32
Bethesda, MD 20892 (301) 496-5133

## HORMONE THERAPY

Office of Technology Assessment
600 Pennsylvania Ave., SE
Washington, DC 20510-8025 (202) 224-8996

## HOSPICE CARE

National Institute on Aging Information Center
P.O. Box 8057
Bethesda, MD 20898-8057 (800) 222-2225

National Cancer Institute
Bldg. 31, Room 10A16
Bethesda, MD 20892 (800) 4-CANCER

## HOSPITAL COMPLAINTS

Health Resource Service Administration
5600 Fishers Lane
Room 11-25, Parklawn Bldg. (800) 638-0742
Rockville, MD 20857 (800) 492-0359 in MD

## HOSPITAL INFECTIONS

National Institute of Allergy and Infectious Diseases
Bldg. 31, Room 7A50
Bethesda, MD 20892 (301) 496-5717

## HOUSEHOLD HAZARDS

RCRA Hotline
Environmental Protection Agency
401 M St., SW, Mail Stop 5305 (703) 920-9810
Washington, DC 20460 (800) 424-9346

## HUMAN GROWTH HORMONE

National Institute of Child Health and Human Development
Bldg. 31, Room 2A32
Bethesda, MD 20892 (301) 496-5133

## HUMAN PAPILLOMA VIRUS

National Cancer Institute
Bldg. 31, Room 10A16
Bethesda, MD 20892 (800) 4-CANCER

National Institute of Allergy and Infectious Diseases
Bldg. 31, Room 7A50
Bethesda, MD 20892 (301) 496-5717

## HUNT'S DISEASE

National Institute of Neurological Disorders and Stroke
Building 31, Room 8A16
Bethesda, MD 20892 (301) 496-5751
(800) 352-9424

## HUNTER'S SYNDROME

National Institute of Diabetes and Digestive and Kidney Diseases
Bldg. 31, Room 9A04
Bethesda, MD 20892 (301) 496-3583

## HUNTINGTON'S CHOREA

National Institute of Neurological Disorders and Stroke
Bldg. 31, Room 8A16
Bethesda, MD 20892 (301) 496-5751
(800) 352-9424

## HURLER'S SYNDROME

National Institute of Child Health and Human Development
Bldg. 31, Room 2A32
Bethesda, MD 20892 (301) 496-5133

## HYALINE MEMBRANE DISEASE

National Institute of Child Health and Human Development
Bldg. 31, Room 2A32
Bethesda, MD 20892 (301) 496-5133

## HYDROCEPHALUS

National Institute of Neurological Disorders and Stroke
Bldg. 31, Room 8A16 (301) 496-5751
Bethesda, MD 20892 (800) 352-9424

## HYDROXYUREA

National Cancer Institute
Bldg. 31, Room 10A16
Bethesda, MD 20892 (800) 4-CANCER

## HYPERACTIVITY

National Institute of Mental Health
5600 Fishers Lane, Room 7C-02
Rockville, MD 20857 (301) 443-4515

## HYPERBARIC OXYGENATION

National Heart, Lung, and Blood Institute Information Center
P.O. Box 30105
Bethesda, MD 20824-0105 (301) 251-1222

## HYPERBILIRUBINEMIA

National Institute of Child Health and Human Development

Bldg. 31, Room 2A32
Bethesda, MD 20892 (301) 496-5133

## HYPERCALCEMIA

*See also Paget's Disease*

National Institute of Diabetes and Digestive and Kidney Diseases
Bldg. 31, Room 9A04
Bethesda, MD 20892 (301) 496-3583

## HYPERCALCIURIA

*See also Osteoporosis*

National Institute of Diabetes and Digestive and Kidney Diseases
Bldg. 31, Room 9A04
Bethesda, MD 20892 (301) 496-3583

## HYPERCHOLESTEROLEMIA

*See Cholesterol*

## HYPERGLYCEMIA

National Institute of Diabetes and Digestive and Kidney Diseases
Bldg. 31, Room 9A04
Bethesda, MD 20892 (301) 496-3583

## HYPERKINESIS

National Institute of Mental Health
5600 Fishers Ln., Room 7C-02
Rockville, MD 20857 (301) 443-4515

## HYPERLIPIDEMIA

National Heart, Lung, and Blood Institute
Information Center
P.O. Box 30105
Bethesda, MD 20824-0105 (301) 251-1222

## HYPERLIPOPROTEINEMIA

National Heart, Lung, and Blood Institute
Information Center
P.O. Box 30105
Bethesda, MD 20824-0105 (301) 251-1222

## HYPERPARATHYROIDISM

National Institute of Diabetes and Digestive and Kidney Diseases
Bldg. 31, Room 9A04
Bethesda, MD 20892 (301) 496-3583

## HYPERPYREXIA

National Institute on Aging
Information Center
P.O. Box 8057
Gaithersburg, MD 20898-8057 (800) 222-2225

## HYPERSENSITIVITY PNEUMONITIS

National Institute of Allergy and Infectious Diseases
Bldg. 31, Room 7A50
Bethesda, MD 20892 (301) 496-5717

## HYPERTENSION

*See High Blood Pressure*

## HYPERTHERMIA

National Institute on Aging
Information Center
P.O. Box 8057
Gaithersburg, MD 20898-8057 (800) 222-2225

## HYPERTHYROIDISM

National Institute of Diabetes and Digestive
and Kidney Diseases
Bldg. 31, Room 9A04
Bethesda, MD 20892 (301) 496-3583

## HYPERTRIGLYCERIDEMIA

National Heart, Lung, and Blood Institute
Information Center
P.O. Box 30105
Bethesda, MD 20824-0105 (301) 251-1222

## HYPERURICEMIA

National Institute of Diabetes and Digestive
and Kidney Diseases
Bldg. 31, Room 9A04
Bethesda, MD 20892 (301) 496-3583

## HYPERVENTILATION

National Heart, Lung, and Blood Institute
Information Center
P.O. Box 30105
Bethesda, MD 20824-0105 (301) 251-1222

## HYPOBETALIPOPROTEINEMIA

National Heart, Lung, and Blood Institute
Information Center
P.O. Box 30105
Bethesda, MD 20824-0105 (301) 251-1222

## HYPOCOMPLEMENTEMIC GLOMERULONEPHRITIS

National Institute of Allergy and Infectious Diseases
Bldg. 31, Room 7A50
Bethesda, MD 20892 (301) 496-5717

## HYPOGLYCEMIA

National Heart, Lung, and Blood Institute
Information Center
P.O. Box 30105
Bethesda, MD 20824-0105 (301) 251-1222

## HYPOGONADISM

National Institute of Diabetes and Digestive and Kidney Diseases
Building 31, Room 9A04
Bethesda, MD 20892 (301) 496-3583

## HYPOKALEMIA

National Heart, Lung, and Blood Institute
Information Center
P.O. Box 30105
Bethesda, MD 20824-0105 (301) 251-1222

## HYPOKALEMIC PERIODIC PARALYSIS

National Institute of Neurological Disorders and Stroke
Building 31, Room 8A16
Bethesda, MD 20892 (301) 496-5751
(800) 352-9424

## HYPOLIPOPROTEINEMIA

National Heart, Lung, and Blood Institute
Information Center
P.O. Box 30105
Bethesda, MD 20824-0105 (301) 251-1222

## HYPOPARATHYROIDISM

National Institute of Diabetes and Digestive
and Kidney Diseases
Building 31, Room 9A04
Bethesda, MD 20892 (301) 496-3583

## HYPOPITUITARISM

National Institute of Diabetes and Digestive
and Kidney Diseases
Bldg. 31, Room 9A04
Bethesda, MD 20892 (301) 496-3583

## HYPOSPADIAS

National Institute of Child Health and Human Development
Bldg. 31, Room 2A32
Bethesda, MD 20892 (301) 496-5133

## HYPOTENSION

*See Low Blood Pressure*

## HYPOTHALAMUS

National Institute of Diabetes and Digestive and Kidney Diseases
Bldg. 31, Room 9A04
Bethesda, MD 20892 (301) 496-3583

## HYPOTHERMIA

National Institute on Aging
Information Center
P.O. Box 8057
Gaithersburg, MD 20898-8057 (800) 222-2225

## HYPOTHYROIDISM

National Institute of Diabetes and Digestive and Kidney Diseases
Bldg. 31, Room 9A04
Bethesda, MD 20892 (301) 496-3583

## HYPOTONIA

National Institute of Neurological Disorders and Stroke

Bldg. 31, Room 8A16
Bethesda, MD 20892 (301) 496-5751
(800) 352-9424

## HYPOVENTILATION

National Heart, Lung, and Blood Institute
Information Center
P.O. Box 30105
Bethesda, MD 20824-0105 (301) 251-1222

## HYPOXIA

National Heart, Lung, and Blood Institute
Information Center
P.O. Box 30105
Bethesda, MD 20824-0105 (301) 251-1222

## HYPSARRHYTHMIA

National Institute of Neurological Disorders and Stroke
Building 31, Room 8A16
Bethesda, MD 20892 (301) 496-5751
(800) 352-9424

# - I -

## IBD AND IBS

*See Irritable Bowel Syndrome*

## ICELAND DISEASE

National Institute of Neurological Disorders and Stroke
Bldg. 31, Room 8A16 (301) 496-5751
Bethesda, MD 20892 (800) 352-9424

## ICHTHYOSIS

National Institute of Arthritis and Musculoskeletal and Skin Diseases
1 AMS Way
Bethesda, MD 20892 (301) 495-4484

## IDENTICAL TWINS

*See Twins*

## IDIOPATHIC HYPERTROPHIC SUBAORTIC STENOSIS

National Heart, Lung, and Blood Institute Information Center
P.O. Box 30105
Bethesda, MD 20824-0105 (301) 251-1222

## IDIOPATHIC INFLAMMATORY MYOPATHY

National Institute of Neurological Disorders and Stroke
Bldg. 31, Room 8A16 (301) 496-5751
Bethesda, MD 20892 (800) 352-9424

## IDIOPATHIC THROMBOCYTOPENIC PURPURA

National Heart, Lung, and Blood Institute
Information Center

P.O. Box 30105
Bethesda, MD 20824-0105 (301) 251-1222

## ILEITIS

National Institute of Diabetes and Digestive and Kidney Diseases
Bldg. 31, Room 9A04
Bethesda, MD 20892 (301) 496-3583

## IMMUNE DEFICIENCY DISEASE

National Institute of Allergy and Infectious Diseases
Bldg. 31, Room 7A50
Bethesda, MD 20892 (301) 496-5717

## IMMUNE THROMBOCYTOPENIC PURPURA

National Heart, Lung, and Blood Institute
Information Center
P.O. Box 30105
Bethesda, MD 20824-0105 (301) 251-1222

## IMMUNIZATIONS

Centers for Disease Control
1600 Clifton Road
Atlanta, GA 30333 (404) 332-4445

## IMPOTENCE

National Institute of Mental Health
5600 Fishers Ln., Room 7C-02
Rockville, MD 20857 (301) 443-4515

National Kidney and Urological Diseases Information Clearinghouse
3 Information Way
Bethesda, MD 20892 (301) 654-4415

## INAPPROPRIATE ANTIDIURETIC SUBAORTIC STENOSIS

National Heart, Lung, and Blood Institute Information Center
P.O. Box 30105
Bethesda, MD 20824-0105 (301) 251-1222

## INBORN HEART DEFECTS

National Heart, Lung, and Blood Institute Information Center
P.O. Box 30105
Bethesda, MD 20824-0105 (301) 251-1222

## INCONTINENCE

National Kidney and Urological Diseases Information Clearinghouse
3 Information Way
Bethesda, MD 20892 (301) 654-4415

## INCONTINENTIA PIGMENTI

National Institute of Neurological Disorders and Stroke
Bldg. 31, Room 8A16 (301) 496-5751
Bethesda, MD 20892 (800) 352-9424

## INDOOR AIR POLLUTION

Indoor Air Quality Information Clearinghouse
P.O. Box 37133
Washington, DC 20013-4318 (800) 438-4318

## INDUCED MOVEMENT DISORDERS

National Institute of Neurological Disorders and Stroke
Bldg. 31, Room 8A16 (301) 496-5751
Bethesda, MD 20892 (800) 352-9424

## INFANT HEALTH

National Maternal and Child Health Clearinghouse
8201 Greensboro Drive, Suite 600
McLean, VA 22102-3810 (703) 821-8955, ext. 254

National Center for Clinical Infant Programs
2000 14th Street, North, Suite 380
Arlington, VA 22201 (800) 899-4301

National Institute of Child Health and Human Development
Bldg. 31, Room 2A32
Bethesda, MD 20892 (301) 496-5133

National Information Clearinghouse for Infants with
Disabilities and Life-Threatening Conditions
Benson Building, First Floor (800) 922-9234
Columbia, SC 29208 (800) 922-1107 in SC

## INFANT NUTRITION

National Maternal and Child Health Clearinghouse
8201 Greensboro Drive, Suite 600
McLean, VA 22102-3810 (703) 821-8955, ext. 254

## INFANTS WITH DISABILITIES

National Information Clearinghouse for Infants with
Disabilities and Life-Threatening Conditions
Benson Building, First Floor (800) 922-9234
Columbia, SC 29208 (800) 922-1107 (in SC)

## INFECTIOUS ARTHRITIS

National Institute of Arthritis and Musculoskeletal
and Skin Diseases
1 AMS Way
Bethesda, MD 20892 (301) 495-4484

## INFECTIOUS DISEASES

National Institute of Allergy and Infectious Diseases
Bldg. 31, Room 7A50
Bethesda, MD 20892 (301) 496-5717

## INFECTIOUS EYE DISEASES

National Eye Institute
Bldg. 31, Room 6A32
Bethesda, MD 20892 (301) 496-5248

## INFERTILITY

National Institute of Child Health and Human Development
Reproductive Sciences Branch
Center for Population Research
Bldg. 61E, Room 8B01
Bethesda, MD 20892 (301) 496-5133

## INFLAMMATORY BOWEL DISEASE

National Institute of Diabetes and Digestive
and Kidney Diseases
Bldg. 31, Room 9A04
Bethesda, MD 20892 (301) 496-3583

## INFLUENZA

*See Flu*

## INSECT STINGS

National Institute of Allergy and Infectious Diseases
Building 31, Room 7A50
Bethesda, MD 20892 (301) 496-5717

## INSOMNIA

National Institute of Mental Health
5600 Fishers Lane
Room 7C-02
Rockville, MD 20857 (301) 443-4515

## INSULIN-DEPENDENT DIABETES

*See also Diabetes*

National Diabetes Information Clearinghouse
1 Information Way
Bethesda, MD 20892 (301) 654-3810

## INSULINOMAS

National Institute of Diabetes and Digestive
and Kidney Diseases
Bldg. 31, Room 9A04
Bethesda, MD 20892 (301) 496-3583

## INTERFERON

National Institute of Allergy and Infectious Diseases
Bldg. 31, Room 7A50
Bethesda, MD 20892 (301) 496-5717

## INTERLEUKIN-2 THERAPY

National Cancer Institute
Bldg. 31, Room 10A16
Bethesda, MD 20892 (800) 4-CANCER

## INTERSTITIAL CYSTITIS

National Institute of Diabetes and Digestive
and Kidney Diseases
Bldg. 31, Room 9A04
Bethesda, MD 20892 (301) 496-3583

## INTESTINAL MALABSORPTION SYNDROME

National Institute of Diabetes and Digestive
and Kidney Diseases
Building 31, Room 9A04
Bethesda, MD 20892 (301) 496-3583

## INTRACRANIAL ANEURYSM

National Institute of Neurological Disorders and Stroke
Building 31, Room 8A16
Bethesda, MD 20892 (301) 496-5751
(800) 352-9424

## INTRAOCULAR LENSES

National Eye Institute
Building 31, Room 6A32
Bethesda, MD 20892 (301) 496-5248

## INTRAUTERINE GROWTH RETARDATION

National Institute of Child Health and Human Development
Building 31, Room 2A32
Bethesda, MD 20892 (301) 496-5133

## INVASIVE DENTAL PROCEDURES

National Institute of Dental Research
Bldg. 31, Room 2C35
31 Center Drive, MSC-2290
Bethesda, MD 20892-2290 (301) 496-4261

## IN VITRO FERTILIZATION

*See also Artificial Insemination*

National Institute of Child Health and Human Development
Bldg. 31, Room 2A32
Bethesda, MD 20892 (301) 496-5133

## IRIDOCYCLITIS

National Eye Institute
Bldg. 31, Room 6A32
Bethesda, MD 20892 (301) 496-5248

## IRITIS

National Eye Institute
Bldg. 31, Room 6A32
Bethesda, MD 20892 (301) 496-5248

## IRON DEFICIENCY

National Institute of Diabetes and Digestive and Kidney Diseases
Bldg. 31, Room 9A04
Bethesda, MD 20892 (301) 496-3583

## IRRADIATION

*See Food Irradiation*

## IRRITABLE BOWEL SYNDROME

*See also Bowel Disease*

National Institute of Diabetes and Digestive and Kidney Diseases
Bldg. 31, Room 9A04
Bethesda, MD 20892 (301) 496-3583

## ISCADOR

National Cancer Institute
Bldg. 31, Room 10A16
Bethesda, MD 20892 (800) 4-CANCER

## ISCHEMIA

National Heart, Lung, and Blood Institute
Information Center

P.O. Box 30105
Bethesda, MD 20824-0105 (301) 251-1222

## ISLET CELL HYPERPLASIA

National Institute of Diabetes and Digestive and Kidney Diseases
Bldg. 31, Room 9A04
Bethesda, MD 20892 (301) 496-3583

## ISOLATED IGA DEFICIENCY

National Cancer Institute
Bldg. 31, Room 10A16
Bethesda, MD 20892 (800) 4-CANCER

# - J -

## JAKOB-CREUTZFELDT DISEASE

National Institute of Neurological Disorders and Stroke
Bldg. 31, Room 8A16 (301) 496-5751
Bethesda, MD 20892 (800) 352-9424

## JOINT REPLACEMENT

National Institute of Arthritis and Musculoskeletal and Skin Diseases
1 AMS Way
Bethesda, MD 20892 (301) 495-4484

## JOSEPH'S DISEASE

National Institute of Neurological Disorders and Stroke
Building 31, Room 8A16 (301) 496-5751
Bethesda, MD 20892 (800) 352-9424

## JUICING

Food and Nutrition Information Center
National Agricultural Library
10301 Baltimore Blvd.
Beltsville, MD 20705 (301) 504-5719

## JUVENILE DELINQUENCY

National Institute of Mental Health
5600 Fishers Lane
Room 7C-02
Rockville, MD 20857 (301) 443-4515

## JUVENILE DIABETES

National Institute of Diabetes and Digestive
and Kidney Diseases
Bldg. 31, Room 9A04
Bethesda, MD 20892 (301) 496-3583

## JUVENILE RHEUMATOID ARTHRITIS

National Institute of Arthritis and Musculoskeletal
and Skin Diseases
1 AMS Way
Bethesda, MD 20892 (301) 495-4484

## JUXTAGLOMERULAR HYPERPLASIA

National Heart, Lung, and Blood Institute
Information Center
P.O. Box 30105
Bethesda, MD 20824-0105 (301) 251-1222

# - K -

## KANNER'S SYNDROME

National Institute of Neurological Disorders and Stroke
Bldg. 31, Room 8A16
Bethesda, MD 20892 (301) 496-5751
(800) 352-9424

## KAPOSI'S SARCOMA

National Cancer Institute
Bldg. 31, Room 10A16
Bethesda, MD 20892 (800) 4-CANCER

## KAWASAKI DISEASE

National Institute of Allergy and Infectious Diseases
Bldg. 31, Room 7A50
Bethesda, MD 20892 (301) 496-5717

## KEARNS-SAYRE SYNDROME

National Institute of Neurological Disorders and Stroke
Bldg. 31, Room 8A16
Bethesda, MD 20892 (301) 496-5751
(800) 352-9424

## KERATITIS

National Eye Institute
Bldg. 31, Room 6A32
Bethesda, MD 20892 (301) 496-5248

## KERATOCONUS

National Eye Institute
Building 31
Room 6A32
Bethesda, MD 20892 (301) 496-5248

## KERATOMILEUSIS

National Eye Institute
Building 31
Room 6A32
Bethesda, MD 20892 (301) 496-5248

## KERATOPLASTY

National Eye Institute
Building 31
Room 6A32
Bethesda, MD 20892 (301) 496-5248

## KERATOSIS PALMARIS ET PLANTARIS

National Cancer Institute
Building 31, Room 10A16
Bethesda, MD 20892 (800) 4-CANCER

## KIDNEY CANCER

National Cancer Institute
Building 31, Room 10A16
Bethesda, MD 20892 (800) 4-CANCER

## KIDNEY DISEASE

National Kidney and Urological Diseases
Information Clearinghouse
3 Information Way
Bethesda, MD 20892 (301) 654-4415

## KIDNEY STONES

National Kidney and Urological Diseases
Information Clearinghouse
3 Information Way
Bethesda, MD 20892 (301) 654-4415

## KIDNEY TRANSPLANTS

National Institute of Diabetes and Digestive
and Kidney Diseases
Building 31, Room 9A04
Bethesda, MD 20892 (301) 496-3583

## KLEINE-LEVIN SYNDROME

National Institute of Allergy and Infectious Diseases
Building 31, Room 7A50
Bethesda, MD 20892 (301) 496-5717

## KLEPTOMANIA

National Institute of Mental Health
5600 Fishers Lane
Room 7C-02
Rockville, MD 20857 (301) 443-4515

## KLINEFELTER'S SYNDROME

National Institute of Child Health and Human Development
Bldg. 31, Room 2A32
Bethesda, MD 20892 (301) 496-5133

## KOCH ANTITOXINS

National Cancer Institute
Bldg. 31, Room 10A16
Bethesda, MD 20892 (800) 4-CANCER

## KRABBE'S DISEASE

National Institute of Allergy and Infectious Diseases
Bldg. 31, Room 7A50
Bethesda, MD 20892 (301) 496-5717

## KREBIOZEN

National Cancer Institute
Bldg. 31, Room 10A16
Bethesda, MD 20892 (800) 4-CANCER

## KUGELBERG-WELANDER DISEASE

National Institute of Allergy and Infectious Diseases
Building 31, Room 7A50
Bethesda, MD 20892 (301) 496-5717

## KURU

National Institute of Allergy and Infectious Diseases
Building 31

Room 7A50
Bethesda, MD 20892 (301) 496-5717

# - L -

## LABORATORY TESTING

Food and Drug Administration
(HFE-88), 5600 Fishers Lane
Rockville, MD 20857 (301) 443-3170

## LABYRINTHITIS

National Institute on Deafness and Other Communication Disorders
1 Communication Avenue (800) 241-1044
Bethesda, MD 20892-3456 (800) 241-1055 (TDD)

National Institute of Neurological Disorders and Stroke
Bldg. 31, Room 8A16 (301) 496-5751
Bethesda, MD 20892 (800) 352-9424

## LACRIMAL GLANDS

National Eye Institute
Building 31, Room 6A32
Bethesda, MD 20892 (301) 496-5248

## LACTATION

National Maternal and Child Health Clearinghouse
8201 Greensboro Drive
Suite 600
McLean, VA 22102-3810 (703) 821-8955, ext. 254

## LACTOSE DEFICIENCY

*See Lactose Intolerance*

## LACTOSE INTOLERANCE

National Digestive Diseases Information Clearinghouse
2 Information Way
Bethesda, MD 20892 (301) 654-3810

## LAETRILE

National Cancer Institute
Bldg. 31, Room 10A16
Bethesda, MD 20892 (800) 4-CANCER

## LAMAZE METHOD OF CHILDBIRTH

*See Childbirth*

## LANGUAGE DISORDERS

National Institute on Deafness and Other Communication Disorders
1 Communication Avenue (800) 241-1044
Bethesda, MD 20892-3456 (800) 241-1055 (TDD)

## LARYNX CANCER

National Cancer Institute
Bldg. 31, Room 10A16
Bethesda, MD 20892 (800) 4-CANCER

## LASER SURGERY

National Health Information Center
P.O. Box 1133
Washington, DC 20013 (301) 565-4167 (DC area)
(800) 336-4797

## LASSA FEVER

National Institute of Allergy and Infectious Diseases
Bldg. 31, Room 7A50
Bethesda, MD 20892 (301) 496-5717

## LAURENCE-MOON-BARDET-BIEDL SYNDROME

National Institute of Neurological Disorders and Stroke
Bldg. 31, Room 8A16
Bethesda, MD 20892 (301) 496-5751
(800) 352-9424

## LEAD POISONING

National Institute of Environmental Health Sciences
P.O. Box 12233
Research Triangle Park, NC 27709 (919) 541-3345

National Heart, Lung, and Blood Institute
Information Center
P.O. Box 30105
Bethesda, MD 20824-0105 (301) 251-1222

National Institute of Neurological Disorders and Stroke
Bldg. 31, Room 8A16
Bethesda, MD 20892 (301) 496-5751
(800) 352-9424

## LEARNING DISABILITIES

National Institute of Child Health and Human Development
Bldg. 31, Room 2A32
Bethesda, MD 20892 (301) 496-5133

## LEBER'S DISEASE

National Eye Institute
Bldg. 31, Room 6A32
Bethesda, MD 20892 (301) 496-5248

## LEGG-PERTHES DISEASE

National Institute of Arthritis and Musculoskeletal and Skin Diseases
1 AMS Way
Bethesda, MD 20892 (301) 495-4484

## LEGIONELLA PNEUMOPHILA

National Institute of Allergy and Infectious Diseases
Building 31, Room 7A50
Bethesda, MD 20892 (301) 496-5717

## LEGIONNAIRE'S DISEASE

National Institute of Allergy and Infectious Diseases
Building 31, Room 7A50
Bethesda, MD 20892 (301) 496-5717

## LEIGH'S DISEASE

National Institute of Neurological Disorders and Stroke

Bldg. 31, Room 8A16 — (301) 496-5751
Bethesda, MD 20892 — (800) 352-9424

## LEISHMANIASIS

National Institute of Allergy and Infectious Diseases
Bldg. 31, Room 7A50
Bethesda, MD 20892 — (301) 496-5717

## LENNOX-GASTAUT SYNDROME

National Institute of Neurological Disorders and Stroke
Bldg. 31, Room 8A16 — (301) 496-5751
Bethesda, MD 20892 — (800) 352-9424

## LENS IMPLANTS

National Eye Institute
Bldg. 31, Room 6A32
Bethesda, MD 20892 — (301) 496-5248

## LEPROSY

Gillis W. Long Hansen's Disease Center
Carville, LA 70721 — (504) 642-4722

National Institute of Allergy and Infectious Diseases
Bldg. 31, Room 7A50
Bethesda, MD 20892 — (301) 496-5717

## LESCH-NYHAN DISEASE

National Institute of Diabetes and Digestive and Kidney Diseases
Bldg. 31, Room 9A04
Bethesda, MD 20892 — (301) 496-3583

## LEUKEMIA

National Cancer Institute
Bldg. 31, Room 10A16
Bethesda, MD 20892 — (800) 4-CANCER

## LEUKOARAIOSIS

National Institute of Neurological Disorders and Stroke
Building 31, Room 8A16
Bethesda, MD 20892 — (301) 496-5751
(800) 352-9424

## LEUKODYSTROPHY

National Institute of Neurological Disorders and Stroke
Building 31, Room 8A16
Bethesda, MD 20892 — (301) 496-5751
(800) 352-9424

## LEUKOENCEPHALOPATHY

National Institute of Neurological Disorders and Stroke
Building 31, Room 8A16
Bethesda, MD 20892 — (301) 496-5751
(800) 352-9424

## LEUKOPLAKIA

National Institute of Dental Research
Building 31, Room 2C35
31 Center Drive, MSC-2290
Bethesda, MD 20892-2290 — (301) 496-4261

## LICE

National Institute of Allergy and Infectious Diseases
Building 31, Room 7A50
Bethesda, MD 20892 (301) 496-5717

## LICHEN PLANUS

National Institute of Dental Research
Building 31, Room 2C35
31 Center Drive, MSC-2290
Bethesda, MD 20892-2290 (301) 496-4261

## LIFE CYCLE

National Institute on Aging
Information Center
P.O. Box 8057
Gaithersburg, MD 20898-8057 (800) 222-2225

## LIFE EXPECTANCY

Centers for Disease Control
6525 Belcrest Rd., Room 1064
Hyattsville, MD 20782 (301) 436-8500

National Institute on Aging Information Center
P.O. Box 8057
Gaithersburg, MD 20898-8057 (800) 222-2225

## LIFESTYLE

Office of Clinical Center Communications
Bldg. 10, Room 1C255
Bethesda, MD 20892 (301) 496-2563

## LIFE-SUSTAINING TECHNOLOGIES

*See Living Wills*

## LIPID RESEARCH

National Heart, Lung, and Blood Institute
Information Center
P.O. Box 30105
Bethesda, MD 20824-0105 (301) 251-1222

## LIPID STORAGE DISEASES

National Institute of Neurological Disorders and Stroke
Bldg. 31, Room 8A16
Bethesda, MD 20892 (301) 496-5751
(800) 352-9424

## LIPID TRANSPORT DISORDERS

National Heart, Lung, and Blood Institute
Information Center
P.O. Box 30105
Bethesda, MD 20824-0105 (301) 251-1222

## LIPIDEMIA

National Heart, Lung, and Blood Institute
Information Center
P.O. Box 30105
Bethesda, MD 20824-0105 (301) 251-1222

## LIPIDOSIS

National Institute of Neurological Disorders and Stroke
Building 31, Room 8A16 (301) 496-5751
Bethesda, MD 20892 (800) 352-9424

## LISTERIOSIS

National Institute of Allergy and Infectious Diseases
Building 31, Room 7A50
Bethesda, MD 20892 (301) 496-5717

## LITHOTRIPSY

National Institute of Diabetes and Digestive and Kidney Diseases
Bldg. 31, Room 9A04
Bethesda, MD 20892 (301) 496-3583

## LIVER DISORDERS

National Institute of Diabetes and Digestive and Kidney Diseases
Building 31, Room 9A04
Bethesda, MD 20892 (301) 496-3583

## LIVING WILLS

*See Aging*

## LOCKED-IN SYNDROME

National Institute of Neurological Disorders and Stroke
Building 31, Room 8A16 (301) 496-5751
Bethesda, MD 20892 (800) 352-9424

## LOCKJAW (Tetanus)

National Institute of Allergy and Infectious Diseases
Bldg. 31, Room 7A50
Bethesda, MD 20892 (301) 496-5717

## LOEFFLER'S SYNDROME

National Institute of Allergy and Infectious Diseases
Bldg. 31, Room 7A50
Bethesda, MD 20892 (301) 496-5717

## LOMUSTINE

National Cancer Institute
Bldg. 31, Room 10A16
Bethesda, MD 20892 (800) 4-CANCER

## LONGEVITY

Centers for Disease Control
6525 Belcrest Rd., Room 1064
Hyattsville, MD 20782 (301) 436-8500

National Institute on Aging
Information Center
P.O. Box 8057
Gaithersburg, MD 20898-8057 (800) 222-2225

## LONG-TERM CARE

*See also Aging; Gerontology; Nursing Homes*

National Institute on Aging
Information Center

P.O. Box 8057
Gaithersburg, MD 20898-8057 (800) 222-2225

## LOU GEHRIG'S DISEASE

National Institute of Neurological Disorders and Stroke
Bldg. 31, Room 8A16 (301) 496-5751
Bethesda, MD 20892 (800) 352-9424

## LOWER BACK PAIN

National Institute of Arthritis and Musculoskeletal and Skin Diseases
1 AMS Way
Bethesda, MD 20892 (301) 495-4484

National Institute of Neurological Disorders and Stroke
Bldg. 31, Room 8A16
Bethesda, MD 20892 (301) 496-5751
(800) 352-9424

## LOW BIRTHWEIGHT

National Institute of Child Health and Human Development
Bldg. 31, Room 2A32
Bethesda, MD 20892 (301) 496-5133

National Maternal and Child Health Clearinghouse
8201 Greensboro Drive, Suite 600
McLean, VA 22102-3810 (703) 821-8955, ext. 254

## LOW BLOOD PRESSURE

National Heart, Lung, and Blood Institute
Information Center
P.O. Box 30105
Bethesda, MD 20824-0105 (301) 251-1222

## LOW DENSITY LIPOPROTEINS

National Heart, Lung, and Blood Institute
Information Center
P.O. Box 30105
Bethesda, MD 20824-0105 (301) 251-1222

## LOW-FAT DIET

*See also Food*

Food and Nutrition Information Center
National Agricultural Library, Room 304
10301 Baltimore Blvd.
Beltsville, MD 20705 (301) 504-5719

## LOW-INCOME MOTHERS

National Clearinghouse for Primary Care Information
8201 Greensboro Drive, Suite 600
McLean, VA 22102 (703) 821-8955, ext. 248

## LOWE'S SYNDROME

National Institute of Child Health and Human Development
Building 31, Room 2A32
Bethesda, MD 20892 (301) 496-5133

## LUNG CANCER

National Cancer Institute
Bldg. 31, Room 10A16
Bethesda, MD 20892 (800) 4-CANCER

## LUNG DISEASE

National Institute of Allergy and Infectious Diseases
Building 31, Room 7A50
Bethesda, MD 20892 (301) 496-5717

National Heart, Lung, and Blood Institute Information Center
P.O. Box 30105
Bethesda, MD 20824-0105 (301) 251-1222

## LUPUS

National Institute of Arthritis and Musculoskeletal and Skin Diseases
1 AMS Way
Bethesda, MD 20892 (301) 495-4484

National Institute of Neurological Disorders and Stroke
Bldg. 31, Room 8A16
Bethesda, MD 20892 (800) 352-9424

## LYME DISEASE

National Institute of Allergy and Infectious Diseases
Building 31, Room 7A50
Bethesda, MD 20892 (301) 496-5717

Centers for Disease Control
Information Resources Management Office
1600 Clifton Road
Atlanta, GA 30333 (404) 332-4555

## LYMPHADENOPATHY SYNDROME

National Institute of Allergy and Infectious Diseases
Bldg. 31, Room 7A50
Bethesda, MD 20892 (301) 496-5717

## LYMPHEDEMA

National Cancer Institute
Building 31, Room 10A16
Bethesda, MD 20892 (800) 4-CANCER

## LYMPHOBLASTIC LYMPHOSARCOMA

National Cancer Institute
Building 31, Room 10A16
Bethesda, MD 20892 (800) 4-CANCER

## LYMPHOMA

National Cancer Institute
Bldg. 31, Room 10A16
Bethesda, MD 20892 (800) 4-CANCER

## LYMPHOSARCOMA

National Cancer Institute
Bldg. 31, Room 10A16
Bethesda, MD 20892 (800) 4-CANCER

# - M -

## MACROGLOBULINEMIA AND MYELOMA

National Cancer Institute
Bldg. 31, Room 10A16
Bethesda, MD 20892 (800) 4-CANCER

## MACULAR DEGENERATION

National Eye Institute
Bldg. 31, Room 6A32
Bethesda, MD 20892 (301) 496-5248

## MAKARI TEST

National Cancer Institute
Bldg. 31, Room 10A16
Bethesda, MD 20892 (800) 4-CANCER

## MALABSORPTIVE DISEASE

National Institute of Diabetes and Digestive and Kidney Diseases
Building 31, Room 9A04
Bethesda, MD 20892 (301) 496-3583

## MALARIA

National Institute of Allergy and Infectious Diseases
Bldg. 31, Room 7A50
Bethesda, MD 20892 (301) 496-5717

Centers for Disease Control
Information Resources Management Office
1600 Clifton Road
Atlanta, GA 30333 (404) 332-4555

## MALIGNANCIES

National Cancer Institute
Bldg. 31, Room 10A16
Bethesda, MD 20892 (800) 4-CANCER

## MALNUTRITION

National Institute of Diabetes and Digestive and Kidney Diseases
Bldg. 31, Room 9A04
Bethesda, MD 20892 (301) 496-3583

## MALOCCLUSION

National Institute of Dental Research
Bldg. 31, Room 2C35
31 Center Drive, MSC-2290
Bethesda, MD 20892-2290 (301) 496-4261

## MAMMOGRAMS

*See also Breast Cancer*

National Cancer Institute
Bldg. 31, Room 10A16
Bethesda, MD 20892 (800) 4-CANCER

## MANDIBLE DISORDERS

National Institute of Dental Research
Bldg. 31, Room 2C35
31 Center Drive, MSC-2290
Bethesda, MD 20892 (301) 496-4261

## MANIA

National Institute of Mental Health
5600 Fishers Lane, Room 7C-02
Rockville, MD 20857 (301) 443-4515

## MANIC-DEPRESSIVE PSYCHOSIS

National Institute of Mental Health
5600 Fishers Lane
Room 7C-02
Rockville, MD 20857 (301) 443-4515

## MAPLE SYRUP URINE DISEASE

National Institute of Diabetes and Digestive
 and Kidney Diseases
Bldg. 31, Room 9A04
Bethesda, MD 20892 (301) 496-3583

## MARBLE BONE DISEASE

*See Osteopetrosis*

## MARBURG VIRUS DISEASE

National Institute of Allergy and Infectious Diseases
Building 31
Room 7A50
Bethesda, MD 20892 (301) 496-5717

## MARFAN SYNDROME

National Institute of Allergy and Infectious Diseases
Building 31
Room 7A50
Bethesda, MD 20892 (301) 496-5717

## MARIJUANA

*See also Drug Abuse*

National Clearinghouse for Alcohol and Drug Information
P.O. Box 2345
Rockville, MD 20852 (800) 729-6686

## MASTECTOMIES

*See also Breast Cancer*

National Cancer Institute
Building 31, Room 10A16
Bethesda, MD 20892 (800) 4-CANCER

## MASTOCYTOSIS

National Institute of Allergy and Infectious Diseases
Building 31, Room 7A50
Bethesda, MD 20892 (301) 496-5717

## MATERNAL AND CHILD HEALTH

National Maternal and Child Health Clearinghouse
8201 Greensboro Drive, Suite 600
McLean, VA 22101-3810 (703) 821-8955, ext. 254

## MCARDLE'S DISEASE

National Institute of Neurological Disorders and Stroke
Building 31, Room 8A16
Bethesda, MD 20892 (301) 496-5751
(800) 352-9424

## MEASLES

*See also Immunizations*

National Institute of Allergy and Infectious Diseases
Bldg. 31, Room 7A50
Bethesda, MD 20892 (301) 496-5717

## MEAT AND POULTRY

U.S. Department of Agriculture
Food Safety and Inspection Service
Room 1165-S
Washington, DC 20205 (800) 535-4555

## MECHLORETHAMINE

National Cancer Institute
Bldg. 31, Room 10A16
Bethesda, MD 20892 (800) 4-CANCER

## MECONIUM ASPIRATION SYNDROME

National Institute of Child Health and Human Development
Building 31, Room 2A32
Bethesda, MD 20892 (301) 496-5133

## MEDICAL DEVICES

Center for Devices and Radiological Health
Food and Drug Administration (HFZ-220)
5600 Fishers Ln.
Rockville, MD 20857 (301) 443-4690

## MEDICAL IMAGING

Center for Devices and Radiological Health
Food and Drug Administration (HFE-220)
5600 Fishers Ln.
Rockville, MD 20857 (301) 443-4690

## MEDICAL TESTING

Food and Drug Administration (HFE-88)
5600 Fishers Lane
Rockville, MD 20857 (301) 443-3170

## MEDICARE AND MEDICAID

Health Care Financing Administration
6325 Security Blvd.
Baltimore, MD 21201 (800) 638-6833

## MEDICATIONS

*See also Drug Approval Process; Drug Evaluation*

Drug Information Clearinghouse
Center for Drug Evaluation and Research
Food and Drug Administration (HFD-8)
5600 Fishers Lane
Rockville, MD 20857 (301) 594-1012

Office of Consumer Affairs
Food and Drug Administration (HFE-88)
5600 Fishers Lane
Rockville, MD 20857 (301) 443-3170

## MEDICINAL PLANTS

Science & Technology Division
Reference Section
Library of Congress
Washington, DC 20540 (202) 707-5580

## MEDITERRANEAN FEVER

National Institute of Allergy and Infectious Diseases
Building 31, Room 7A50
Bethesda, MD 20892 (301) 496-5717

## MEGALOBLASTIC ANEMIA

*See Anemia*

## MEGAVITAMIN THERAPY

Food and Nutrition Information Service
National Agricultural Library, Room 304
10301 Baltimore Blvd.
Beltsville, MD 20705 (301) 504-5719

## MEIGE'S SYNDROME (Facial Dystonia)

National Institute on Deafness and
Other Communication Disorders
1 Communication Avenue
Bethesda, MD 20892-3456 (800) 241-1044
(800) 241-1055 (TDD)

## MELANOMA

*See also Cancer*

National Cancer Institute
Building 31, Room 10A16
Bethesda, MD 20892 (800) 4-CANCER

## MELKERSON'S SYNDROME

National Institute of Neurological Disorders and Stroke
Building 31, Room 8A16
Bethesda, MD 20892 (301) 496-5751
(800) 352-9424

## MELPHALAN

National Cancer Institute
Bldg. 31, Room 10A16
Bethesda, MD 20892 (800) 4-CANCER

## MEMORY LOSS

National Institute of Mental Health
5600 Fishers Ln., Room 7C-02
Rockville, MD 20857 (301) 443-4515

## MENIER'S DISEASE

National Institute of Neurological Disorders and Stroke
Bldg. 31, Room 8A16
Bethesda, MD 20892 (301) 496-5751
(800) 352-9424

## MENINGITIS

National Institute of Allergy and Infectious Diseases
Bldg. 31, Room 7A50
Bethesda, MD 20892 (301) 496-5717

## MENINGOCELE

National Institute of Child Health and Human Development
Building 31, Room 2A32
Bethesda, MD 20892 (301) 496-5133

## MENKE'S DISEASE

National Institute of Neurological Disorders and Stroke
Building 31, Room 8A16
Bethesda, MD 20892 (301) 496-5751
(800) 352-9424

## MENOPAUSE

*See also Estrogen*

National Institute on Aging
Information Center
P.O. Box 8057
Gaithersburg, MD 20898-8057 (800) 222-2225

## MENSTRUATION

National Institute of Child Health and Human Development
Building 31, Room 2A32
Bethesda, MD 20892 (301) 496-5133

## MENTAL HEALTH IN CHILDREN

National Institute of Mental Health (NIMH)
5600 Fishers Lane, Room 7C-02
Rockville, MD 20857 (301) 443-4515

## MENTAL ILLNESS

National Institute of Mental Health
5600 Fishers Lane, Room 7C-02
Rockville, MD 20857 (301) 443-4515

National Institute on Aging
Information Center
P.O. Box 8057
Gaithersburg, MD 20898-8057 (800) 222-2225

## MENTAL RETARDATION

President's Committee on Mental Retardation
330 Independence Ave., SW, Room 5325
North Building
Washington, DC 20201 (202) 619-0634

## MERCAPTOPURINE

National Cancer Institute
Bldg. 31, Room 10A16
Bethesda, MD 20892 (800) 4-CANCER

## MERCURY POISONING

*See also Seafood Inspection*

National Institute of Neurological Disorders and Stroke

Bldg. 31, Room 8A16 (301) 496-5751
Bethesda, MD 20892 (800) 352-9424

## MERCURY VAPOR LAMPS

Center for Devices and Radiological Health
Food and Drug Administration (HFZ-210)
5600 Fishers Ln.
Rockville, MD 20857 (301) 443-4690

## METABOLIC DISORDERS

National Institute of Diabetes and Digestive and Kidney Diseases
Bldg. 31, Room 9A04
Bethesda, MD 20892 (301) 496-3583

## METASTATIC TUMORS

*See also Cancer*

National Institute of Neurological Disorders and Stroke
Building 31, Room 8A16 (301) 496-5751
Bethesda, MD 20892 (800) 352-9424

## METHADONE

Food and Drug Administration
5600 Fishers Lane
Rockville, MD 20857 (301) 443-3170

## METHOTREXATE

National Cancer Institute
Bldg. 31, Room 10A16
Bethesda, MD 20892 (800) 4-CANCER

## MICROCEPHALY

National Institute of Child Health and Human Development
Building 31, Room 2A32
Bethesda, MD 20892 (301) 496-5133

## MICROTROPIA

National Eye Institute
Building 31, Room 6A32
Bethesda, MD 20892 (301) 496-5248

## MICROVASCULAR SURGERY

National Institute of Neurological Disorders and Stroke
Building 31, Room 8A16
Bethesda, MD 20892 (301) 496-5751
(800) 352-9424

## MICROWAVES

Center for Devices and Radiological Health
Food and Drug Administration (HFZ-210)
5600 Fishers Lane
Rockville, MD 20857 (301) 443-4690

## MIDDLE EAR INFECTIONS

National Institute on Deafness and
Other Communication Disorders
1 Communication Avenue
Bethesda, MD 20892-3456 (800) 241-1044
(800) 241-1055 (TDD)

## MIGRAINES

National Institute of Neurological Disorders and Stroke
Bldg. 31, Room 8A16
Bethesda, MD 20892
(301) 496-5751
(800) 352-9424

## MILK

*See also Lactose Intolerance*

Food and Nutrition Information Center
National Agricultural Library, Room 304
10301 Baltimore Blvd.
Beltsville, MD 20705
(301) 504-5719

## MINORITY HEALTH CARE

Office of Minority Health Resource Center
P.O. Box 37337
Washington, DC 20013
(800) 444-6472

## MINORITY HEALTH PROFESSIONALS

Division of Disadvantaged Assistance
Bureau of Health Professions
5600 Fishers Lane, Room 8A-09
Rockville, MD 20857
(301) 443-3843

## MITOCHONDRIAL MYOPATHIES

National Institute of Neurological Disorders and Stroke
Bldg. 31, Room 8A16
Bethesda, MD 20892
(800) 352-9424

## MITOMYCIN

National Cancer Institute
Bldg. 31, Room 10A16
Bethesda, MD 20892 (800) 4-CANCER

## MITOTANE

National Cancer Institute
Bldg. 31, Room 10A16
Bethesda, MD 20892 (800) 4-CANCER

## MITRAL VALVE PROLAPSE

National Heart, Lung, and Blood Institute Information Center
P.O. Box 30105
Bethesda, MD 20824-0105 (301) 251-1222

## MIXED CONNECTIVE TISSUE DISEASE

National Institute of Arthritis and Musculoskeletal and Skin Diseases
1 AMS Way
Bethesda, MD 20892 (301) 495-4484

## MOLDS

National Institute of Allergy and Infectious Diseases
Bldg. 31, Room 7A50
Bethesda, MD 20892 (301) 496-5717

## MONGOLISM

*See Down Syndrome*

## MONONUCLEOSIS

National Institute of Allergy and Infectious Diseases
Bldg. 31, Room 7A50
Bethesda, MD 20892 (301) 496-5717

## MONOZYGOTIC TWINS

*See Twins*

## MORTALITY RATE

National Center for Health Statistics
6525 Belcrest Rd., Room 1064
Hyattsville, MD 20782 (301) 436-8500

## MOTOR NEURON DISEASE

National Institute of Neurological Disorders and Stroke
Bldg. 31, Room 8A16 (301) 496-5751
Bethesda, MD 20892 (800) 352-9424

## MOVEMENT DISORDERS

National Institute of Neurological Disorders and Stroke
Bldg. 31, Room 8A16 (301) 496-5751
Bethesda, MD 20892 (800) 352-9424

## MOYA-MOYA DISEASE

National Institute of Neurological Disorders and Stroke
Bldg. 31, Room 8A16 (301) 496-5751
Bethesda, MD 20892 (800) 352-9424

## MRI

Center for Devices and Radiological Health
Food and Drug Administration (HFZ-210)
5600 Fishers Ln.
Rockville, MD 20857 (301) 443-4690

## MSG

*See Chinese Restaurant Syndrome*

## MUCOPOLY-SACCHARIDOSIS

National Institute of Arthritis and Musculoskeletal and Skin Diseases
1 AMS Way
Bethesda, MD 20892 (301) 495-4484

## MULTI-INFARCT DEMENTIA

*See also Aging*

National Institute on Aging
Information Center
P.O. Box 8057
Gaithersburg, MD 20898-8057 (800) 222-2225

## MULTIPLE SCLEROSIS

National Institute of Neurological Disorders and Stroke
Building 31, Room 8A16
Bethesda, MD 20892 (301) 496-5751
(800) 352-9424

## MUMPS

*See also Immunizations*

National Institute of Allergy and Infectious Diseases
Bldg. 31, Room 7A50
Bethesda, MD 20892 (301) 496-5717

## MUSCULAR DYSTROPHY

National Institute of Neurological Disorders and Stroke
Bldg. 31, Room 8A16
Bethesda, MD 20892 (301) 496-5751
(800) 352-9424

## MUSCULAR FATIGUE

National Institute of Neurological Disorders and Stroke
Bldg. 31, Room 8A16
Bethesda, MD 20892 (301) 496-5751
(800) 352-9424

## MYASTHENIA GRAVIS

National Institute of Neurological Disorders and Stroke
Bldg. 31, Room 8A16
Bethesda, MD 20892 (301) 496-5751
(800) 352-9424

## MYCOBACTERIAL INFECTIONS

National Institute of Allergy and Infectious Diseases
Bldg. 31, Room 7A50
Bethesda, MD 20892 (301) 496-5717

## MYCOSES

National Institute of Allergy and Infectious Diseases
Bldg. 31, Room 7A50
Bethesda, MD 20892 (301) 496-5717

## MYCOSIS FUNGOIDES

National Cancer Institute
Bldg. 31, Room 10A16
Bethesda, MD 20892 (800) 4-CANCER

## MYCOTOXINS

National Institute of Environmental Health Sciences
P.O. Box 12233
Research Triangle Park, NC 27709 (919) 541-3345

## MYELODYSPLASTIC SYNDROMES

National Heart, Lung, and Blood Institute
Information Center
P.O. Box 30105
Bethesda, MD 20824-0105 (301) 251-1222

## MYELOFIBROSIS

National Institute of Arthritis and Musculoskeletal
and Skin Diseases
1 AMS Way
Bethesda, MD 20892 (301) 495-4484

## MYELOMA

National Cancer Institute
Bldg. 31, Room 10A16
Bethesda, MD 20892 (800) 4-CANCER

## MYOCARDIAL INFARCTION

*See also Heart Disease*

National Heart, Lung, and Blood Institute
Information Center
P.O. Box 30105
Bethesda, MD 20824-0105 (301) 251-1222

## MYOCLONUS

National Institute of Neurological Disorders and Stroke
Bldg. 31, Room 8A16
Bethesda, MD 20892 (301) 496-5751
(800) 352-9424

## MYOFASCIAL PAIN SYNDROME

National Institute of Arthritis and Musculoskeletal and Skin Diseases
1 AMS Way
Bethesda, MD 20892 (301) 495-4484

## MYOPIA

National Eye Institute
Bldg. 31, Room 6A32
Bethesda, MD 20892 (301) 496-5248

## MYOSITIS

National Institute of Arthritis and Musculoskeletal and Skin Diseases
1 AMS Way
Bethesda, MD 20892 (301) 495-4484

## MYOTONIA

National Institute of Arthritis and Musculoskeletal and Skin Diseases
1 AMS Way
Bethesda, MD 20892 (301) 495-4484

# - N -

## NARCOLEPSY

National Institute of Neurological Disorders and Stroke
Bldg. 31, Room 8A16
Bethesda, MD 20892 (301) 496-5751
(800) 352-9424

## NATIONAL HEALTH INSURANCE

*See Health Insurance*

## NATIVE AMERICANS

*See also Minority Health Care*

Indian Health Service
5600 Fishers Lane
Rockville, MD 20857 (301) 443-3593

## NATURAL CHILDBIRTH

*See Childbirth*

## NEARSIGHTEDNESS

National Eye Institute
Building 31, Room 6A32
Bethesda, MD 20892 (301) 496-5248

## NEMALINE MYOPATHY

National Institute of Neurological Disorders and Stroke
Building 31, Room 8A16
Bethesda, MD 20892 (301) 496-5751
(800) 352-9424

## NEOPLASIA

National Institute of Diabetes and Digestive
and Kidney Diseases
Building 31, Room 9A04
Bethesda, MD 20892 (301) 496-3583

## NEONATAL ASPHYXIA

National Institute of Neurological Disorders and Stroke
Bldg. 31, Room 8A16
Bethesda, MD 20892 (301) 496-5751
(800) 352-9424

## NEONATAL RESPIRATORY DISTRESS SYNDROME

National Heart, Lung and Blood Institute
Information Center
P.O. Box 30105
Bethesda, MD 20824-0105 (301) 251-1222

## NEPHRITIS

National Institute of Diabetes and Digestive
and Kidney Diseases
Building 31, Room 9A04
Bethesda, MD 20892 (301) 496-3583

## NEPHROCALCINOSIS

National Institute of Diabetes and Digestive
and Kidney Diseases
Bldg. 31, Room 9A04
Bethesda, MD 20892 (301) 496-3583

## NEPHROLITHIASIS

National Institute of Diabetes and Digestive
and Kidney Diseases
Bldg. 31, Room 9A04
Bethesda, MD 20892 (301) 496-3583

## NEPHROTIC SYNDROME

National Institute of Diabetes and Digestive and Kidney Diseases
Bldg. 31, Room 9A04
Bethesda, MD 20892 (301) 496-3583

## NERVE DAMAGE

National Institute of Neurological Disorders and Stroke
Bldg. 31, Room 8A16
Bethesda, MD 20892 (301) 496-5751
(800) 352-9424

## NEURAL TUBE DEFECTS

*See also Birth Defects*

National Institute of Neurological Disorders and Stroke
Bldg. 31, Room 8A16
Bethesda, MD 20892 (301) 496-5751
(800) 352-9424

## NEURALGIA

National Institute of Neurological Disorders and Stroke
Bldg. 31, Room 8A16
Bethesda, MD 20892 (301) 496-5751
(800) 352-9424

## NEURODERMATITIS

National Arthritis and Musculoskeletal and Skin Diseases
Information Clearinghouse
1 AMS Way
Bethesda, MD 20892 (301) 495-4484

## NEURO-OPHTHALMOLOGY

National Eye Institute
Building 31, Room 6A32
Bethesda, MD 20892 (301) 496-5248

## NEUROAXONAL DYSTROPHY

National Institute of Neurological Disorders and Stroke
Building 31, Room 8A16
Bethesda, MD 20892 (301) 496-5751
(800) 352-9424

## NEUROBLASTOMA

National Cancer Institute
Bldg. 31, Room 10A16
Bethesda, MD 20892 (800) 4-CANCER

## NEUROFIBROMATOSIS

National Institute on Deafness and Other Communication Disorders
1 Communication Avenue
Bethesda, MD 20892-1044 (800) 241-1044
(800) 241-1055 (TDD)

## NEUROGENIC ARTHROPATHY

National Institute of Neurological Disorders and Stroke
Building 31, Room 8A16
Bethesda, MD 20892 (301) 496-5751
(800) 352-9424

## NEUROLOGICAL DISORDERS

National Institute of Neurological Disorders and Stroke
Building 31, Room 8A16
Bethesda, MD 20892 (301) 496-5751
(800) 352-9424

## NEUROPATHIES

National Institute of Neurological Disorders and Stroke
Bldg. 31, Room 8A16
Bethesda, MD 20892
(301) 496-5751
(800) 352-9424

## NEUROSCIENCE

Office of Technology Assessment
600 Pennsylvania Ave., SE
Washington, DC 20510
(202) 224-8996

## NEUROSCLEROSIS

National Institute of Neurological Disorders and Stroke
Bldg. 31, Room 8A16
Bethesda, MD 20892
(301) 496-5751
(800) 352-9424

## NEUROTOXICITY

National Institute of Neurological Disorders and Stroke
Bldg. 31, Room 8A16
Bethesda, MD 20892
(301) 496-5751
(800) 352-9424

## NEWBORN SCREENING

National Maternal and Child Health Clearinghouse
8201 Greensboro Drive, Suite 600
McLean, VA 22102-3810
(703) 821-8955, ext. 254

## NIEMANN-PICK DISEASE

National Institute of Neurological Disorders and Stroke
Building 31, Room 8A16
Bethesda, MD 20892 (301) 496-5751
(800) 352-9424

## NIGHT BLINDNESS

National Eye Institute
Bldg. 31, Room 6A32
Bethesda, MD 20892 (301) 496-5248

## NOISE, EFFECTS OF

National Institute of Environmental Health Sciences
P.O. Box 12233
Research Triangle Park, NC 27709 (919) 541-3345

National Institute on Deafness and Other Communication Disorders
1 Communication Avenue (800) 241-1044
Bethesda, MD 20892-3456 (800) 241-1055 (TDD)

## NONGONOCOCCAL URETHRITIS

National Sexually Transmitted Diseases Hotline
P.O. Box 13827
Research Triangle Park, NC 27709 (800) 227-8922

## NONPRESCRIPTION DRUGS

Center for Drug Evaluation and Research
Food and Drug Administration (HFD-8)
5600 Fishers Ln.
Rockville, MD 20857 (301) 594-1012

## NORPLANT

*See also Contraception*

Office of Consumer Inquiries
Food and Drug Administration, HFD-88
5600 Fishers Road
Rockville, MD 20857 (301) 443-3170

## NOSEBLEEDS

National Heart, Lung, and Blood Institute
Information Center
P.O. Box 30105
Bethesda, MD 20824-0105 (301) 251-1222

## NUCLEAR MEDICINE

Center for Devices and Radiological Health
Food and Drug Administration (HFZ-210)
5600 Fishers Lane
Rockville, MD 20857 (301) 443-4690

## NURSING HOMES

*See also Long-Term Care*

National Institute on Aging
P.O. Box 8057
Gaithersburg, MD 20898-8057 (800) 222-2225

## NUTRITION

Food and Nutrition Information Center
National Agricultural Library, Room 304

10301 Baltimore Blvd.
Beltsville, MD 20705 (301) 504-5719

National Maternal and Child Health Clearinghouse
8201 Greensboro Drive, Suite 600
McLean, VA 22102-3810 (703) 821-8955, ext. 254

Human Nutrition Information Service
U.S. Department of Agriculture
6505 Belcrest Road, Room 363
Hyattsville, MD 20782 (301) 436-8617

Food and Nutrition Service
3101 Park Center Drive
Park Office Bldg.
Alexandria, VA 22302 (703) 305-2554

## NUTRITIONAL LABELING

*See Food Labeling*

## NYSTAGMUS

National Eye Institute
Building 31, Room 6A32
Bethesda, MD 20892 (301) 496-5248

# - O -

## OBESITY

*See also Dieting*

National Institute of Diabetes and Digestive and Kidney Diseases
National Institutes of Health

Building 31, Room 9A04
Bethesda, MD 20892 (301) 496-5877

## OBSESSIVE-COMPULSIVE

National Institute of Mental Health
5600 Fishers Lane
Room 7C-02
Rockville, MD 20857 (301) 443-4515

## OCCUPATIONAL SAFETY AND HEALTH

Technical Information Branch
National Institute for Occupational Safety and Health
4676 Columbia Parkway
Cincinnati, OH 45226 (800) 35-NIOSH

## OCULAR HYPERTENSION

National Eye Institute
Bldg. 31, Room 6A32
Bethesda, MD 20892 (301) 496-5248

## ODOR DISORDERS

National Institute on Deafness and
Other Communication Disorders
1 Communication Ave.
Bethesda, MD 20892-3456 (800) 241-1044
(800) 241-1055 (TDD)

National Institute of Neurological Disorders and Stroke
Bldg. 31, Room 8A16
Bethesda, MD 20892 (301) 496-5751
(800) 352-9424

## OLIVOPONTOCEREBELLAR ATROPHY

National Institute of Neurological Disorders and Stroke
Bldg. 31, Room 8A16
Bethesda, MD 20892 (301) 496-5751
(800) 352-9424

## ONCHOCERCIASIS

National Eye Institute
Bldg. 31, Room 6A32
Bethesda, MD 20892 (301) 496-5248

## ONCOLOGY

*See also Cancer*

National Cancer Institute
Bldg. 31, Room 10A16
Bethesda, MD 20892 (800) 4-CANCER

## OPHTHALMIA NEONATORUM

National Eye Institute
Bldg. 31, Room 6A32
Bethesda, MD 20892 (301) 496-5248

## OPPENHEIM'S DISEASE

National Institute of Neurological Disorders and Stroke
Bldg. 31, Room 8A16
Bethesda, MD 20892 (301) 496-5751
(800) 352-9424

## OPTIC ATROPHY

National Eye Institute
Bldg. 31, Room 6A32
Bethesda, MD 20892 (301) 496-5248

## OPTIC NEURITIS

National Eye Institute
Bldg. 31, Room 6A32
Bethesda, MD 20892 (301) 496-5248

## ORAL CANCER

*See also Cancer*

National Institute of Dental Research
Bldg. 31, Room 2C35
31 Center Dr., MSC-2290
Bethesda, MD 20892-2290 (301) 496-4261

## ORAL CONTRACEPTIVES

*See also Contraception*

National Institute of Child Health and Human Development
Bldg. 31, Room 2A32
31 Center Dr., MSC-2290
Bethesda, MD 20892-2290 (301) 496-5133

Center for Drug Evaluation and Research
Food and Drug Administration
7520 Standish Place, Room 201
Rockville, MD 20855 (301) 594-1012

## ORAL HEALTH

National Institute of Dental Research
Bldg. 31, Room 2C35
31 Center Dr., MSC-2290
Bethesda, MD 20892-2290 (301) 496-4261

## ORGAN TRANSPLANTS

Bureau of Health Resources Development
Health Resources and Services Administration
5600 Fishers Lane, Room 718
Rockville, MD 20857 (301) 443-7577

## OROTIC ACIDURIA

National Institute of Arthritis and Musculoskeletal
and Skin Diseases
1 AMS Way
Bethesda, MD 20892 (301) 495-4484

## ORPHAN DISEASES

National Information Center for Orphan Drugs
and Rare Diseases
5600 Fishers Lane, Room 873
Rockville, MD 20857 (800) 300-7469

## ORPHAN DRUGS

National Information Center for Orphan Drugs
and Rare Diseases
5600 Fishers Lane, Room 873
Rockville, MD 20857 (800) 300-7469

## ORTHODONTICS

National Institute of Dental Research
Building 31, Room 2C35
31 Center Dr., MSC-2290
Bethesda, MD 20892-2290 (301) 496-4261

## ORTHOGNATHIC SURGERY

National Institute of Dental Research
Bldg. 31, Room 2C35
31 Center Dr., MSC-2290
Bethesda, MD 20892-2290 (301) 496-4261

## ORTHOKERATOLOGY

National Eye Institute
Bldg. 31, Room 6A32
Bethesda, MD 20892 (301) 496-5248

## ORTHOPEDICS

National Institute of Arthritis and Musculoskeletal
and Skin Diseases
1 AMS Way
Bethesda, MD 20892 (301) 495-4484

## ORTHOPEDIC IMPLANTS

National Institute of Arthritis and Musculoskeletal
and Skin Diseases
1 AMS Way
Bethesda, MD 20892 (301) 495-4484

## ORTHOSTATIC HYPOTENSION

National Heart, Lung, and Blood Institute
Information Center
P.O. Box 30105
Bethesda, MD 20824-0105 (301) 251-1222

## ORTHOTICS

National Institute of Arthritis and Musculoskeletal and Skin Diseases
1 AMS Way
Bethesda, MD 20892 (301) 495-4484

## OSTEITIS DEFORMANS

National Institute of Arthritis and Musculoskeletal and Skin Diseases
1 AMS Way
Bethesda, MD 20892 (301) 495-4484

## OSTEOARTHRITIS

National Institute of Arthritis and Musculoskeletal and Skin Diseases
1 AMS Way
Bethesda, MD 20892 (301) 495-4484

## OSTEOGENESIS

National Institute of Arthritis and Musculoskeletal and Skin Diseases
1 AMS Way
Bethesda, MD 20892 (301) 495-4484

## OSTEOGENIC SARCOMA

National Cancer Institute
Bldg. 31, Room 10A16
Bethesda, MD 20892 (800) 4-CANCER

## OSTEOMALACIA

National Institute of Arthritis and Musculoskeletal and Skin Diseases
1 AMS Way
Bethesda, MD 20892 (301) 495-4484

## OSTEOMYELITIS

National Institute of Allergy and Infectious Diseases
Building 31, Room 7A50
Bethesda, MD 20892 (301) 496-5717

## OSTEOPETROSIS

National Institute of Child Health and Human Development
Building 31, Room 2A32
Bethesda, MD 20892 (301) 496-5133

## OSTEOPOROSIS

National Institute on Aging
P.O. Box 8057
Gaithersburg, MD 20892-8057 (800) 222-2225

National Arthritis and Musculoskeletal and Skin Diseases
Information Clearinghouse
1 AMS Way
Bethesda, MD 20892 (301) 495-4484

## OSTEOSARCOMA

*See also Papilloma Virus*

National Cancer Institute
Bldg. 31, Room 10A16
Bethesda, MD 20892 (800) 4-CANCER

## OSTEOSCLEROSIS

National Institute of Child Health and Human Development
Bldg. 31, Room 2A32
Bethesda, MD 20892 (301) 496-5133

## OTITIS MEDIA

*See Ear Infections*

## OTOSCLEROSIS

National Institute on Deafness and
Other Communication Disorders
1 Communication Ave. (800) 241-1044
Bethesda, MD 20892-3456 (800) 241-1055 (TDD)

National Institute of Neurological Disorders and Stroke
Bldg. 31, Room 8A16 (301) 496-5751
Bethesda, MD 20892 (800) 352-9424

## OVARIAN CANCER

*See also Cancer*

National Cancer Institute

Building 31, Room 10A16
Bethesda, MD 20892 (800) 4-CANCER

## OVER-THE-COUNTER DRUGS

*See also Medications*

Over-the Counter Drug Evaluation Division
Center for Drug Evaluation and Research
Food and Drug Administration
7520 Standish Place, Room 201
Rockville, MD 20855 (301) 594-5000

## OVULATION

National Institute of Child Health and Human Development
Building 31, Room 2A32
Bethesda, MD 20892 (301) 496-5133

# - P -

## PACEMAKERS

National Heart, Lung, and Blood Institute
Information Center
P.O. Box 30105
Bethesda, MD 20824-0105 (301) 251-1222

## PAGET'S DISEASE

National Institute of Arthritis and Musculoskeletal and Skin Diseases
1 AMS Way
Bethesda, MD 20892 (301) 495-4484

## PAIN

National Cancer Institute
Bldg. 31, Room 10A16
Bethesda, MD 20892 (800) 4-CANCER

## PALPITATIONS

National Heart, Lung, and Blood Institute
Information Center
P.O. Box 30105
Bethesda, MD 20824-0105 (301) 251-1222

## PALSY

National Institute of Neurological Disorders and Stroke
Bldg. 31, Room 8A16
Bethesda, MD 20892 (301) 496-5751
(800) 352-9424

## PANCREATIC CANCER

*See also Cancer*

National Cancer Institute
Bldg. 31, Room 10A16
Bethesda, MD 20892 (800) 4-CANCER

## PANCREATITIS

National Digestive Diseases Information Clearinghouse
2 Information Way
Bethesda, MD 20892 (301) 654-3810

## PANIC ATTACKS

National Institute of Mental Health
5600 Fishers Lane, Room 7C-02
Rockville, MD 20857 (301) 443-4515

## PANENCEPHALITIS

National Institute of Neurological Disorders and Stroke
Bldg. 31, Room 8A16
Bethesda, MD 20892 (301) 496-5751
(800) 352-9424

## PANNICULITIS

National Institute of Diabetes and Digestive and Kidney Diseases
Bldg. 31, Room 9A04
Bethesda, MD 20892 (301) 496-3583

## PAP TESTS

National Cancer Institute
Bldg. 31, Room 10A16
Bethesda, MD 20892 (800) 4-CANCER

## PAPILLOMA VIRUS

*See also Cancer*

National Cancer Institute
Bldg. 31, Room 10A16
Bethesda, MD 20892 (800) 4-CANCER

## PARALYSIS AGITANS

National Institute of Neurological Disorders and Stroke
Bldg. 31, Room 8A16
Bethesda, MD 20892 (301) 496-5751
(800) 352-9424

## PARAMYOTONIA CONGENITA

National Institute of Neurological Disorders and Stroke
Bldg. 31, Room 8A16
Bethesda, MD 20892 (301) 496-5751
(800) 352-9424

## PARANOIA

National Institute of Mental Health
5600 Fishers Lane, Room 7C-02
Rockville, MD 20857 (301) 443-4515

## PARAPLEGIA

National Institute of Neurological Disorders and Stroke
Bldg. 31, Room 8A16
Bethesda, MD 20892 (301) 496-5751
(800) 352-9424

## PARASITIC DISEASE

National Institute of Allergy and Infectious Diseases
Bldg. 31, Room 7A50
Bethesda, MD 20892 (301) 496-5717

## PARATHYROID DISORDERS

National Institute of Diabetes and Digestive
and Kidney Diseases
Bldg. 31, Room 9A04
Bethesda, MD 20892 (301) 496-3583

## PARKINSON'S DISEASE

National Institute of Neurological Disorders and Stroke
Bldg. 31, Room 8A16
Bethesda, MD 20892 (301) 496-5751
(800) 352-9424

## PAROXYSMAL ATRIAL TACHYCARDIA

National Heart, Lung, and Blood Institute
Information Center
P.O. Box 30105
Bethesda, MD 20824-0105 (301) 251-1222

## PAROXYSMAL NOCTURNAL HEMOGLOBINURIA

National Heart, Lung, and Blood Institute
Information Center
P.O. Box 30105
Bethesda, MD 20824-0105 (301) 251-1222

## PARS PLANITIS

National Eye Institute
Bldg. 31, Room 6A32
Bethesda, MD 20892 (301) 496-5248

## PARVOVIRUS INFECTIONS

National Institute of Allergy and Infectious Diseases
Bldg. 31, Room 7A50
Bethesda, MD 20892 (301) 496-5717

## PASSIVE SMOKING

*See also Smoking*

Office on Smoking and Health
Centers for Disease Control
4770 Buford Hwy, NE, MS K-50
Atlanta, GA 30341 (404) 488-5705

## PCP

*See also Drug Abuse*

National Clearinghouse for Alcohol and Drug Information
P.O. Box 2345
Rockville, MD 20852 (301) 468-2600
(800) 729-6686

## PECTUS EXCAVATUM

National Heart, Lung, and Blood Institute
Information Center
P.O. Box 30105
Bethesda, MD 20824-0105 (301) 251-1222

## PEDIATRIC AIDS

*See AIDS*

## PEDICULOSIS

*See Lice*

## PEDODONTICS

National Institute of Dental Research
31 Center Dr., MSC-2290
Bldg. 31, Room 2C35
Bethesda, MD 20892-2290 (301) 496-4261

## PELIZAEOUS-MERZBACHER DISEASE

National Institute of Neurological Disorders and Stroke
Bldg. 31, Room 8A16 (301) 496-5751
Bethesda, MD 20892 (800) 352-9424

## PELVIC INFLAMMATORY DISEASE

National Institute of Allergy and Infectious Diseases
Bldg. 31, Room 7A50
Bethesda, MD 20892 (301) 496-5717

## PEMPHIGOID

National Cancer Institute
Bldg. 31, Room 10A16
Bethesda, MD 20892 (800) 4-CANCER

## PENICILLIN

Food and Drug Administration
5600 Fishers Lane (HFE-88)
Rockville, MD 20857 (301) 443-3170

## PEPTIC ULCERS

National Institute of Diabetes and Digestive
and Kidney Diseases
Building 31, Room 9A04
Bethesda, MD 20892 (301) 496-3583

## PERIARTERITIS NODOSA

National Heart, Lung, and Blood Institute
Information Center
P.O. Box 30105
Bethesda, MD 20824-0105 (301) 251-1222

## PERICARDITIS

National Heart, Lung, and Blood Institute
Information Center
P.O. Box 30105
Bethesda, MD 20824-0105 (301) 251-1222

## PERICARDIAL TAMPONADE

National Heart, Lung, and Blood Institute
Information Center
P.O. Box 30105
Bethesda, MD 20824-0105 (301) 251-1222

## PERINATAL SERVICES

*See Prenatal*

## PERIODONTAL DISEASE

National Institute of Dental Research
Building 31, Room 2C35
31 Center Dr., MSC-2290
Bethesda, MD 20892-2290 (301) 496-4261

## PERIPHERAL NEUROPATHY

National Institute of Neurological Disorders and Stroke
Bldg. 31, Room 8A16
Bethesda, MD 20892 (301) 496-5751
(800) 352-9424

## PERIPHERAL VASCULAR DISEASE

National Heart, Lung, and Blood Institute
Information Center
P.O. Box 30105
Bethesda, MD 20824-0105 (301) 251-1222

## PERNICIOUS ANEMIA

National Institute of Diabetes and Digestive and Kidney Diseases
Bldg. 31, Room 9A04
Bethesda, MD 20892 (301) 496-3583

## PERSONALITY DISORDERS

National Institute of Mental Health
5600 Fishers Lane, Room 7C-02
Rockville, MD 20857 (301) 443-4515

## PERTUSSIS

*See also Immunizations*

National Institute of Allergy and Infectious Diseases
Bldg. 31, Room 7A50
Bethesda, MD 20892 (301) 496-5717

## PERVASIVE DEVELOPMENTAL DISORDERS

*See also Developmental Disabilities*

National Institute of Neurological Disorders and Stroke
Bldg. 31, Room 8A16 (301) 496-5751
Bethesda, MD 20892 (800) 352-9424

## PESTICIDES

National Pesticide Telecommunications Network
Texas Tech University
Health Sciences Center
Lubbock, TX 79430 (800) 858-7378

National Institute of Environmental Health Sciences
P.O. Box 12233
Research Triangle Park, NC 27709 (919) 541-3345

## PEYRONIE'S DISEASE

National Institute of Diabetes and Digestive and Kidney Diseases
Bldg. 31, Room 9A04
Bethesda, MD 20892 (301) 496-3583

## PHARMACEUTICALS

*See Medications; Drug Approval Process; Drug Evaluation*

## PHARMACOLOGY

National Institute of General Medical Sciences
National Institutes of Health
Building 31, Room 4A52
Bethesda, MD 20892 (301) 496-7301

## PHARYNGEAL DISABILITIES

National Institute of Dental Research
Bldg. 31, Room 2C35
31 Center Dr., MSC-2290
Bethesda, MD 20892-2290 (301) 496-4261

## PHENYLKETONURIA

*See PKU*

## PHEOCHROMOCYTOMA

National Heart, Lung, and Blood Institute
Information Center
P.O. Box 30105
Bethesda, MD 20824-0105 (301) 251-1222

## PHLEBITIS

National Heart, Lung, and Blood Institute
Information Center
P.O. Box 30105
Bethesda, MD 20824-0105 (301) 251-1222

## PHLEBOTHROMBOSIS

National Heart, Lung, and Blood Institute
Information Center
P.O. Box 30105
Bethesda, MD 20824-0105 (301) 251-1222

## PHOBIAS

National Institute of Mental Health
5600 Fishers Lane, Room 7C-02
Rockville, MD 20857 (301) 443-4515

## PHYSICAL FITNESS

*See Exercise*

## PICK'S DISEASE

National Institute of Neurological Disorders and Stroke
Bldg. 31, Room 8A16 (301) 496-5751
Bethesda, MD 20892 (800) 352-9424

## THE PILL

*See Oral Contraceptives*

## PI-MESONS

National Cancer Institute
Bldg. 31, Room 10A16
Bethesda, MD 20892 (800) 4-CANCER

## PIMPLES

*See Acne*

## PINK EYE

National Eye Institute
Bldg. 31, Room 6A32
Bethesda, MD 20892 (301) 496-5248

## PINTA

National Arthritis and Musculoskeletal and Skin Diseases Clearinghouse
1 AMS Way
Bethesda, MD 20892 (301) 495-4484

## PINWORMS

National Institute of Allergy and Infectious Diseases
Bldg. 31, Room 7A50
Bethesda, MD 20892 (301) 496-5717

## PITUITARY TUMORS

National Institute of Neurological Disorders and Stroke
Bldg. 31, Room 8A16 (301) 496-5751
Bethesda, MD 20892 (800) 352-9424

## PITYRIASIS

National Institute of Arthritis and Musculoskeletal and Skin Diseases
1 AMS Way
Bethesda, MD 20892 (301) 495-4484

## PKD

*See Polycystic Kidney Disease*

## PKU (Phenylketonuria)

National Institute of Child Health and Human Development
Building 31, Room 2A32
Bethesda, MD 20892 (301) 496-5133

## PLACENTA DISORDERS

National Institute of Child Health and Human Development
Bldg. 31, Room 2A32
Bethesda, MD 20892 (301) 496-5133

## PLAQUE

National Institute of Dental Research
Bldg. 31, Room 2C35
31 Center Dr., MSC-2290
Bethesda, MD 20892-2290 (301) 496-4261

## PLASMA CELL CANCER

National Cancer Institute
Bldg. 31, Room 10A16
Bethesda, MD 20892 (800) 4-CANCER

## PLASTIC SURGERY

*See Face Lifts*

## PLAYGROUND SAFETY

National Maternal and Child Health Clearinghouse
8201 Greensboro Dr., Suite 600
McLean, VA 22102-3810 (703) 821-8955, ext. 254

## PLEURISY

National Heart, Lung, and Blood Institute
Information Center
P.O. Box 30105
Bethesda, MD 20824-0105 (301) 251-1222

## PLICAMYCIN

National Cancer Institute
Bldg. 31, Room 10A16
Bethesda, MD 20892 (800) 4-CANCER

## PMS

National Institute of Child Health and Human Development
Bldg. 31, Room 2A32
Bethesda, MD 20892 (301) 496-5133

National Institute of Mental Health
5600 Fishers Lane, Room 7C-02
Rockville, MD 20857 (301) 443-4515

## PNEUMOCOCCAL INFECTIONS

National Institute of Allergy and Infectious Diseases
Bldg. 31, Room 7A50
Bethesda, MD 20892 (301) 496-5717

National Heart, Lung, and Blood Institute
Information Center
P.O. Box 30105
Bethesda, MD 20824-0105 (301) 251-1222

## PNEUMOTHORAX

National Heart, Lung, and Blood Institute
Information Center
P.O. Box 30105
Bethesda, MD 20824-0105 (301) 251-1222

## POISONING

**Alabama**
Alabama Poison Center (205) 345-0600
AL only: (800) 462-0800

**Arizona**
Arizona Poison Control and Drug Information System (602) 626-7899
Tucson: (602) 626-6016
Phoenix: (602) 253-3334
AZ only: (800) 362-0101

**California**
Los Angeles Regional Drug and Poison Information Center
(213) 222-3212
(800) 777-6476

San Diego Regional Poison Center (619) 543-6000

San Francisco Bay Area Regional Poison Control Center (415) 206-5265
(800) 523-2222

**Colorado**
Rocky Mountain Poison Center Denver: (303) 629-1123
CO only: (800) 332-3073
MT only: (800) 525-5042

**Florida**

Tampa Bay Regional Control System (813) 253-4444
(800) 282-3171

**Georgia**

Georgia Poison Control Center (404) 616-9000
GA only: (800) 282-5846
TTY: (404) 616-9287

**Kentucky**

Kentucky Regional Poison Center of Kosair Children's Hospital
(502) 589-8222
KY only (TDD): (800) 722-5725

**Louisiana**

Louisiana Regional Poison Control Center LA only: (800) 256-9822

**Maryland**

Maryland Poison Center Montgomery County: (202) 625-3333
MD only: (800) 492-2414

**Massachusetts**

Massachusetts Poison Control System (617) 735-6607
Emergency: (617) 232-2120
MD only: (800) 682-9211

**Michigan**

Michigan Poison Control Center (313) 745-5711
remainder of MI: (800) POISIN-1

**Minnesota**

Hennepin Regional Poison Center (612) 347-3144
Emergency: (612) 347-3141
TTY: (612) 337-7474
(800) 222-1222

**Missouri**

Cardinal Glennon Children's Hospital
Regional Poison Center (314) 772-8300
(314) 772-5200
MO only: (800) 336-8888

**Nebraska**
Mid-Plains Poison Center (402) 390-5434
NE only: (800) 955-9119

**New Jersey**
New Jersey Poison Information and Education System (201) 926-7443
NJ only: (800) POISIN-1

**New Mexico**
New Mexico Poison and Drug Information Center (505) 277-4261
Albuquerque: (505) 843-2551
NM only: (800) 432-6866

**New York**
New York City Poison Control Center (212) 340-4494

Long Island Regional Poison Control Center (516) 542-2323

**North Carolina**
Duke University Poison Control Center (919) 684-4438
(919) 684-8111
NC only (Emergency): (800) 672-1697

**Ohio**
Central Ohio Poison Center (614) 722-2636
(614) 228-1323
(800) 682-7625

Southwest Ohio Regional Poison Control System (513) 558-5111
OH only: (800) 872-5111

**Oregon**
Oregon Poison Control and Drug Information Center (503) 594-8968
(800) 452-7165

**Pennsylvania**
Pittsburgh Poison Center (412) 681-6669

**Texas**
Texas State Poison Center (409) 772-3332
TX only: (800) 764-7661

North Texas Poison Center (214) 590-5000
TX only: (800) 764-7661

**Utah**
Utah Poison Control Center (801) 581-7504
Emergency: (801) 581-2151
UT only: (800) 662-0062

**West Virginia**
West Virginia Poison Center (304) 347-1212
Emergency: (304) 348-4211
WV only: (800) 642-3625

**Washington, D.C.**
Washington DC (202) 625-3333

## POISON IVY

National Institute of Allergy and Infectious Diseases
Bldg. 31, Room 7A50
Bethesda, MD 20892 (301) 496-5717

## POLIOENCEPHALITIS

National Institute of Neurological Disorders and Stroke
Bldg. 31, Room 8A16
Bethesda, MD 20892 (301) 496-5751
(800) 352-9424

## POLIOMYELITIS

National Institute of Allergy and Infectious Diseases
Bldg. 31, Room 7A50
Bethesda, MD 20892 (301) 496-5717

## POLLEN ALLERGY

National Institute of Allergy and Infectious Diseases
Bldg. 31, Room 7A50
Bethesda, MD 20892 (301) 496-5717

## POLYARTERITIS

National Heart, Lung, and Blood Institute
Information Center
P.O. Box 30105
Bethesda, MD 20824-0105 (301) 251-1222

## POLYCYSTIC KIDNEY DISEASE (PKD)

National Kidney and Urologic Diseases
Information Clearinghouse
3 Information Way
Bethesda, MD 20892 (301) 654-4415

## POLYCYSTIC OVARY SYNDROME

National Institute of Child Health and Human Development
Bldg. 31, Room 2A32
Bethesda, MD 20892 (301) 496-5133

## POLYCYTHEMIA

National Heart, Lung, and Blood Institute
Information Center
P.O. Box 30105
Bethesda, MD 20824-0105 (301) 251-1222

## POLYMYALGIA RHEUMATICA

National Institute of Arthritis and Musculoskeletal and Skin Diseases
1 AMS Way
Bethesda, MD 20892 (301) 495-4484

## POLYMYOSITIS

National Institute of Arthritis and Musculoskeletal and Skin Diseases
1 AMS Way
Bethesda, MD 20892 (301) 495-4484

## POLYNEURITIS

National Institute of Arthritis and Musculoskeletal and Skin Diseases
1 AMS Way
Bethesda, MD 20892 (301) 495-4484

## POLYOSTOTIC FIBROUS DYSPLASIA

National Institute of Arthritis and Musculoskeletal and Skin Diseases
1 AMS Way
Bethesda, MD 20892 (301) 495-4484

## POLYPS

National Cancer Institute
Bldg. 31, Room 10A16
Bethesda, MD 20892 (800) 4-CANCER

## POLYSEROSITIS

National Institute of Allergy and Infectious Diseases

Bldg. 31, Room 7A50
Bethesda, MD 20892 (301) 496-5717

## POMPE'S DISEASE

National Institute of Neurological Disorders and Stroke
Bldg. 31, Room 8A16
Bethesda, MD 20892 (301) 496-5751
(800) 352-9424

## POPULATION CONTROL

National Institute of Child Health and Human Development
Bldg. 31, Room 2A32
Bethesda, MD 20892 (301) 496-5133

## PORPHYRIA

National Institute of Arthritis and Musculoskeletal and Skin Diseases
1 AMS Way
Bethesda, MD 20892 (301) 495-4484

## POSITRON EMISSION TOMOGRAPHY

National Institute of Neurological Disorders and Stroke
Bldg. 31, Room 7A50 (301) 496-5751
Bethesda, MD 20892 (800) 352-9424

## POSTNATAL CARE

*See also Childbirth; Child Health*

National Institute of Child Health and Human Development
Bldg. 31, Room 2A32
Bethesda, MD 20892 (301) 496-5133

National Maternal and Child Health Clearinghouse
8201 Greensboro Dr.
McLean, VA 22102-3810
(703) 821-8955, ext. 254

## POST-POLIO SYNDROME

National Institute of Neurological Disorders and Stroke
Building 31, Room 8A16
Bethesda, MD 20892 (301) 496-5751
(800) 352-9424

## POSTURAL HYPOTENSION

National Heart, Lung, and Blood Institute
Information Center
P.O. Box 30105
Bethesda, MD 20824-0105 (301) 251-1222

## POTASSIUM

*See also Food*

National Heart, Lung, and Blood Institute
Information Center
P.O. Box 30105
Bethesda, MD 20824-0105 (301) 251-1222

## POTT'S DISEASE

National Institute of Neurological Disorders and Stroke
Bldg. 31, Room 8A16
Bethesda, MD 20892 (301) 496-5751
(800) 352-9424

## POULTRY INSPECTION

*See also Meat & Poultry*

Food Safety and Inspection Service
U.S. Department of Agriculture
Room 1165-S
Washington, DC 20205 (800) 535-4555

## POWER LINES

Center for Devices and Radiological Health
Food and Drug Administration (HFZ-210)
5600 Fishers Lane
Rockville, MD 20857 (301) 443-4190

## PRADER-WILLI SYNDROME

National Institute of Child Health and Human Development
Bldg. 31, Room 2A32
Bethesda, MD 20892 (301) 496-5133

## PREDNISONE

National Cancer Institute
Bldg. 31, Room 10A16
Bethesda, MD 20892 (800) 4-CANCER

## PREGNANCY

*See also Amniocentesis*

National Institute of Child Health and Human Development
Bldg. 31, Room 2A32
Bethesda, MD 20892 (301) 496-5133

National Maternal and Child Health Clearinghouse
8201 Greensboro Dr.
McLean, VA 22102-3810 (703) 821-8955, ext. 254

Office on Smoking Health Centers for Disease Control
Mail Stop K-50, 4770 Buford Hwy NE
Atlanta, GA 30341-3724 (404) 488-5705

## PREGNANCY AND ALCOHOL

*See also Alcoholism; Drug Abuse*

National Clearinghouse for Alcohol and Drug Information
P.O. Box 2345
Rockville, MD 20852 (800) 729-6686

## PREMATURE BABIES

National Institute of Child Health and Human Development
Bldg. 31, Room 2A32
Bethesda, MD 20892 (301) 496-5133

National Maternal and Child Health Clearinghouse
8201 Greensboro Dr.
McLean, VA 22102-3810
(703) 821-8955, ext. 254

## PREMENSTRUAL SYNDROME

*See PMS*

## PRENATAL CARE

National Institute of Child Health and Human Development
Bldg. 31, Room 2A32
Bethesda, MD 20892 (301) 496-5133

National Maternal and Child Health Clearinghouse
8201 Greensboro Dr.
McLean, VA 22102-3810 (703) 821-8955, ext. 254

## PRESBYCUSIS

National Institute on Deafness and
Other Communication Disorders
1 Communication Ave.
Bethesda, MD 20892-3456 (800) 241-1044
(800) 241-1055 (TDD)

## PRESBYOPIA

National Eye Institute
Building 31, Room 6A32
Bethesda, MD 20892 (301) 496-5248

## PRESCRIPTION DRUGS

*See also Medications*

## PRESENILE DEMENTIA

*See also Dementia; Alzheimer's Disease*

National Institute on Aging
Information Center
P.O. Box 8057
Gaithersburg, MD 20898-8057 (800) 222-2225

National Institute of Neurological Disorders and Stroke
Bldg. 31, Room 8A16
Bethesda, MD 20892 (301) 496-5751
(800) 352-9424

National Institute of Mental Health
Information and Inquiries Branch, Room 7C-02
5600 Fishers Lane
Bethesda, MD 20857 (301) 443-4515

## PRESERVATIVES

*See Food Preservatives*

## PRIMARY CARE

National Clearinghouse for Primary Care Information
8201 Greensboro Drive, Suite 600
McLean, VA 22102 (703) 821-8955, ext. 248

## PRIMARY LATERAL SCLEROSIS

National Institute of Neurological Disorders and Stroke
Bldg. 31, Room 8A16
Bethesda, MD 20892 (301) 496-5751
(800) 352-9424

## PRIMARY OVARIAN FAILURE

National Institute of Child Health and Human Development
Bldg. 31, Room 2A32
Bethesda, MD 20892 (301) 496-5133

## PROCARBAZINE

National Cancer Institute
Bldg. 31, Room 10A16
Bethesda, MD 20892 (800) 4-CANCER

## PROGERIA

National Institute on Aging
Information Center
P.O. Box 8057
Gaithersburg, MD 20898-8057 (800) 222-2225

## PROGESTINS

National Institute of Child Health and Human Development
Building 31, Room 2A32
Bethesda, MD 20892 (301) 496-5133

## PROGRESSIVE MULTIFOCAL LEUKOENCEPHALOPATHY

National Institute of Neurological Disorders and Stroke
Building 31, Room 8A16 (301) 496-5751
Bethesda, MD 20892 (800) 352-9424

## PROGRESSIVE SUPRANUCLEAR PALSY

National Institute of Neurological Disorders and Stroke
Building 31, Room 8A16 (301) 496-5751
Bethesda, MD 20892 (800) 352-9424

## PROSTATE CANCER

*See also Cancer*

National Cancer Institute
Building 31, Room 8A16
Bethesda, MD 20892 (800) 4-CANCER

## PROSTATE PROBLEMS

National Institute of Diabetes and Digestive and Kidney Diseases
Bldg. 31, Room 9A04
Bethesda, MD 20892 (301) 496-3583

## PROSTHESES

National Center for Medical Rehabilitation Research
National Institutes of Health
Building 31, Room 2A03
6100 Executive Blvd., MSC 7510
Bethesda, MD 20892-7510 (301) 402-2242

## PROSTHODONTICS

National Institute of Dental Research
Bldg. 31, Room 2C35
31 Center Dr., MSC-2290
Bethesda, MD 20892-2290 (301) 496-4261

## PRURIGO NODULARIS

National Institute of Arthritis and Musculoskeletal
and Skin Diseases
1 AMS Way
Bethesda, MD 20892 (301) 495-4484

## PRURITUS

National Arthritis and Musculoskeletal and
Skin Diseases Clearinghouse
1 AMS Way
Bethesda, MD 20892 (301) 495-4484

## PSEUDOGOUT

National Institute of Arthritis and Musculoskeletal and Skin Diseases
1 AMS Way
Bethesda, MD 20892 (301) 495-4484

## PSEUDOHYPERTROPHIC DYSTROPHY

*See Muscular Dystrophy*

## PSEUDOHYPOPARATHYROIDISM

National Institute of Diabetes and Digestive and Kidney Diseases
Building 31, Room 9A04
Bethesda, MD 20892 (301) 496-3583

## PSEUDOMONAS INFECTIONS

National Institute of Allergy and Infectious Diseases
Building 31, Room 7A50
Bethesda, MD 20892 (301) 496-5717

## PSEUDOSENILITY

National Institute on Aging Information Center
P.O. Box 8057
Gaithersburg, MD 20898-8057 (800) 222-2225

## PSEUDOTUMOR CEREBRI

National Eye Institute
Bldg. 31, Room 6A32
Bethesda, MD 20892 (301) 496-5248

## PSEUDOXANTHOMA ELASTICUM

National Heart, Lung, and Blood Institute
Information Center
P.O. Box 30105
Bethesda, MD 20824-0105 (301) 251-1222

## PSITTACOSIS

National Institute of Allergy and Infectious Diseases
Building 31, Room 7A50
Bethesda, MD 20892 (301) 496-5717

## PSORIASIS

National Institute of Arthritis and Musculoskeletal
and Skin Diseases
1 AMS Way
Bethesda, MD 20892 (301) 495-4484

## PSORIATIC ARTHRITIS

National Institute of Arthritis and Musculoskeletal
and Skin Diseases
1 AMS Way
Bethesda, MD 20892 (301) 495-4484

## PSYCHOTIC EPISODES

National Institute of Mental Health
5600 Fishers Lane
Room 7C-02
Rockville, MD 20857 (301) 443-4515

## PTERYGIUM

National Eye Institute
Building 31, Room 6A32
Bethesda, MD 20892 (301) 496-5248

## PTOSIS

National Eye Institute
Building 31, Room 6A32
Bethesda, MD 20892 (301) 496-5248

## PUBERTY

*See also Adolescent Health; Teenagers*

National Institute of Child Health and Human Development
Building 31, Room 2A32
Bethesda, MD 20892 (301) 496-5133

## PULMONARY ALVEOLAR PROTEINOSIS

National Heart, Lung, and Blood Institute
Information Center
P.O. Box 30105
Bethesda, MD 20824-0105 (301) 251-1222

## PULMONARY DISEASE

National Heart, Lung, and Blood Institute
Information Center
P.O. Box 30105
Bethesda, MD 20824-0105 (301) 251-1222

## PULMONARY TOXICANTS

Office of Technology Assessment
600 Pennsylvania Ave., SE
Washington, DC 20510-8025 (202) 224-8996

## PURE RED CELL APLASIA

National Heart, Lung, and Blood Institute
Information Center
P.O. Box 30105
Bethesda, MD 20824-0105 (301) 251-1222

## PURPURA

National Institute of Arthritis and Musculoskeletal
and Skin Diseases
1 AMS Way
Bethesda, MD 20892 (301) 495-4484

## PYELONEPHRITIS

National Institute of Diabetes and Digestive
and Kidney Diseases
Bldg. 31, Room 9A04
Bethesda, MD 20892 (301) 496-3583

## PYOGENIC INFECTIONS

National Institute of Allergy and Infectious Diseases
Bldg. 31, Room 7A50
Bethesda, MD 20892 (301) 496-5717

## PYORRHEA

National Institute of Dental Research
Building 31, Room 2C35
31 Center Dr., MSC-2290
Bethesda, MD 20892-2290 (301) 496-4261

# - Q -

## QUADRIPLEGIA

National Institute of Neurological Disorders and Stroke
Bldg. 31, Room 8A16 (301) 496-5751
Bethesda, MD 20892 (800) 352-9424

# - R -

## RABIES

National Institute of Allergy and Infectious Diseases
Bldg. 31, Room 7A50
Bethesda, MD 20892 (301) 496-5717

Centers for Disease Control
Information Resources Management Office
1600 Clifton Drive
Atlanta, GA 30341 (404) 332-4555

## RADIAL KERATOTOMY

National Eye Institute
Bldg. 31, Room 6A32
Bethesda, MD 20892 (301) 496-5248

## RADIATION

National Cancer Institute
Bldg. 31, Room 10A16
Bethesda, MD 20892 (800) 4-CANCER

National Institute of Environmental Health Sciences
P.O. Box 12233
Research Triangle Park, NC 27709 (919) 541-3345

Center for Devices and Radiological Health
Food and Drug Administration (HF2-210)
5600 Fishers Lane
Rockville, MD 20857 (301) 443-4190

## RADON

National Radon Hotline
Box 16622
Alexandria, VA 22302 (800) 767-7236

Public Information Center PM3404-B
Environmental Protection Agency
401 M St., SW
Washington, DC 20460 (202) 260-7751

## RAMSEY HUNT SYNDROME

National Institute of Neurological Disorders and Stroke
Bldg. 31, Room 8A16 (301) 496-5751
Bethesda, MD 20892 (800) 352-9424

## RAPE

National Institute of Mental Health
5600 Fishers Lane

Room 7C-02
Rockville, MD 20857 (301) 443-4515

## RARE DISEASES

National Information Center for Orphan Drugs and Rare Diseases
450 5th St., NW, Room 873
Washington, DC 20857 (800) 443-4903

## RASHES

National Institute of Allergy and Infectious Diseases
Building 31, Room 7A50
Bethesda, MD 20892 (301) 496-5717

## RAYNAUD'S DISEASE

National Heart, Lung, and Blood Institute
Information Center
P.O. Box 30105
Bethesda, MD 20824-0105 (301) 251-1222

## READING DISORDERS

National Institute of Child Health and Human Development
Bldg. 31, Room 2A32
Bethesda, MD 20892 (301) 496-5133

National Institute on Deafness and Other Communication Disorders
1 Communication Avenue (800) 241-1044
Bethesda, MD 20892-3456 (800) 241-1055 (TDD)

## READ METHOD OF CHILDBIRTH

*See Childbirth*

## RECURRENT FEVER

National Institute of Allergy and Infectious Diseases
Bldg. 31, Room 7A50
Bethesda, MD 20892 (301) 496-5717

## REFLEX SYMPATHETIC DYSTROPHY SYNDROME

National Institute of Arthritis and Musculoskeletal
and Skin Diseases
Bldg. 31, Room 4C05
Bethesda, MD 20892 (301) 495-4484

## REFLUX NEPHROPATHY

National Institute of Diabetes and Digestive and Kidney Diseases
Bldg. 31, Room 9A04
Bethesda, MD 20892 (301) 496-3583

## REFRACTORY ANEMIA

National Heart, Lung, and Blood Institute
Information Center
P.O. Box 30105
Bethesda, MD 20824-0105 (301) 251-1222

## REFSUM'S DISEASE

National Institute of Neurological Disorders and Stroke
Bldg. 31, Room 8A16
Bethesda, MD 20892 (301) 496-5751
(800) 352-9424

## REGIONAL ENTERITIS

*See Crohn's Disease*

## REHABILITATION

*See also Disabilities*

National Rehabilitation Information Center
8455 Colesville Road, Suite 935
Silver Spring, MD 20910 (800) 346-2742 (voice and TDD)

## REITER'S SYNDROME

National Institute of Arthritis and Musculoskeletal and Skin Diseases
Bldg. 31, Room 4C05
Bethesda, MD 20892 (301) 495-4484

## RELAXATION

National Institute of Mental Health
5600 Fishers Lane, Room 7C-02
Rockville, MD 20857 (301) 443-4515

## RENAL DISORDERS

National Institute of Diabetes and Digestive and Kidney Diseases
Bldg. 31, Room 9A04
Bethesda, MD 20892 (301) 496-3583

## RENOVASCULAR HYPERTENSION

National Institute of Diabetes and Digestive and Kidney Diseases

Bldg. 31, Room 9A04
Bethesda, MD 20892 (301) 496-3583

## REPETITIVE STRESS SYNDROME

National Institute of Occupational Safety and Health
4676 Columbia Parkway, MS C-13
Cincinnati, OH 45226 (800) 35-NIOSH

## REPRODUCTIVE DISORDERS

National Institute of Child Health and Human Development
Bldg. 31, Room 2A32
Bethesda, MD 20892 (301) 496-5133

## RESPIRATORY DISEASES

National Institute of Allergy and Infectious Diseases
Bldg. 31, Room 7A50
Bethesda, MD 20892 (301) 496-5717

## RESPIRATORY DISTRESS SYNDROME

National Heart, Lung, and Blood Institute
Information Center
P.O. Box 30105
Bethesda, MD 20824-0105 (301) 251-1222

## RESPIRATORY SYNCYTIAL VIRUS

National Institute of Allergy and Infectious Diseases
Building 31, Room 7A50
Bethesda, MD 20892 (301) 496-5717

## RESTLESS LEG SYNDROME

National Institute of Neurological Disorders and Stroke
Bldg. 31, Room 8A16 (301) 496-5751
Bethesda, MD 20892 (800) 352-9424

## RETARDATION

*See Mental Retardation*

## RETINAL DISEASE

National Eye Institute
Bldg. 31, Room 6A32
Bethesda, MD 20892 (301) 496-5248

## RETT'S SYNDROME

National Institute of Neurological Disorders and Stroke
Bldg. 31, Room 8A16 (301) 496-5751
Bethesda, MD 20892 (800) 352-9424

## REYE'S SYNDROME

National Institute of Neurological Disorders and Stroke
Bldg. 31, Room 8A16 (301) 496-5751
Bethesda, MD 20892 (800) 352-9424

## RH FACTOR

National Heart, Lung, and Blood Institute
Information Center

P.O. Box 30105
Bethesda, MD 20824-0105 (301) 251-1222

## RHABDOMYOSARCOMA

National Cancer Institute
Bldg. 31, Room 10A16
Bethesda, MD 20892 (800) 4-CANCER

## RHEUMATIC FEVER

National Institute of Allergy and Infectious Diseases
Building 31, Room 7A50
Bethesda, MD 20892 (301) 496-5717

## RHEUMATIC HEART

National Heart, Lung, and Blood Institute
Information Center
P.O. Box 30105
Bethesda, MD 20824-0105 (301) 251-1222

## RHEUMATISM

National Institute of Arthritis and Musculoskeletal and Skin Diseases
1 AMS Way
Bethesda, MD 20892 (301) 495-4484

## RHEUMATOID ARTHRITIS

National Institute of Arthritis and Musculoskeletal
and Skin Diseases
1 AMS Way
Bethesda, MD 20892 (301) 495-4484

## RHINITIS

National Institute of Allergy and Infectious Diseases
Building 31, Room 7A50
Bethesda, MD 20892 (301) 496-5717

## RHUS DERMATITIS

National Arthritis and Musculoskeletal and Skin Diseases Clearinghouse
1 AMS Way
Bethesda, MD 20892 (301) 495-4484

## RHYTIDOPLASTY

*See Face Lift*

## RICKETS

National Institute of Diabetes and Digestive and Kidney Diseases
Bldg. 31, Room 9A04
Bethesda, MD 20892 (301) 496-3583

## RILEY-DAY SYNDROME

National Institute of Neurological Disorders and Stroke
Bldg. 31, Room 8A16 (301) 496-5751
Bethesda, MD 20892 (800) 352-9424

## RINGWORM

National Institute of Allergy and Infectious Diseases
Bldg. 31, Room 7A50
Bethesda, MD 20892 (301) 496-5717

## RIVER BLINDNESS

National Eye Institute
Bldg. 31, Room 6A32
Bethesda, MD 20892 (301) 496-5248

## ROCKY MOUNTAIN SPOTTED FEVER

National Institute of Allergy and Infectious Diseases
Bldg. 31, Room 7A50
Bethesda, MD 20892 (301) 496-5717

## ROOT CARIES

National Institute of Dental Research
Bldg. 31, Room 2C35
31 Center Drive, MSC-2290
Bethesda, MD 20892-2290 (301) 496-4261

## ROSACEAE

National Arthritis and Musculoskeletal and Skin Diseases Clearinghouse
1 AMS Way
Bethesda, MD 20892 (301) 495-4484

## ROTAVIRUS

National Institute of Allergy and Infectious Diseases
Bldg. 31, Room 7A50
Bethesda, MD 20892 (301) 496-5717

## ROTHMUND-THOMPSON SYNDROME

National Cancer Institute

Bldg. 31, Room 10A16
Bethesda, MD 20892 (800) 4-CANCER

## RUBELLA

*See also Immunizations*

National Institute of Allergy and Infectious Diseases
Bldg. 31, Room 7A50
Bethesda, MD 20892 (301) 496-5717

## RUNAWAY HOTLINE

National Runaway Hotline
3080 N. Lincoln Avenue
Chicago, IL 60657 (800) 621-4000

# - S -

## SAFE SEX

*See also AIDS; Sexually Transmitted Diseases*

National AIDS Information Clearinghouse
P.O. Box 6003
Rockville, MD 20850 (800) 458-5231

## SALIVARY SYSTEM DISEASES

National Institute of Dental Research
Bldg. 31, Room 2C35
31 Center Drive, MSC-2290
Bethesda, MD 20892-2290 (301) 496-4261

## SALMONELLA INFECTIONS

National Institute of Allergy and Infectious Diseases
Bldg. 31, Room 7A50
Bethesda, MD 20892 (301) 496-5717

## SALT

Food and Nutrition Information Center
National Agricultural Library, Room 304
10301 Baltimore Blvd.
Beltsville, MD 20705 (301) 504-5719

## SANTAVUORI DISEASE

National Institute of Neurological Disorders and Stroke
Bldg. 31, Room 8A16 (301) 496-5751
Bethesda, MD 20892 (800) 352-9424

## SARCOIDOSIS

National Institute of Allergy and Infectious Diseases
Bldg. 31, Room 7A50
Bethesda, MD 20892 (301) 496-5717

## SARCOMA

National Cancer Institute
Bldg. 31, Room 10A16
Bethesda, MD 20892 (800) 4-CANCER

## SATURATED FAT

Food and Nutrition Information Center

National Agricultural Library, Room 304
10301 Baltimore Blvd.
Beltsville, MD 20705 (301) 504-5719

## SCABIES

National Institute of Allergy and Infectious Diseases
Bldg. 31, Room 7A50
Bethesda, MD 20892 (301) 496-5717

## SCARLET FEVER

National Institute of Allergy and Infectious Diseases
Bldg. 31, Room 7A50
Bethesda, MD 20892 (301) 496-5717

## SCHILDER'S DISEASE

National Institute of Neurological Disorders and Stroke
Bldg. 31, Room 8A16
Bethesda, MD 20892 (301) 496-5751
(800) 352-9424

## SCHISTOSOMIASIS

National Institute of Allergy and Infectious Diseases
Bldg. 31, Room 7A50
Bethesda, MD 20892 (301) 496-5717

## SCHIZOPHRENIA

National Institute of Mental Health
5600 Fishers Lane
Room 7C-02
Rockville, MD 20857 (301) 443-4515

## SCHOOL HEALTH

Office of the Secretary
U.S. Department of Education
400 Maryland Ave., SW, Room 4145
Washington, DC 20202-0100 (202) 401-3030

## SCHWANNOMA

National Cancer Institute
Bldg. 31, Room 10A16
Bethesda, MD 20892 (800) 4-CANCER

## SCIATICA

*See also Back Problems*

National Institute of Arthritis and Musculoskeletal and Skin Diseases
1 AMS Way
Bethesda, MD 20892 (301) 495-4484

## SCLERODERMA

National Institute of Arthritis and Musculoskeletal and Skin Diseases
1 AMS Way
Bethesda, MD 20892 (301) 495-4484

## SCLEROSIS

National Institute of Neurological Disorders and Stroke
Bldg. 31, Room 8A16
Bethesda, MD 20892 (301) 496-5751
(800) 352-9424

## SCOLIOSIS

National Institute of Arthritis and Musculoskeletal
and Skin Diseases
1 AMS Way
Bethesda, MD 20892 (301) 495-4484

## SEAFOOD INSPECTION

Office of Seafood (HFS-400)
Center for Food Safety and Applied Nutrition
200 C Street, SW
Washington, DC 20204 (202) 418-3133

## SELF-HELP

National Clearinghouse for Alcohol and Drug Information
P.O. Box 2345
Rockville, MD 20852 (800) 729-6686

## SEGAWA'S DYSTONIA

National Institute of Neurological Disorders and Stroke
Building 31, Room 8A16 (301) 496-5751
Bethesda, MD 20892 (800) 352-9424

## SEIZURES

*See also Epilepsy*

National Institute of Neurological Disorders and Stroke
Building 31, Room 8A16 (301) 496-5751
Bethesda, MD 20892 (800) 352-9424

## SEMINOMA

*See Testicular Cancer*

## SENILITY

*See also Aging; Alzheimer's Disease*

National Institute on Aging
P.O. Box 8057
Gaithersburg, MD 20898-8057 (800) 222-2225

## SENILE MACULAR DEGENERATION

National Eye Institute
Building 31, Room 67A50
Bethesda, MD 20892 (301) 496-5248

## SEPTAL DEFECTS

National Heart, Lung, and Blood Institute
Information Center
P.O. Box 30105
Bethesda, MD 20824-0105 (301) 251-1222

## SEX CHANGES

National Institute of Child Health and Human Development
Bldg. 31, Room 27A50
Bethesda, MD 20892 (301) 496-5133

## SEX DETERMINATION

National Institute of Child Health and Human Development
Bldg. 31, Room 27A50
Bethesda, MD 20892 (301) 496-5133

## SEX HORMONES

National Institute of Child Health and Human Development
Bldg. 31, Room 27A50
Bethesda, MD 20892 (301) 496-5133

## SEXUAL ABUSE

*See also Child Abuse; Family Violence*

Clearinghouse on Child Abuse and Neglect Information
P.O. Box 1182
Washington, DC 20013 (800) FYI-3366

## SEXUALITY

National Institute of Child Health and Human Development
Building 31, Room 27A50
Bethesda, MD 20892 (301) 496-5133

## SEXUALLY TRANSMITTED DISEASES

*See also Safe Sex*

National AIDS Information Clearinghouse
P.O. Box 6003
Rockville, MD 20850 (800) 342-AIDS

Sexually Transmitted Diseases Hotline
P.O. Box 13827
Research Triangle Park, NC 27709 (800) 227-8922

National Institute of Allergy and Infectious Diseases
Bldg. 31, Room 7A50
Bethesda, MD 20892 (301) 496-5717

## SEZARY SYNDROME

National Cancer Institute
Building 31, Room 10A16
Bethesda, MD 20892 (800) 4-CANCER

## SHAKEN BABY SYNDROME

Clearinghouse on Child Abuse and Neglect Information
P.O. Box 1182
Washington, DC 20013 (800) FYI-3366
(800) 394-3366

## SHINGLES

National Institute of Neurological Disorders and Stroke
Building 31, Room 8A16
Bethesda, MD 20892 (301) 496-5751
(800) 352-9424

## SHOCK

National Heart, Lung, and Blood Institute
Information Center
P.O. Box 30105
Bethesda, MD 20824-0105 (301) 251-1222

## SHORT STATURE

National Institute of Child Health and Human Development
Bldg. 31, Room 7A32
Bethesda, MD 20892 (301) 496-5133

## SHY-DRAGER SYNDROME

National Institute of Neurological Disorders and Stroke
Bldg. 31, Room 8A16 (301) 496-5751
Bethesda, MD 20892 (800) 352-9424

## SIAMESE TWINS

*See Twins*

## SICK BUILDINGS

Indoor Air Quality Information Clearinghouse
P.O. Box 37133
Washington, DC 20013-7133 (800) 438-4318

## SICKLE CELL

National Heart, Lung, and Blood Institute
Information Center
P.O. Box 30105
Bethesda, MD 20824-0105 (301) 251-1222

## SIDEROBLASTIC ANEMIA

National Heart, Lung, and Blood Institute
Information Center

P.O. Box 30105
Bethesda, MD 20824-0105 (301) 251-1222

## SILICONE IMPLANTS

*See Breast Implants*

## SINUSITIS

National Institute of Allergy and Infectious Diseases
Bldg. 31, Room 7A50
Bethesda, MD 20892 (301) 496-5717

## SJOGREN'S SYNDROME

National Institute of Arthritis and Musculoskeletal
and Skin Diseases
1 AMS Way
Bethesda, MD 20892 (301) 495-4484

## SKIN AND AGING

National Institute on Aging
Information Center
P.O. Box 30105
Bethesda, MD 20824-0105 (800) 222-2225

## SKIN CANCER

National Cancer Institute
Bldg. 31, Room 10A16
Bethesda, MD 20892 (800) 4-CANCER

## SKIN CONDITIONS

National Institute of Arthritis and Musculoskeletal and Skin Diseases
1 AMS Way
Bethesda, MD 20892 (301) 495-4484

## SLEEP APNEA

National Institute of Neurological Disorders and Stroke
Bldg. 31, Room 8A16
Bethesda, MD 20892 (301) 496-5751
(800) 352-9424

## SLEEP DISORDERS

National Institute of Neurological Disorders and Stroke
Bldg. 31, Room 8A16
Bethesda, MD 20892 (301) 496-5751
(800) 352-9424

## SLOW VIRUSES

National Institute of Neurological Disorders and Stroke
Bldg. 31, Room 8A16
Bethesda, MD 20892 (301) 496-5751
(800) 352-9424

## SMALLPOX

National Institute of Allergy and Infectious Diseases
Bldg. 31, Room 7A50
Bethesda, MD 20892 (301) 496-5717

## SMELL DISORDERS

National Institute on Deafness and Other Communication Disorders
1 Communication Avenue
Bethesda, MD 20892-3456 (800) 241-1044
(800) 241-1055 (TDD)

## SMOKELESS TOBACCO

*See also Smoking*

Office on Smoking and Health, Centers for Disease Control
1600 Clifton Rd., NE, MS K-50
Atlanta, GA 30333 (404) 488-5705

## SMOKING

Office on Smoking and Health, Centers for Disease Control
1600 Clifton Rd., NE, MS K-50
Atlanta, GA 30333 (404) 488-5705

National Cancer Institute
Bldg. 31, Room 8A16
Bethesda, MD 20892 (800) 4-CANCER

National Heart, Lung, and Blood Institute
Information Center
P.O. Box 30105
Bethesda, MD 20824-0105 (301) 251-1222

## SNACKING

Food and Nutrition Information Center
National Agricultural Library, Room 304
10301 Baltimore Blvd.
Beltsville, MD 20705 (301) 504-5719

## SOCIAL SECURITY

Social Security Administration
Office of Public Affairs
P.O. Box 17743
Baltimore, MD 21235 — (410) 965-0945
(800) 772-1213

## SODIUM

*See Salt*

## SOLAR BURNS

National Eye Institute
Building 31, Room 67A50
Bethesda, MD 20892 — (301) 496-5248

## SPASMODIC DYSPHONIA

National Institute on Deafness and Other Communication Disorders
1 Communication Avenue
Bethesda, MD 20892-3456 — (800) 241-1044
(800) 241-1055 (TDD)

## SPASTIC CONDITIONS

National Institute of Neurological Disorders and Stroke
Bldg. 31, Room 8A16
Bethesda, MD 20892 — (301) 496-5751
(800) 352-9424

## SPEECH AND LANGUAGE DISORDERS

National Institute on Deafness and Other
Communication Disorders
1 Communication Avenue
Bethesda, MD 20892-3456
(800) 241-1044
(800) 241-1055 (TDD)

## SPHINGOLIPIDOSIS

National Institute of Neurological Disorders and Stroke
Bldg. 31, Room 8A16
Bethesda, MD 20892
(301) 496-5751
(800) 352-9424

## SPIELMEYER-SJOGREN'S DISEASE

National Institute of Neurological Disorders and Stroke
Bldg. 31, Room 8A16
Bethesda, MD 20892
(301) 496-5751
(800) 352-9424

## SPINA BIFIDA

National Institute of Neurological Disorders and Stroke
Bldg. 31, Room 8A16
Bethesda, MD 20892
(301) 496-5751
(800) 352-9424

## SPINAL ARACHNOIDITIS

National Institute of Neurological Disorders and Stroke
Bldg. 31, Room 8A16
Bethesda, MD 20892
(301) 496-5751
(800) 352-9424

## SPINAL CORD INJURIES

National Rehabilitation Information Center
8455 Colesville Rd., Suite 935
Silver Spring, MD 20910 (301) 588-9284
(800) 346-2742 (Voice and TDD)

National Institute of Neurological Disorders and Stroke
Bldg. 31, Room 8A16
Bethesda, MD 20892 (301) 496-5751
(800) 352-9424

## SPINAL CORD TUMORS

National Institute of Neurological Disorders and Stroke
Bldg. 31, Room 8A16
Bethesda, MD 20892 (301) 496-5751
(800) 352-9424

## SPINE CURVATURE

*See Scoliosis*

## SPINAL MUSCULAR ATROPHY

National Institute of Arthritis and Musculoskeletal and Skin Diseases
1 AMS Way
Bethesda, MD 20892 (301) 495-4484

## SPINE JOINTS

*See Ankylosis Spondylitis*

## SPINOCEREBELLAR DEGENERATION

National Institute of Neurological Disorders and Stroke
Building 31, Room 8A16 (301) 496-5751
Bethesda, MD 20892 (800) 352-9424

## SPORTS MEDICINE

National Institute of Arthritis and Musculoskeletal and Skin Diseases
1 AMS Way
Bethesda, MD 20892 (301) 495-4484

## SPORTS NUTRITION

Food and Nutrition Information Center
National Agricultural Library, Room 304
10301 Baltimore Blvd.
Beltsville, MD 20705 (301) 504-5719

## SPOUSAL ABUSE

*See Battered Spouses; Family Violence*

## SQUAMOUS CELL

National Cancer Institute
Bldg. 31, Room 10A16
Bethesda, MD 20892 (800) 4-CANCER

## STAINED TEETH

National Institute of Dental Research
Bldg. 31, Room 2C35

31 Center Drive, MSC-2290
Bethesda, MD 20892-2290 (301) 496-4261

## STAPHYLOCOCCAL (STAPH) INFECTIONS

National Institute of Allergy and Infectious Diseases
Building 31, Room 7A50
Bethesda, MD 20892 (301) 496-5717

## STEELE-RICHARDSON DISEASE

National Institute of Neurological Disorders and Stroke
Building 31, Room 8A16 (301) 496-5751
Bethesda, MD 20892 (800) 352-9424

## STEINERTS DISEASE

*See Muscular Dystrophy*

## STERILIZATION

*See also Vasectomies*

Contraceptive Development Branch
National Institute of Child Health and Human Development
6100 Executive Blvd., (MSC-7510)
Bethesda, MD 20892-7510 (301) 496-1661

National Institute of Child Health and Human Development
Bldg. 31, Room 2A32
Bethesda, MD 20892 (301) 496-5133

## STEROID CONTRACEPTIVES

National Institute of Child Health and Human Development
Bldg. 31, Room 2A32
Bethesda, MD 20892 (301) 496-5133

## STEROID HYPERTENSION

National Heart, Lung, and Blood Institute
Information Center
P.O. Box 30105
Bethesda, MD 20824-0105 (301) 251-1222

## STEROIDS

Food and Drug Administration
5600 Fishers Lane, HFD-88
Rockville, MD 20857 (301) 443-3170

National Clearinghouse for Alcohol and Drug Information
P.O. Box 2345 (301) 468-2600
Rockville, MD 20852 (800) 729-6686

## STEVENS-JOHNSON SYNDROME

National Institute of Allergy and Infectious Diseases
Bldg. 31, Room 7A50
Bethesda, MD 20892 (301) 496-5717

## STIFF MAN SYNDROME

National Institute of Neurological Disorders and Stroke
Bldg. 31, Room 8A16 (301) 496-5751
Bethesda, MD 20892 (800) 352-9424

## STILL'S DISEASE

National Institute of Arthritis and Musculoskeletal
and Skin Diseases
1 AMS Way
Bethesda, MD 20892 (301) 495-4484

## STOMACH CANCER

National Cancer Institute
Bldg. 31, Room 10A16
Bethesda, MD 20892 (800) 4-CANCER

## STOMATITIS

National Institute of Dental Research
Bldg. 31, Room 2C35
31 Center Drive, MSC-2290
Bethesda, MD 20892-2290 (301) 496-4261

## STRABISMUS

National Eye Institute
Bldg. 31, Room 67A50
31 Center Drive, MSC-2290
Bethesda, MD 20892-2290 (301) 496-5248

## STREPTOCOCCAL (STREP) INFECTIONS

National Institute of Allergy and Infectious Diseases
Bldg. 31, Room 7A50
Bethesda, MD 20892 (301) 496-5717

## STREPTOKINASE

National Heart, Lung, and Blood Institute
Information Center
P.O. Box 30105
Bethesda, MD 20824-0105 (301) 251-1222

## STRESS

National Institute of Mental Health
5600 Fishers Lane, Room 7C-02
Rockville, MD 20857 (301) 443-4515

## STRIATONIGRAL DEGENERATION

National Institute of Neurological Disorders and Stroke
Bldg. 31, Room 8A16
Bethesda, MD 20892 (301) 496-5751
(800) 352-9424

## STROKE

National Institute of Neurological Disorders and Stroke
Building 31, Room 8A16
Bethesda, MD 20892 (301) 496-5751
(800) 352-9424

## STRONGYLOIDIASIS (Roundworm)

National Institute of Allergy and Infectious Diseases
Building 31, Room 7A50
Bethesda, MD 20892 (301) 496-5717

## STURGE-WEBER SYNDROME

National Institute of Neurological Disorders and Stroke
Bldg. 31, Room 8A16
Bethesda, MD 20892 (301) 496-5751
(800) 352-9424

## STUTTERING

National Institute on Deafness and Other
Communication Disorders
1 Communication Avenue
Bethesda, MD 20892-3456 (800) 241-1044
(800) 241-1055 (TDD)

## STYE

National Eye Institute
Bldg. 31, Room 67A50
Bethesda, MD 20892 (301) 496-5248

## SUDDEN CARDIAC DEATH

National Heart, Lung, and Blood Institute
Information Center
P.O. Box 30105
Bethesda, MD 20824-0105 (301) 251-1222

## SUDDEN INFANT DEATH SYNDROME

National Sudden Infant Death Syndrome Clearinghouse
8201 Greensboro Dr., Suite 600
McLean, VA 22102 (703) 821-8955

## SUICIDE

National Institute of Mental Health
5600 Fishers Lane, Room 7C-02
Rockville, MD 20857 (301) 443-4515

## SULFITES

Food and Nutrition Information Center
National Agricultural Library, Room 304
10301 Baltimore Blvd.
Beltsville, MD 20705 (301) 504-5719

## SURGERY

Health Care Financing Administration
ORD-ES, Room 2230-OM
6325 Security Blvd.
Baltimore, MD 21207 (410) 966-6584

## SWEAT GLAND DISORDERS

*See also Anaphoresis*

National Institute of Arthritis and Musculoskeletal and Skin Diseases
1 AMS Way
Bethesda, MD 20892 (301) 495-4484

## SWINE FLU

*See also Flu*

National Institute of Allergy and Infectious Diseases
Bldg. 31, Room 7A50
Bethesda, MD 20892 (301) 496-5717

## SYDENHAM'S CHOREA

National Institute of Neurological Disorders and Stroke
Bldg. 31, Room 8A16 (301) 496-5751
Bethesda, MD 20892 (800) 352-9424

## SYNCOPE

*See also Fainting*

National Heart, Lung, and Blood Institute Information Center
P.O. Box 30105
Bethesda, MD 20824-0105 (301) 251-1222

## SYNOVITIS

National Institute of Arthritis and Musculoskeletal and Skin Diseases
1 AMS Way
Bethesda, MD 20892 (301) 495-4484

## SYPHILIS

National Sexually Transmitted Diseases Hotline
P.O. Box 13827
Research Triangle Park, NC 27709 (800) 227-8922

National Institute of Allergy and Infectious Diseases
Bldg. 31, Room 7A50
Bethesda, MD 20892 (301) 496-5717

## SYRINGOMYELIA

National Institute of Neurological Disorders and Stroke
Building 31, Room 8A16 (301) 496-5751
Bethesda, MD 20892 (800) 352-9424

## SYSTEMIC LUPUS ERYTHEMATOSUS

*See Lupus*

## SYSTEMIC SCLEROSIS

National Institute of Neurological Disorders and Stroke
Bldg. 31, Room 8A16
Bethesda, MD 20892 (301) 496-5751
(800) 352-9424

National Institute of Arthritis and Musculoskeletal and Skin Diseases
1 AMS Way
9000 Rockville Pike
Bethesda, MD 20892 (301) 495-4484

## SYSTOLIC HYPERTENSION

National Heart, Lung, and Blood Institute
Information Center
P.O. Box 30105
Bethesda, MD 20824-0105 (301) 251-1222

# - T -

## TACHYCARDIA

National Heart, Lung, and Blood Institute
Information Center
P.O. Box 30105
Bethesda, MD 20824-0105 (301) 251-1222

## TAKAYASU'S ARTERITIS

National Institute of Allergy and Infectious Diseases
Information Center
Building 31, Room 7A50
P.O. Box 30105
Bethesda, MD 20824-0105 (301) 251-1222

## TAMOXIFEN

National Cancer Institute
Building 31
Room 10A16
Bethesda, MD 20892 (800) 4-CANCER

## TANGIER DISEASE

National Heart, Lung, and Blood Institute
Information Center
P.O. Box 30105
Bethesda, MD 20824-0105 (301) 251-1222

National Institute of Neurological Disorders and Stroke
Bldg. 31, Room 8A16
Bethesda, MD 20892 (301) 496-5751
(800) 352-9424

## TANNING

Center for Devices and Radiological Health
Food and Drug Administration (HFZ-210)
5600 Fishers Lane
Rockville, MD 20857 (301) 443-4690

## TAPEWORM INFECTION

National Institute of Allergy and Infectious Diseases
Bldg. 31, Room 7A50
Bethesda, MD 20892 (301) 496-5717

## TARDIVE DYSKINESIA

National Institute of Mental Health
5600 Fishers Lane
Room 7C-02
Rockville, MD 20857 (301) 443-4515

## TASTE DISORDERS

National Institute on Deafness and
Other Communication Disorders
1 Communication Avenue
Bethesda, MD 20892-3456 (800) 241-1044
(800) 241-1055 (TDD)

## TATTOO REMOVAL

National Institute of Arthritis and Musculoskeletal
and Skin Diseases
1 AMS Way
Bethesda, MD 20892 (301) 495-4484

## TAY-SACH'S DISEASE

National Institute of Neurological Disorders and Stroke
Bldg. 31, Room 8A16
Bethesda, MD 20892 (301) 496-5751
(800) 352-9424

## TEENAGERS

*See also Adolescent Health*

National Institute of Child Health and Human Development
Bldg. 31, Room 2A32
Bethesda, MD 20892 (301) 496-5133

## TEEN PREGNANCY

National Institute of Child Health and Human Development
Bldg. 31, Room 2A32
Bethesda, MD 20892 (301) 496-5133

## TEETH PROBLEMS

National Institute of Dental Research
Bldg. 31, Room 2C35
31 Center Drive, MSC-2290
Bethesda, MD 20892-2290 (301) 496-4261

## TEMPORAL ARTERITIS

National Eye Institute
Bldg. 31, Room 6A32
Bethesda, MD 20892 (301) 496-5248

## TENDONITIS

National Institute of Arthritis and Musculoskeletal
and Skin Diseases
1 AMS Way
Bethesda, MD 20892 (301) 495-4484

## TENNIS ELBOW

National Arthritis and Musculoskeletal
and Skin Diseases
Information Clearinghouse
1 AMS Way
Bethesda, MD 20892 (301) 495-4484

## TEST TUBE BABIES

National Institute of Child Health and Human Development
Bldg. 31, Room 2A32
Bethesda, MD 20892 (301) 496-5133

## TESTICULAR CANCER

*See also Cancer*

National Cancer Institute
Bldg. 31, Room 10A16
Bethesda, MD 20892 (800) 4-CANCER

## TETANUS

National Institute of Allergy and Infectious Diseases
Bldg. 31, Room 7A32
Bethesda, MD 20892 (301) 496-5717

## TETRALOGY OF FALLOT

National Heart, Lung, and Blood Institute
Information Center
P.O. Box 30105
Bethesda, MD 20824-0105 (301) 251-1222

## THALASSEMIA

National Heart, Lung, and Blood Institute
Information Center
P.O. Box 30105
Bethesda, MD 20824-0105 (301) 251-1222

## THERAPEUTIC ENDOSCOPY

National Digestive Diseases
Information Clearinghouse
2 Information Way
Bethesda, MD 20892 (301) 654-3810

## THORACIC-OUTLET SYNDROME

National Institute of Neurological Disorders and Stroke
Bldg. 31, Room 8A16
Bethesda, MD 20892 (301) 496-5751
(800) 352-9424

## THROMBASTHENIA

National Institute of Diabetes and Digestive
and Kidney Diseases
Bldg. 31, Room 9A04
Bethesda, MD 20892 (301) 496-3583

## THROMBOCYTOPENIA

National Institute of Diabetes and Digestive
and Kidney Diseases
Building 31, Room 9A04
Bethesda, MD 20892 (301) 496-3583

## THROMBOLYSIS

National Heart, Lung, and Blood Institute
Information Center
P.O. Box 30105
Bethesda, MD 20824-0105 (301) 251-1222

## THROMBOPHLEBITIS

National Heart, Lung, and Blood Institute
Information Center
P.O. Box 30105
Bethesda, MD 20824-0105 (301) 251-1222

## THROMBOSIS

National Heart, Lung, and Blood Institute
Information Center
P.O. Box 30105
Bethesda, MD 20824-0105 (301) 251-1222

## THYROID DISORDERS

National Institute of Diabetes and Digestive
and Kidney Diseases
Bldg. 31, Room 9A04
Bethesda, MD 20892 (301) 496-3583

## THYMOMA

National Cancer Institute
Bldg. 31, Room 10A16
Bethesda, MD 20892 (800) 4-CANCER

## THYROTOXIC MYOPATHY

National Institute of Neurological Disorders and Stroke
Bldg. 31, Room 8A16
Bethesda, MD 20892
(301) 496-5751
(800) 352-9424

## THYROTOXIC PERIODIC PARALYSIS

National Institute of Neurological Disorders and Stroke
Building 31, Room 8A16
Bethesda, MD 20892
(301) 496-5751
(800) 352-9424

## TIC DOULOUREUX

National Institute of Neurological Disorders and Stroke
Bldg. 31, Room 8A16
Bethesda, MD 20892
(301) 496-5751
(800) 352-9424

## TICKS

National Institute of Allergy and Infectious Diseases
Building 31, Room 7A50
Bethesda, MD 20892
(301) 496-5717

## TINNITUS

National Institute on Deafness and
Other Communication Disorders
1 Communication Avenue
Bethesda, MD 20892-3456
(800) 241-1044
(800) 241-1055 (TDD)

National Institute of Neurological Disorders and Stroke
Bldg. 31, Room 8A16
Bethesda, MD 20892
(301) 496-5751
(800) 352-9424

## TOBACCO

*See Passive Smoking; Smoking; Smokeless Tobacco*

## TONGUE TIED

National Institute on Deafness and Other Communication Disorders
1 Communication Avenue (800) 241-1044
Bethesda, MD 20892-3456 (800) 241-1055 (TDD)

## TORSION DYSTONIA

National Institute of Neurological Disorders and Stroke
Bldg. 31, Room 8A16 (301) 496-5751
Bethesda, MD 20892 (800) 352-9424

## TORTICOLLIS

National Institute of Neurological Disorders and Stroke
Bldg. 31, Room 8A16 (301) 496-5751
Bethesda, MD 20892 (800) 352-9424

## TOURETTE SYNDROME

National Institute of Neurological Disorders and Stroke
Bldg. 31, Room 8A16 (301) 496-5751
Bethesda, MD 20892 (800) 352-9424

## TOXICS

National Pesticide Telecommunication Network (NPTN)
Texas Tech University

Health Sciences Center
Lubbock, TX 79430 (800) 858-PEST

Division of Environmental Health Laboratory Sciences
Centers for Disease Control
1600 Clifton Rd.
Atlanta, GA 30333 (404) 488-4132

## TOXIC SHOCK

Center for Devices and Radiological Health
Food and Drug Administration
5600 Fishers Lane (HFZ-210)
Rockville, MD 20857 (301) 443-4690

## TOXOCARIASIS

National Eye Institute
Building 31, Room 6A32
Bethesda, MD 20892 (301) 496-5248

## TOXOPLASMOSIS

National Institute of Allergy and Infectious Diseases
Building 31, Room 7A50
Bethesda, MD 20892 (301) 496-5717

## TRACE ELEMENTS

Grand Forks Human Nutrition Research Center
P.O. Box 9034
University Station
Grand Forks, ND 58202-7166 (701) 795-8456

## TRACHOMA

National Eye Institute
Bldg. 31, Room 6A32
Bethesda, MD 20892 (301) 496-5248

## TRANQUILIZERS

National Institute of Mental Health
5600 Fishers Lane, Room 7C-02
Rockville, MD 20857 (301) 443-4515

## TRANSDERMAL DELIVERY OF DRUGS

Center for Drug Evaluation and Research
Food and Drug Administration
5600 Fishers Lane
Rockville, MD 20857 (301) 443-2894

## TRANSFUSIONS

Center for Biologics Evaluation and Research
Food and Drug Administration
Woodmont Office Center
Suite 200 (HFM-12)
1401 Rockville Pike
Rockville, MD 20852-1448 (301) 594-1800

## TRANSFUSIONAL HEMOSIDEROSIS

National Heart, Lung, and Blood Institute
Information Center
P.O. Box 30105
Bethesda, MD 20824-0105 (301) 251-1222

## TRANSIENT ISCHEMIC ATTACKS

National Institute of Neurological Disorders and Stroke
Building 31, Room 8A16
Bethesda, MD 20892
(301) 496-5751
(800) 352-9424

## TRANSPLANTS

National Heart, Lung, and Blood Institute
Information Center
P.O. Box 30105
Bethesda, MD 20824-0105
(301) 251-1222

National Eye Institute
Bldg. 31, Room 6A32
Bethesda, MD 20892
(301) 496-5248

National Institute of Diabetes and Digestive
and Kidney Diseases
Bldg. 31, Room 9A04
Bethesda, MD 20892
(301) 496-3583

## TRANSVERSE MYELITIS

National Institute of Neurological Disorders and Stroke
Bldg. 31, Room 8A16
Bethesda, MD 20892
(301) 496-5751
(800) 352-9424

## TRAUMATIC BRAIN INJURIES

*See also Head Injuries*

National Rehabilitation Information Center
8455 Colesville Rd, Suite 935
Silver Spring, MD 20910
(301) 588-9284
(800) 346-2742 (Voice and TDD)

## TRAVELERS' HEALTH

Centers for Disease Control
Information Resources Management Office
Mail Stop C-13
1600 Clifton Rd., NE
Atlanta, GA 30333 (404) 332-4555

## TREMORS

National Institute of Neurological Disorders and Stroke
Bldg. 31, Room 8A16
Bethesda, MD 20892 (301) 496-5751
(800) 352-9424

## TRENCH MOUTH

National Institute of Dental Research
Bldg. 31, Room 2C35
31 Center Drive, MSC-2290
Bethesda, MD 20892-2290 (301) 496-4261

## TRICHINOSIS

National Institute of Allergy and Infectious Diseases
Bldg. 31, Room 7A50
Bethesda, MD 20892 (301) 496-5717

## TRICHOMONIASIS

National Institute of Allergy and Infectious Diseases
Bldg. 31, Room 7A50
Bethesda, MD 20892 (301) 496-5717

## TRICHURIASIS

*See Strongyloidiasis*

## TRIGEMINAL NEURALGIA

National Institute of Neurological Disorders and Stroke
Bldg. 31, Room 8A16 (301) 496-5751
Bethesda, MD 20892 (800) 352-9424

## TROPHOBLASTIC CANCER

National Cancer Institute
Bldg. 31, Room 10A16
Bethesda, MD 20892 (800) 4-CANCER

## TROPICAL DISEASES

National Institute of Allergy and Infectious Diseases
Building 31, Room 7A50
Bethesda, MD 20892 (301) 496-5717

## TROPICAL OILS

Food and Nutrition Information Center
National Agricultural Library, Room 304
Beltsville, MD 20705 (301) 504-5719

## TRUNCUS ARTERIOSUS

National Heart, Lung, and Blood Institute
Information Center

P.O. Box 30105
Bethesda, MD 20824-0105 (301) 251-1222

## TRYPANOSOMIASIS

National Institute of Allergy and Infectious Diseases
Building 31, Room 7A50
Bethesda, MD 20892 (301) 496-5717

## TRYPSINOGEN DEFICIENCY

National Institute of Diabetes and Digestive
and Kidney Diseases
Building 31, Room 9A04
Bethesda, MD 20892 (301) 496-3583

## TUBAL LIGATION

*See Contraception; Sterilization*

## TUBERCULOSIS

National Institute of Allergy and Infectious Diseases
Bldg. 31, Room 7A50
Bethesda, MD 20892 (301) 496-5717

## TUBEROUS SCLEROSIS

National Institute of Neurological Disorders and Stroke
Bldg. 31, Room 8A16
Bethesda, MD 20892 (301) 496-5751
(800) 352-9424

## TULAREMIA

National Institute of Allergy and Infectious Diseases
Building 31, Room 7A50
Bethesda, MD 20892 (301) 496-5717

## TUMORS

*See also Cancer*

National Cancer Institute
Bldg. 31, Room 10A16
Bethesda, MD 20892 (800) 4-CANCER

National Institute of Diabetes and Digestive and Kidney Diseases
Bldg. 31, Room 9A04
Bethesda, MD 20892 (301) 496-3583

## TURNER SYNDROME

National Institute of Child Health and Human Development
Bldg. 31, Room 2A32
Bethesda, MD 20892 (301) 496-5133

## TWINS

National Institute of Child Health and Human Development
Bldg. 31, Room 2A32
Bethesda, MD 20892 (301) 496-5133

## TYPHOID FEVER

National Institute of Allergy and Infectious Diseases
Bldg. 31, Room 7A50
Bethesda, MD 20892 (301) 496-5717

# - U -

## ULCERS

*See also Peptic Ulcers*

National Digestive Diseases Information Clearinghouse
2 Information Way
Bethesda, MD 20892 (301) 654-3810

## ULCERATIVE COLITIS

National Institute of Diabetes and Digestive and Kidney Diseases
Bldg. 31, Room 9A04
Bethesda, MD 20892 (301) 496-3583

## ULTRASOUND

National Institute of Child Health and Human Development
Bldg. 31, Room 2A32
Bethesda, MD 20892 (301) 496-5133

## UNCONVENTIONAL MEDICINE PRACTICES

*See Alternative Medicine Practices*

## UREMIA

National Institute of Diabetes and Digestive
and Kidney Diseases
Bldg. 31, Room 9A04
Bethesda, MD 20892 (301) 496-3583

## URINARY INCONTINENCE

*See Incontinence*

## URINARY TRACT DISEASE

National Kidney and Urological Diseases
Information Clearinghouse
3 Information Way
Bethesda, MD 20892 (301) 654-4415

## UROLITHIASIS

National Institute of Diabetes and Digestive
and Kidney Diseases
Bldg. 31, Room 9A04
Bethesda, MD 20892 (301) 496-3583

## URTICARIA

National Institute of Allergy and Infectious Diseases
Bldg. 31, Room 7A50
Bethesda, MD 20892 (301) 496-5717

## UTERINE CANCER

*See also Cancer*

National Cancer Institute
Bldg. 31, Room 10A16
Bethesda, MD 20892 (800) 4-CANCER

## UVEITIS

National Eye Institute
Bldg. 31, Room 6A32
Bethesda, MD 20892 (301) 496-5248

# - V -

## VACCINES

National Institute of Allergy and Infectious Diseases
Bldg. 31, Room 7A50
Bethesda, MD 20892 (301) 496-5717

Center for Biologics Evaluation and Research
Congressional and Consumer Affairs Branch (HFM-12)
Woodmont Office Center, Suite 200 North
1401 Rockville Pike
Rockville, MD 20852-1448 (301) 594-1800

Disease Hotline
Centers for Disease Control
1600 Clifton Road
Atlanta, GA 30333 (404) 332-4555

## VAGINITIS

National Institute of Allergy and Infectious Diseases
Bldg. 31, Room 7A50
Bethesda, MD 20892 (301) 496-5717

## VALVULAR HEART DISEASE

National Heart, Lung, and Blood Institute
Information Center

P.O. Box 30105
Bethesda, MD 20824-0105 (301) 251-1222

## VARICELLA

National Institute of Neurological Disorders and Stroke
Building 31, Room 8A16
Bethesda, MD 20892 (301) 496-5751
(800) 352-9424

## VARICOSE VEINS

National Heart, Lung, and Blood Institute
Information Center
P.O. Box 30105
Bethesda, MD 20824-0105 (301) 251-1222

## VASCULITIS

National Heart, Lung, and Blood Institute
Information Center
P.O. Box 30105
Bethesda, MD 20824-0105 (301) 251-1222

## VASECTOMIES

*See also Contraception; Sterilization*

National Institute of Child Health and Human Development
Building 31, Room 2A32
Bethesda, MD 20892 (301) 496-5133

## VD

*See Venereal Disease*

## VEGETARIANISM

*See also Food; Nutrition*

Food & Nutrition Information Center
National Agricultural Library, Room 304
Beltsville, MD 20705-2351 (301) 504-5719

## VENEREAL DISEASE

National Sexually Transmitted Diseases Hotline
P.O. Box 13827
Research Triangle Park, NC 27709 (800) 227-8922

National Institute of Allergy and Infectious Diseases
Building 31, Room 7A50
Bethesda, MD 20892 (301) 496-5717

## VENEZUELAN EQUINE ENCEPHALITIS

National Institute of Allergy and Infectious Diseases
Building 31, Room 7A50
Bethesda, MD 20892 (301) 496-5717

## VERTIGO

National Institute of Neurological Disorders and Stroke
Building 31, Room 8A16
Bethesda, MD 20892 (301) 496-5751
(800) 352-9424

## VETERAN'S DRUG & ALCOHOL TREATMENT

U.S. Department of Veterans Affairs
Mental Health and Behavioral Sciences Services (111-C-1B)

810 Vermont Ave., NW
Washington, DC 20420 (202) 535-7316

## VETERINARY FOOD AND MEDICINE

Center for Veterinary Medicine
Communication and Education Branch
Food and Drug Administration
7500 Standish Place
Rockville, MD 20855 (301) 594-5909

## VIDEO DISPLAY TERMINALS

National Institute For Occupational Safety and Health
4676 Columbia Parkway
Cincinnati, OH 45226 (800) 356-4674

## VINBLASTINE

National Cancer Institute
Bldg. 31, Room 10A16
Bethesda, MD 20892 (800) 4-CANCER

## VINCENT'S INFECTION

National Institute of Dental Research
Building 31, Room 2C35
31 Center Drive, MSC-2290
Bethesda, MD 20892-2290 (301) 496-4261

## VINCRISTINE

National Cancer Institute
Bldg. 31, Room 10A16
Bethesda, MD 20892 (800) 4-CANCER

## VIRUSES

National Institute of Allergy and Infectious Diseases
Bldg. 31, Room 7A50
Bethesda, MD 20892 (301) 496-5717

## VISION

*See also Eye Care*

National Eye Institute
Bldg. 31, Room 6A32
Bethesda, MD 20892 (301) 496-5248

## VITAL STATISTICS

*See Health Statistics*

## VITAMINS

National Institute on Aging
Information Center
P.O. Box 8057
Gaithersburg, MD 20898-8057 (800) 222-2225

National Heart, Lung, and Blood Institute
Information Center
P.O. Box 30105
Bethesda, MD 20824-0105 (301) 251-1222

## VITILIGO

National Institute of Arthritis and Musculoskeletal and Skin Diseases
1 AMS Way
Bethesda, MD 20892 (301) 495-4484

## VITRECTOMY

National Eye Institute
Bldg. 31, Room 6A32
Bethesda, MD 20892 (301) 496-5248

## VOCAL CHORD PARALYSIS

National Institute of Neurological Disorders and Stroke
Bldg. 31, Room 8A16
Bethesda, MD 20892 (301) 496-5751
(800) 352-9424

## VOGT-KOYANAGI DISEASE

National Eye Institute
Building 31, Room 6A32
Bethesda, MD 20892 (301) 496-5248

## VON RECKLINGHAUSEN'S DISEASE

National Institute of Neurological Disorders and Stroke
Bldg. 31, Room 8A16
Bethesda, MD 20892 (301) 496-5751
(800) 352-9424

## VON WILLEBRAND'S DISEASE

National Heart, Lung, and Blood Institute
Information Center
P.O. Box 30105
Bethesda, MD 20824-0105 (301) 251-1222

# - W -

## WAARDENBURG SYNDROME

National Institute on Deafness and Other Communication Disorders
1 Communication Avenue
Bethesda, MD 20892-3456
(800) 241-1044
(800) 241-1055 (TDD)

## WALDENSTROMS MACROGLOBULINEMIA

National Cancer Institute
Bldg. 31, Room 10A16
Bethesda, MD 20892
(800) 4-CANCER

## WALLEYE

National Eye Institute
Bldg. 31, Room 6A32
Bethesda, MD 20892
(301) 496-5248

## WARTS

National Institute of Allergy and Infectious Diseases
Bldg. 31, Room 7A50
Bethesda, MD 20892
(301) 496-5717

## WATER

*See Drinking Water*

## WEBER-CHRISTIAN DISEASE

National Institute of Arthritis and Musculoskeletal
and Skin Diseases
1 AMS Way
Bethesda, MD 20892 (301) 495-4484

## WEGENER'S GRANULOMATOSIS

National Institute of Arthritis and Musculoskeletal
and Skin Diseases
1 AMS Way
Bethesda, MD 20892 (301) 495-4484

## WEIGHT LOSS

*See Dieting*

## WERDNIG-HOFFMANN DISEASE

National Institute of Neurological Disorders and Stroke
Bldg. 31, Room 8A16
Bethesda, MD 20892 (301) 496-5751
(800) 352-9424

## WERNER'S SYNDROME

National Institute of Diabetes and Digestive
and Kidney Diseases
Bldg. 31, Room 9A04
Bethesda, MD 20892 (301) 496-3583

## WERNICKE'S ENCEPHALOPATHY

National Institute of Neurological Disorders and Stroke
Bldg. 31, Room 8A16 (301) 496-5751
Bethesda, MD 20892 (800) 352-9424

## WHIPLASH

National Institute of Neurological Disorders and Stroke
Building 31, Room 8A16 (301) 496-5751
Bethesda, MD 20892 (800) 352-9424

## WHOOPING COUGH

National Institute of Allergy and Infectious Diseases
Building 31, Room 7A50
Bethesda, MD 20892 (301) 496-5717

## WIFE ABUSE

*See Battered Spouses*

## WILMS' TUMOR

National Cancer Institute
Bldg. 31, Room 10A16
Bethesda, MD 20892 (800) 4-CANCER

## WILSON DISEASE

National Institute of Diabetes and Digestive and Kidney Diseases
Building 31, Room 9A04
Bethesda, MD 20892 (301) 496-3583

## WISKOTT-ALDRICH SYNDROME

National Cancer Institute
Bldg. 31, Room 10A16
Bethesda, MD 20892 (800) 4-CANCER

## WOLFF-PARKINSON-WHITE SYNDROME

National Heart, Lung, and Blood Institute
Information Center
P.O. Box 30105
Bethesda, MD 20824-0105 (301) 251-1222

## WOMEN

*See also Battered Spouses*

National Heart, Lung, and Blood Institute
Information Center
P.O. Box 30105
Bethesda, MD 20824-0105 (301) 251-1222

National Institute on Aging
Information Center
P.O. Box 8057
Gaithersburg, MD 20898-8057 (800) 222-2225

## WORKPLACE DRUG ABUSE

*See also Drug Abuse; Alcoholism*

National Clearinghouse for Alcohol and Drug Information
P.O. Box 2345
Rockville, MD 20852 (800) 729-6686

## WORKPLACE HEALTH AND SAFETY

National Institute for Occupational Safety and Health
4676 Columbia Parkway
Cincinnati, OH 45226 (800) 356-4674

Occupational Safety and Health Administration
U.S. Department of Labor
200 Constitution Ave., NW
Washington, DC 20210 (202) 219-8148

National Resource Center on Worksite Health Promotion
777 North Capitol St., NE, Suite 800
Washington, DC 20002 (202) 408-9320

## WRYNECK

National Institute of Neurological Disorders and Stroke
Building 31, Room 8A16 (301) 496-5751
Bethesda, MD 20892 (800) 352-9424

# - X -

## XANTHINURIA

National Institute of Diabetes and Digestive and Kidney Diseases
Building 31, Room 9A04
Bethesda, MD 20892 (301) 496-3583

## XANTHOMATOSIS

National Heart, Lung, and Blood Institute
Information Center
P.O. Box 30105
Bethesda, MD 20824-0105 (301) 251-1222

## XERODERMA PIGMENTOSUM

National Institute of Arthritis and Musculoskeletal and Skin Diseases
1 AMS Way
Bethesda, MD 20892 (301) 495-4484

## XEROPHTHALMIA

National Eye Institute
Bldg. 31, Room 6A32
Bethesda, MD 20892 (301) 496-5248

## XEROSTOMIA

*See Dry Mouth*

## X-RAYS

*See also Radiation*

Center for Devices and Radiological Health
(HFZ-210), Food and Drug Administration
5600 Fishers Ln.
Rockville, MD 20857 (301) 443-4690

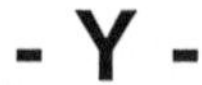


## YEAST INFECTIONS

National Institute of Allergy and Infectious Diseases
Bldg. 31, Room 7A50
Bethesda, MD 20892 (301) 496-5717

## YELLOW FEVER

National Institute of Allergy and Infectious Diseases
Bldg. 31, Room 7A50
Bethesda, MD 20892 (301) 496-5717

Centers for Disease Control
Information Resources Management Office
1600 Clifton Road
Atlanta, GA 30333 (404) 332-4555

# - Z -

## ZOLLINGER-ELLISON SYNDROME

National Institute of Diabetes and Digestive and Kidney Diseases
Bldg. 31, Room 9A04
Bethesda, MD 20892 (301) 496-3583

## ZOONOSES

National Institute of Allergy and Infectious Diseases
Bldg. 31, Room 7A50
Bethesda, MD 20892 (301) 496-5717